Francie Wolgin

# Advanced Skills for Nursing Assistants

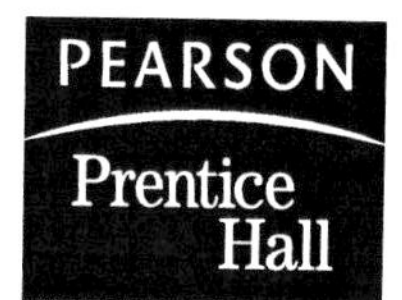


Upper Saddle River, New Jersey 07458

**Library of Congress Cataloging-in-Publication Data**
Wolgin, Francie.
Advanced skills for nursing assistants / Francie Wolgin.
p. ; cm.
Includes index.
Combined chapters from Advanced skills and competency assessment for caregivers.
ISBN 0-13-177985-0
1. Nurses' aides—Standards. 2. Care of the sick—Standards. 3. Nursing—Standards.
[DNLM: 1. Nurses' Aides—standards. 2. Caregivers—standards. 3. Nursing Process—standards. WY 193 W861a 2005] I. Wolgin, Francie. Advanced skills and competency assessment for caregivers. II. Title.
RT84.W645 2005
610.73'06'98—dc22

2004024930

**NOTICE**

The procedures described in this textbook are based on consultation with nursing authorities. The author and publisher have taken care to make certain that these procedures reflect currently accepted clinical practice; however, they cannot be considered absolute recommendations.

The material in this textbook contains the most current information available at the time of publication. However, federal, state, and local guidelines concerning clinical practices, including without limitation, those governing infection control and universal precautions, change rapidly. The reader should note, therefore, that new regulations may require changes in some procedures.

It is the responsibility of the reader to familiarize himself or herself with the policies and procedures set by federal, state, and local agencies, as well as by the institution or agency where the reader is employed. The authors and the publishers of this textbook, and the supplements written to accompany it, disclaim any liability, loss, or risk resulting directly or indirectly from the suggested procedures and theory, from any undetected errors, or from the reader's misunderstanding of the text. It is the reader's responsibility to stay informed of any new changes or recommendations made by any federal, state, and local agencies as well as by his or her employing health care institution or agency.

Publisher: *Julie Levin Alexander*
Assistant to the Publisher: *Regina Bruno*
Editor-in-Chief: *Maura Connor*
Executive Editor: *Barbara Krawiec*
Managing Development Editor: *Marilyn Meserve*
Development Editor: *Maureen Muncaster*
Editorial Assistants: *Jennifer Dwyer and Christopher DiLeo*
Director of Manufacturing and Production: *Bruce Johnson*
Managing Production Editor: *Patrick Walsh*
Production Liaison: *Mary C. Treacy*
Production Editor: *Karen Ettinger, The GTS Companies/York, PA Campus*
Manufacturing Manager: *Ilene Sanford*
Manufacturing Buyer: *Pat Brown*
Design Director: *Cheryl Asherman*
Senior Design Coordinator: *Maria Guglielmo Walsh*
Director of Marketing: *Karen Allman*
Executive Marketing Manager: *Nicole Benson*
Marketing Assistant: *Patricia Linard*
Marketing Coordinator: *Michael Sirinides*
Channel Marketing Manager: *Rachele Strober*
Composition: *The GTS Companies/York, PA Campus*
Cover Printer: *Phoenix Color*
Printer/Binder: *Bind-Rite Graphics, Inc.*

*Dedicated to my parents, Francis and Betty Sullivan, who have always encouraged and valued education and supported my siblings and me in all our varied enterprises and careers.*



Pearson Education LTD.
Pearson Education Singapore, Pte. Ltd
Pearson Education, Canada, Ltd
Pearson Education—Japan
Pearson Education Australia PTY, Limited
Pearson Education North Asia Ltd
Pearson Educación de Mexico, S.A. de C.V.
Pearson Education Malaysia, Pte. Ltd
Pearson Education, Upper Saddle River, New Jersey

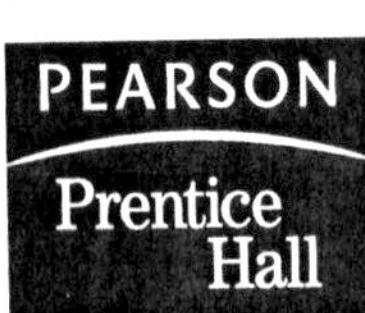


10 9 8 7 6 5
ISBN 0-13-177985-0

# CONTENTS

## CHAPTER 4



## CHAPTER 5



## CHAPTER 6

## CHAPTER 7

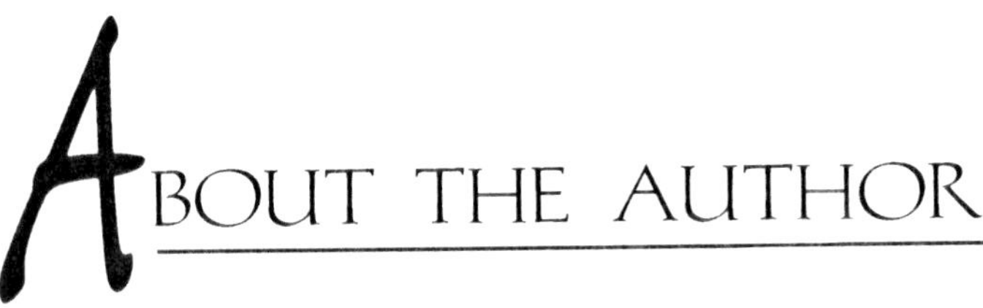

# About the Author

## Francie Wolgin, MSN, RN, CNA

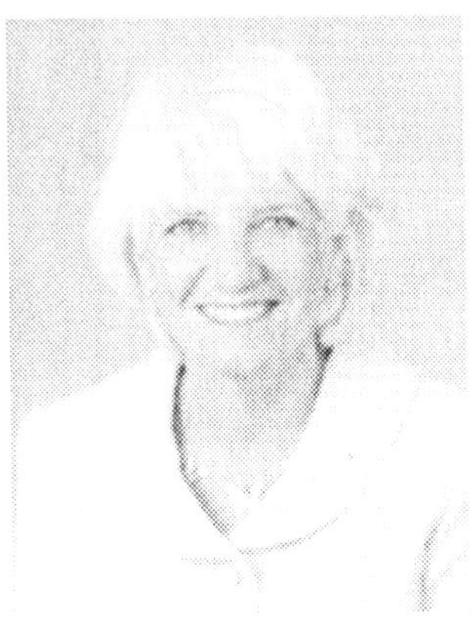

Francie Wolgin serves as Community Health Development Officer for The Health Foundation of Greater Cincinnati. She maintains a relationship with colleagues currently teaching nursing assistants, patient care technicians, and nursing students in several states. She serves on the nursing advisory boards of Cross Country University and Medcom Nursing. She was awarded the University of Cincinnati College of Nursing Distinguished Alumni Award in 1999.

Ms. Wolgin's previous positions include system leader for Education and Employee Development, St. Joseph Mercy Hospital, Ann Arbor, Michigan; president of the National Nursing Staff Development Organization; director of Nursing Practice Development; and clinical associate at the School of Nursing, Duke University Medical Center; several management, staff development, and administrative positions at the University of Cincinnati Hospital; and a faculty appointment at the University of Cincinnati College of Nursing and Health. She wrote *Being a Nursing Assistant*, 9th edition, as well as many articles, and she contributes to books on staff development, competency, and training advanced nursing assistants. Considerable experience as a direct caregiver in a variety of positions and areas gives her both perspective and firsthand knowledge of the challenges and opportunities available throughout the health care continuum.

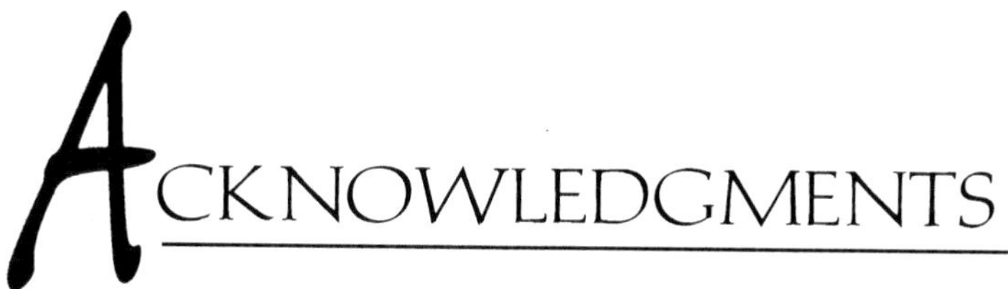

# Acknowledgments

For their contributions to individual chapters, I thank the following:

***Lisa F. Friedman,*** MS, RN, Education Specialist, St. Joseph Mercy Hospital, Ann Arbor, Michigan

***David Micham,*** BS, RRT, Respiratory Therapy Education Coordinator, St. Joseph Mercy Hospital, Ann Arbor, Michigan

***Mary Morochnick,*** BA, RN, Nurse Manager, IV Chemotherapy Team and Rehabilitation Unit, Duke University Medical Center, Durham, North Carolina

***Paula M. Nedela,*** MS, RN, Clinical Nurse Specialist for Neurosurgery and Orthopedics, St. Joseph Mercy Hospital, Ann Arbor, Michigan

***Pat Parr,*** BSN, RN, Director of Staff Development, Chelsea Community Hospital, Chelsea, Michigan

***Gloria Sveller,*** MA, RN, C, Education Coordinator, St. Joseph Mercy Hospital, Ann Arbor, Michigan

## St. Joseph Mercy Hospital, Ann Arbor, MI

Special thanks to Garry Faja, President and CEO of St. Joseph Mercy Health System, and Julie MacDonald, Senior Vice President of St. Joseph Mercy Hospital, for their support throughout the project and for permission to reprint or adapt materials from St. Joseph Mercy Hospital and Home Care. I would also like to thank Joy Stair, former Director of St. Joseph Mercy Home Care and Hospice; Jeanne Christie, Clinical Nurse Manager, Outpatient Oncology Clinic; and her staff, who provided their perspectives and ideas related to care delivery in a variety of settings. Special thanks to everyone who facilitated and participated in the photo shoot, and especially to Volunteer Services for their support.

## Technical Advisers

***Curtis Donald***
Patient Care Technician

***Lisa F. Friedman,*** MS, RN
Education Specialist

***Renee Gallagher***
Patient Care Technician

***David Micham,*** BS, RRT
Respiratory Therapy

***Paula M. Nedela,*** MS, RN
Clinical Nurse Specialist

***Kathy Smith,*** BS, RRT
Respiratory Therapist

***Gloria Sveller,*** MA, RN, C
Education Coordinator

## Reviewers

***Joan S. Braun,*** MA, RNC
Director of Staff Development
Raritan Bay Medical Center
Perth Amboy, New Jersey

***Jeanne Sind Christie,*** MS, ONC
Nurse Manager, Outpatient Oncology Clinic
St. Joseph Mercy Hospital
Ann Arbor, Michigan

***Joanne S. Curtis,*** MSEd, BSN
ViaHealth of Wayne
Sodus, New York

***Patricia DeiTos,*** RN, MSN
Program Developer, Continuing Education and Workforce Development
Northern Virginia Community College
Medical Education Campus
Springfield, Virginia

***Donna Diehl,*** RN, BSN
Staff Development Coordinator
Potomac Valley Hospital
Keyer, Wisconsin

***Cindy Elliott,*** RN, C, BSN
Clinical Nurse Manager
St. Joseph Mercy Home Care
Saline, Michigan

***Brenda Johansson,*** RN, C, MSN, CCRN
Acute Care Educator, Enloe Education Center
Lecturer, California State University
Chico, California

***Robert McClish,*** BA, RRT
Clinical Supervisor, Senior Allied Health Clinical Specialist
University of Michigan Hospitals
Main Hospital Critical Care Support Services
Ann Arbor, Michigan

***Kathleen O'Neill,*** RN, MS
Central Suffolk Hospital
Riverhead, New York

***Martin Redick,*** BS, MS
Instructor, Respiratory Therapy
Washtenaw Community College
Ypsilanti, Michigan

***Carol Sarokas,*** BS, RN
Director of Quality Management
Northside Mental Health Center
Tampa, Florida

***Gloria Sveller,*** MA, RN, C
Education Coordinator
St. Joseph Mercy Hospital
Ann Arbor, Michigan

# INTRODUCTION

Welcome to *Advanced Skills for Nursing Assistants*. This book responds to identified needs and challenges in health care today. Educators are expected to develop programs to cross-train staff and provide orientation for new employees so that they can competently perform a variety of complex skills. Variations in practice patterns and regulated professional nursing practice occur from state to state because there are no consistent national standards. Therefore, educators adhere to the standards and expectations applicable to their practice setting. Educators and caregivers will find that there are frequent changes or advances in health care as a result of research studies, clinical outcome measurements, insights, equipment changes, or new technology. Instructors or preceptors will have the most current knowledge and can change the term *patient* to *client* or *resident* if that is preferred.

This book is designed to assist educators, preceptors, and caregivers by providing a framework for assessing the caregiver's competency in performing advanced skills. There are seven individual chapters that are designed to stand alone for the purpose of cross-training a variety of health care professionals, or they can serve as a foundation for many of the skills required of multifunctional workers or cross-trained registered nurses.

Each individual skill includes a description of its purpose, supplies needed, key terms, pertinent information, and appropriate age-specific implications. To help reinforce retention, the key concept is stressed. The procedure for each skill is frequently complemented by photographs or drawings.

## OVERVIEW

The chapters in this book are designed to expand on the foundation of advanced skills as the learner progresses from chapter to chapter. This foundation is based on a knowledge of age-specific considerations and developmental tasks for infants through older adults, as well as on Standard Precautions and aseptic and sterile techniques. Each of the skills is designed to stand alone or be combined with others specific to your practice.

Procedures tend to have a series of steps that occur in a particular order. There is limited variation in how one employs Standard Precautions or protective equipment, for example. Guidelines, on the other hand, may be seen as more flexible recommendations, and as such may be carried out with more caregiver variation. There may be several correct ways to perform an activity when the outcome is the same.

Skills require the effective application of knowledge, along with ready execution, coordination, or manual dexterity. Each advanced skill is outlined in step-by-step form. Some skills are more easily described than others. For those skills where more in-depth information has been deemed necessary, the information is presented before the skill is described. Examples include neurological observation and pulse oximetry monitoring. Many caregivers have not had exposure to this material and will require time to study and review the information presented. This book is a resource for them to study and review the skill steps. Your instructor or preceptor will require that you successfully demonstrate competence before validating your ability to independently perform advanced skills in your practice setting or place of employment.

All chapters, main sections, and skills are listed in the contents.

## Introduction

A paragraph at the beginning of each chapter highlights the content and skills included in the chapter.

## Purpose

The reason for performing a skill is located at the beginning of each skill. Frequently, patients ask caregivers what they are doing or why it is necessary. The placement of this information at the beginning of the skill provides a framework for what follows. If you do not understand what you are trying to accomplish, it is difficult to describe it to someone else.

## Objectives

Each skill begins with a list of objectives that describes what the caregiver will be able to do in measurable, reachable goals: procedures or tasks to be performed, guidelines or techniques to be followed, and information to be reported or documented.

## Key Terms

Listed in the beginning of each chapter or following the objectives in each skill are key terms that are used in the chapter or skill description. Learning or reviewing the meaning of these terms before reading the chapter will greatly increase your understanding of the content and improve your ability to remember what you learn. Key terms are printed in bold followed by their definition.

## Supplies/Equipment

A list of the supplies or equipment needed to perform a skill is included.

## Pertinent Points

Information, suggestions, or patient considerations to keep in mind are listed in each skill.

## Age-Specific Considerations

All skills include important age-specific information that must be taken into account when performing the skill. When appropriate, these considerations are also included elsewhere in the chapter.

## Key Concept

The key concept is the most vital piece of information to keep in mind as you perform a given skill. Frequently, the patient's safety and well-being or the successful completion of the skill are dependent on the key concept.

## Steps

Each step is listed in order, along with photographs or drawings to assist in the comprehension of a particular aspect of a skill.

# CHAPTER 1
# ADVANCED PATIENT CARE SKILLS

## INTRODUCTION

The caregiver needs a broad range of skills and techniques to care for patients and to meet their needs. This chapter includes advanced skills that require knowledge of aseptic technique, knowledge of patients' growth and development needs, and knowledge related to basic anatomy and physiology. These skills generally require physician's orders or are intended to be implemented following an institution's written protocols for care. Each of these skills requires attention to the patient's response to the procedure. Predetermined outcomes or limits require additional skills and intervention by a nurse or physician. Each of these factors is examined and explained along with the skill.

This chapter prepares caregivers to perform the following skills, which are listed under the relevant section titles:

*Clean and Sterile Dressing Changes and Ostomy Care*

Changing a Clean Dressing

Changing an Ostomy Appliance

Changing a Sterile Dressing

*Urinary Catheterization*

Inserting a Straight Urinary Catheter

Clean Intermittent Catheterization—Home Use Only

Inserting an Indwelling Urinary Catheter

Discontinuing an Indwelling Urinary Catheter

*Staple and Suture Removal*

Removing Staples

Removing Sutures

*Checking Blood Products*

S E C T I O N   O N E

# Clean and Sterile Dressing Changes and Ostomy Care

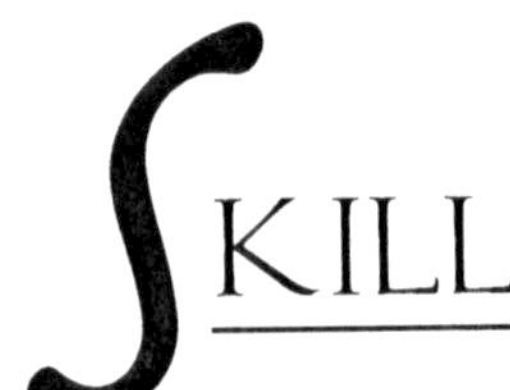

## SKILL

## Changing a Clean Dressing

***Purpose*** Dressings are placed over and in wounds to facilitate healing. They collect drainage from the wound or incision, help keep the wound clean, and help prevent infection. Dressings may also be used if a patient is not able to look at the wound yet and feels more comfortable seeing it covered. Clean dressings are used when the wound or incision is nearly healed or when there is little risk of infection.

### Objectives

**The caregiver demonstrates the ability to do the following:**

1. Gather the correct supplies.
2. Communicate using a style that reduces the patient's anxiety.
3. Ask the patient about any allergies (latex, tape, etc.).
4. Maintain clean technique.
5. Perform the clean dressing change as delegated.
6. Report the results of the procedure to the registered nurse (RN) or preceptor.

### Key Terms

**Dressing** Materials used to cover a wound or incision, including gauze, transparent dressings, and hydrocolloid dressings.

**Clean Technique** A procedure that is clean but not sterile. Supplies do not need to be sterile, but must be clean, not dirty. Clean gloves are worn.

### Supplies/ Equipment

Dressing materials (as ordered) • Tape • Clean gloves • Biohazard bag or container

### Pertinent Points

- A physician's order may be needed for a dressing change. This activity is generally a delegated task, and an RN should be consulted before a dressing is changed.
- A patient may be nervous about having a dressing changed. Explaining the procedure to the patient before beginning may help decrease anxiety.
- Time the dressing change to occur at least 30 minutes after the patient has received pain medication.

### Age-Specific Considerations

Certain types of tape used during dressing application may be irritating to the skin of infants, the elderly, or of patients with very delicate or thin skin. It may be better to use paper tape with such patients. This tape is not as harsh on fragile skin as are other types of tape, and it will help protect the skin from tearing.

Key Concept

*It* is important to always use clean supplies and clean technique when doing a clean dressing change to promote wound healing without infection. If you think your supplies may not be clean, it is essential to dispose of them and get new supplies.

Steps

1. Determine the type, variety, and amount of dressing needed by asking the RN caring for the patient or by checking the physician's order.
2. Gather the supplies.
3. Identify the patient in accordance with institution policy.
4. Explain the procedure to the patient, and ask about any allergies.
5. Wash hands.
6. Position the patient and ensure privacy.
7. Place the dressing supplies on a clean, dry, flat surface.
8. Put on nonsterile (clean) gloves.
9. Remove, inspect, and document the old dressing. Save it for the RN or preceptor to assess, and then discard it in the biohazard bag or container.
10. Ask the RN or preceptor to inspect the wound.
11. Remove and discard gloves, and put on new nonsterile (clean) gloves.
12. Redress the wound using clean technique, and secure as necessary (Figures 1.1 and 1.2).

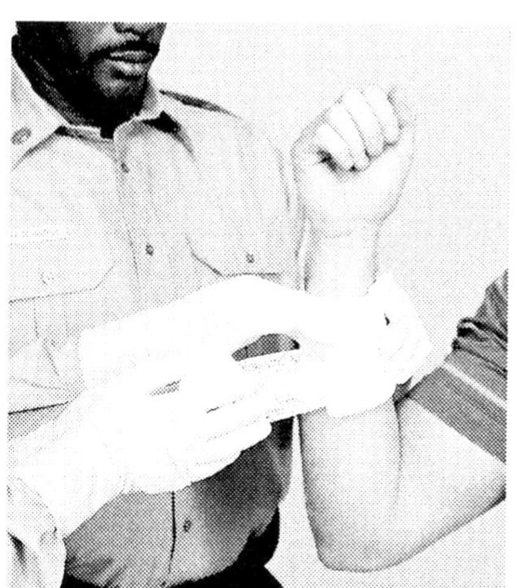

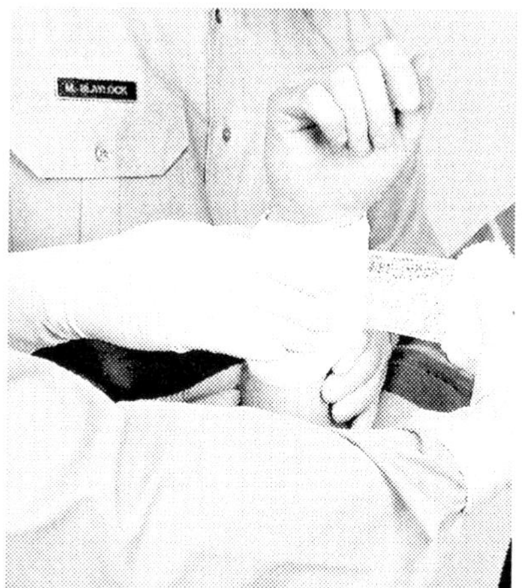

**Figure 1.1** Applying a clean dressing using gauze wrap.

13. Discard waste appropriately, remove gloves, and wash hands.
14. Return the patient to a comfortable position.
15. Document the procedure and observations, and inform the RN of the completion of the task.
16. Provide input to update the care plan as needed.

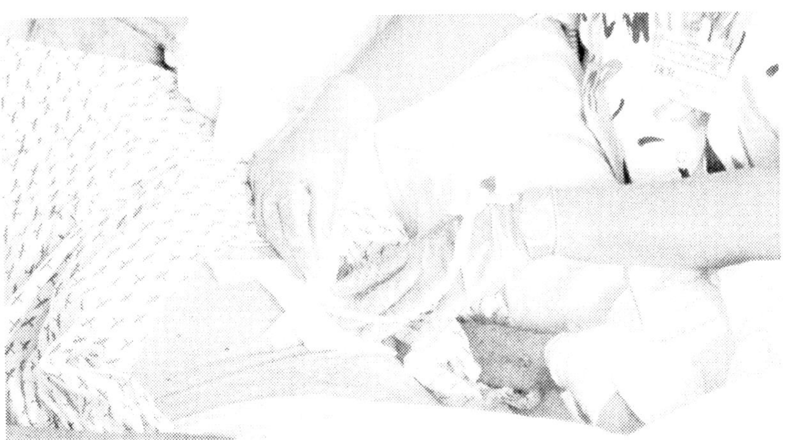

**Figure 1.2** Applying a clean dressing to a feeding tube site.

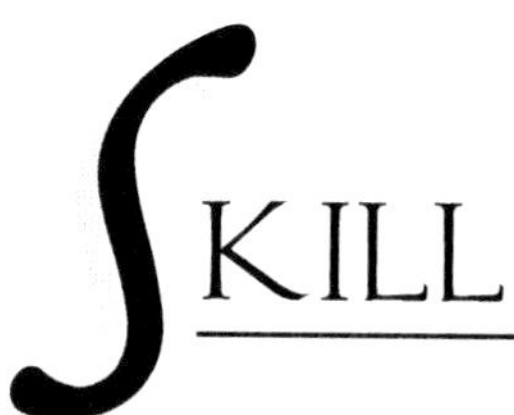

# SKILL

## Changing an Ostomy Appliance

***Purpose*** Ostomies may be temporary or permanent. An ostomy may be performed to divert the patient's feces from the rectum. Ostomies are often performed when treating diseases such as colon cancer, ulcerative colitis, or Crohn's disease. Feces may be temporarily diverted to allow the bowel to rest and heal after injury. An ostomy may also be performed to divert urine when the bladder or kidneys are injured or diseased.

### Objectives

**The caregiver demonstrates the ability to do the following:**

1. Gather the correct supplies.
2. Communicate using a style that reduces the patient's anxiety.
3. Remove the old ostomy appliance.
4. Note the condition of the patient's skin and stoma.
5. Apply a new appliance.
6. Record the amount of drainage and its consistency and color.
7. Report the results of the procedure to the RN or preceptor.

### Key Terms

**Ostomy** A surgical procedure that creates a new opening, usually in the abdomen, for the discharge of wastes (feces or urine) from the body. Examples include colostomy (feces), ileostomy (feces), and ileoconduit (urine).

**Ostomy Appliance** A collection pouch that attaches to the skin around the stoma with some type of adhesive.

**Stoma** A surgically made opening that allows waste to exit the body.

### Supplies/Equipment

Towel • Bed protector • Gloves • Washcloth • Basin of warm water • Wafer with flange (whatever product the patient uses or is supplied within your institution) • New stoma pouch • Stoma adhesive paste

### Pertinent Points

- Stomas are usually red due to the large number of blood vessels located in the tissue.
- When giving care to a stoma, it is not uncommon to note a small amount of bleeding. If you note a large amount or if the bleeding does not stop, notify the RN or preceptor immediately.
- Patients react differently to an ostomy. Feelings of loss, fear, anger, and anxiety are normal when adjusting to changes in body image. Allow patients time to express their feelings when you are caring for them.

### Age-Specific Considerations

The change in body image that results from an ostomy can be frightening to young children, who may see it as body mutilation. For adolescents and adults, the change can bring out fears and concerns related to sexuality and changes in lifestyle. For elderly patients, an ostomy can generate fears that they may not be able to care for themselves. All of these fears can be addressed through the help of enterostomal therapists (nurses who specialize in the care of ostomy patients) and through support groups where patients can talk with others who have successfully made the transition after an ostomy.

## Key Concept

It is crucial to get a good "fit" for the wafer around the patient's stoma. When the fit is poor, feces will irritate the patient's skin and cause it to break down.

## Steps

1. Wash hands.
2. Explain the procedure to the patient.
3. Provide for privacy.
4. Position the patient for comfort.
5. Expose only the appliance (Figure 1.3). Place a towel over the patient's abdomen and a bed protector under the patient's hips to keep the bed clean.
6. Assemble the equipment and put on gloves.
7. Gently remove the old pouch and wafer. Measure the contents, and dispose of contents according to institution policy.
8. Wipe the skin around the stoma with a warm, wet washcloth to remove any stool or urine. Rinse the skin carefully. Pat the area dry with a towel. A washcloth can be placed over the stoma to prevent soiling of the area while the new wafer is prepared.
9. Prepare the new wafer by sizing and cutting it to fit over the stoma. The skin should not show between the stoma and the wafer. Use stoma adhesive if necessary (Figure 1.4a).
10. Hold the wafer between your hands to warm it and make it more flexible. Remove backing and apply the new wafer to the skin (Figure 1.4b). Make sure there are no air pockets under the wafer. Hold it in place for 30 seconds to help the adhesive stick well.
11. Apply stoma pouch to the flange on the wafer. Make sure the pouch is correctly sealed (Figure 1.4c).
12. Remove the towel and bed protector. Clean up the area.
13. Wash hands.
14. Document and report the results and the patient's tolerance to the RN or preceptor.

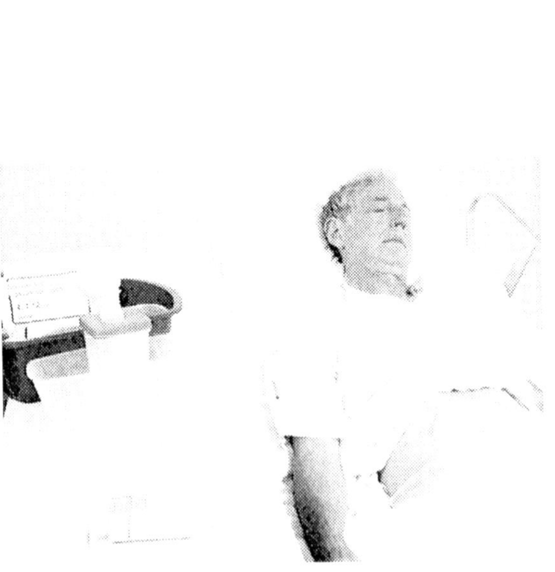

**Figure 1.3** Ostomy appliance in place over stoma.

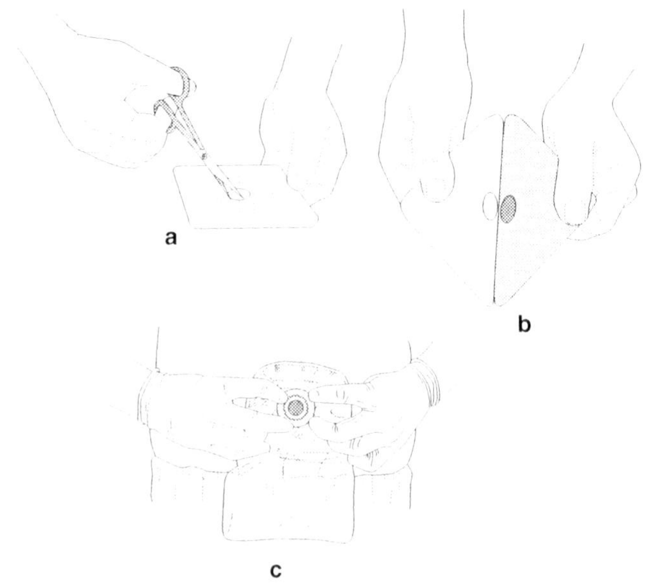


**Figure 1.4** Replacing an ostomy appliance.

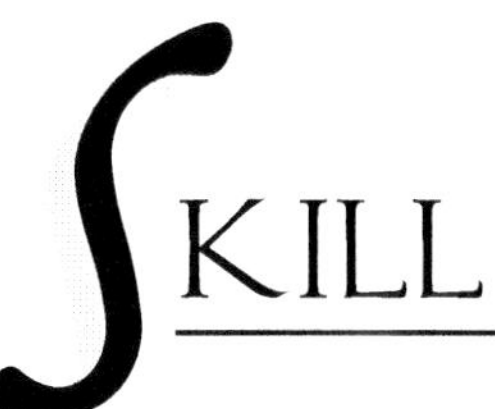

# SKILL

## Changing a Sterile Dressing

**Purpose** Dressings are placed over and in wounds to facilitate healing. They collect drainage from the wound or incision, help keep the wound clean, and help prevent infection. Dressings may also be used if a patient is not able to look at the wound yet and feels more comfortable seeing it covered. Sterile dressings are used when wounds or incisions are just beginning to heal or when the risk of infection is high.

### Objectives

**The caregiver demonstrates the ability to do the following:**

1. Gather the correct supplies.
2. Communicate using a style that reduces the patient's anxiety.
3. Ask the patient about any allergies (latex, tape, etc.).
4. Maintain sterile technique.
5. Perform the sterile dressing change as delegated.
6. Report the results of the procedure to the RN or preceptor.

### Key Terms

**Sterile Technique** A procedure that remains germfree. Sterile supplies are used, and special steps are taken to ensure that the materials remain sterile. Sterile gloves are worn.

### Supplies/Equipment

Dressing materials (as ordered) • Tape • Clean gloves • Sterile gloves • Biohazard bag or container

### Pertinent Points

- A physician's order may be needed for a dressing change. Generally, this activity is a delegated task, and an RN should be consulted before a dressing is changed.
- A patient may be nervous about having a dressing changed.
- Explaining the procedure to the patient before beginning may help decrease anxiety.
- Time the dressing change to occur at least 30 minutes after the patient has received pain medication.

### Age-Specific Considerations

Certain types of tape used during dressing application may be irritating to the skin of infants, the elderly, or patients with very delicate or thin skin. It may be better to use paper tape with such patients. This tape is not as harsh on fragile skin as other types of tape, and it will help protect the skin from tearing.

### Key Concept

It is important to always use sterile supplies and sterile technique when doing a sterile dressing change to promote wound healing without infection. If you think your supplies may not be sterile, it is essential to dispose of them and get new sterile supplies.

## Steps

1. Determine the type, variety, and amount of dressing needed by asking the RN caring for the patient.
2. Gather the supplies.
3. Identify the patient in accordance with institution policy.
4. Explain the procedure to the patient. Instruct the patient that the procedure will be sterile, and explain the importance of not touching any of the supplies being used. Ask about any allergies.
5. Wash hands.
6. Position the patient and ensure privacy.
7. Place the sterile dressing supplies on a clean, dry, flat surface.
8. Put on nonsterile (clean) gloves.
9. Remove and inspect the old dressing. Save it for the RN or preceptor to assess, and then discard it in the biohazard bag or container.
10. Ask the RN or preceptor to inspect the wound.
11. Remove and discard gloves.
12. Open the sterile dressing supplies, maintaining a sterile field.
13. Put on sterile gloves.
14. Redress the wound using sterile technique, and secure as necessary (Figure 1.5).
15. Discard waste appropriately, remove gloves, and wash hands.
16. Return the patient to a comfortable position.
17. Document the procedure and observations, and inform the RN or preceptor of the completion of the task.
18. Provide input to update the care plan as needed.

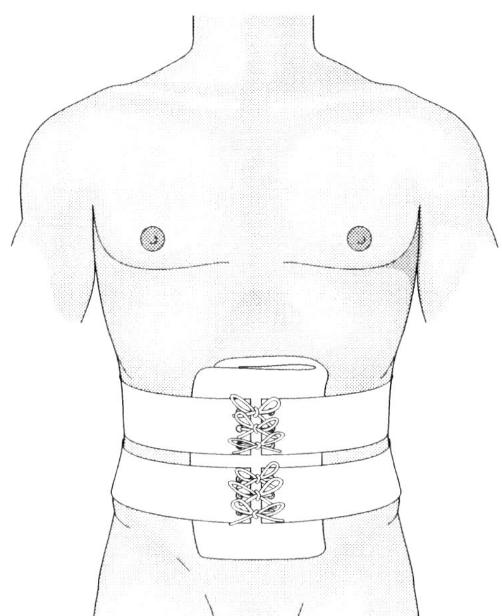

**Figure 1.5** A sterile dressing using montgomery straps.

SECTION TWO

# Urinary Catheterization

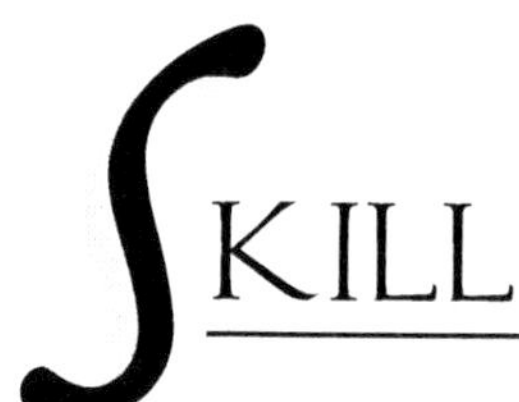

## SKILL

## Inserting a Straight Urinary Catheter

***Purpose*** Straight catheterization is used to drain the bladder of urine. This procedure is often performed for patients who are experiencing urinary retention or are having difficulty emptying their bladder on their own, for patients who must provide sterile urine samples, or for patients who are undergoing bladder retraining. The catheter is inserted into the bladder, the urine is drained, and then the catheter is removed. This procedure is often performed intermittently.

### Objectives

**The caregiver demonstrates the ability to do the following:**

1. Gather the correct supplies.
2. Communicate using a style that reduces the patient's anxiety.
3. Ask the patient about any allergies (latex, rubber, iodine-based products, tape, etc.).
4. Perform the catheterization.
5. Record the amount of urine obtained.
6. Report the results of the procedure to the RN or preceptor.

### Key Terms

**Bladder** A holding vessel for urine.

**Catheterization** The process of passing a tubular instrument into a body cavity to insert or remove fluids or gases.

**Kidneys** The organs that filter the blood to remove waste products and produce urine.

**Retention** A dangerous condition in which urine becomes trapped in the bladder. Retention can lead to loss of bladder tone, development of renal calculi, and urinary infection.

**Ureters** Connecting tubes that run between the kidneys and the bladder.

**Urethra** The normal outlet for urine from the body. The sphincter controls the elimination of urine.

**Urinary Meatus** The external opening of the urethra.

### Supplies/Equipment

Sterile gloves • Fenestrated drape • Cotton balls • Iodine cleansing solution • Water-soluble lubricant • A size 14–16 French urinary straight catheter • Urine collection basin • Sterile urine cup • Forceps

These items are usually contained within a kit (Figure 1.6).

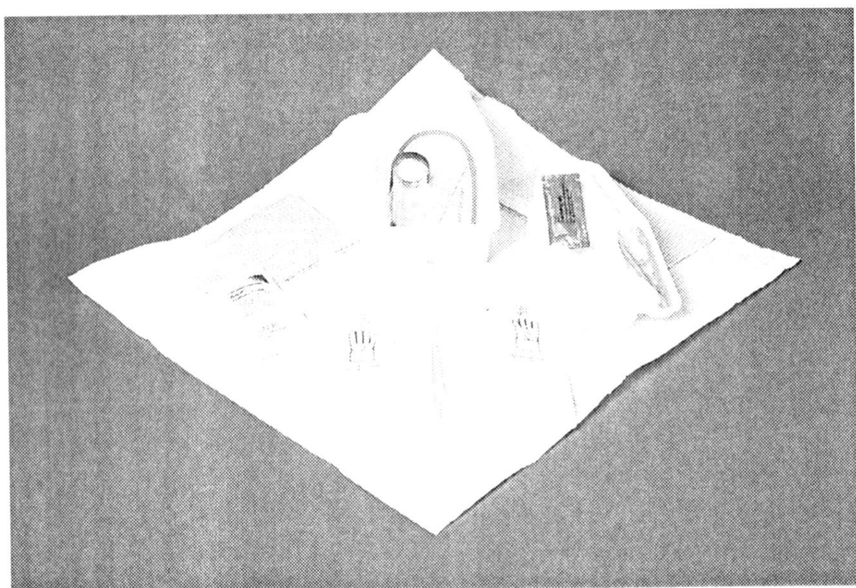

**Figure 1.6** Straight catheter kit.

## Pertinent Points

- Urinary catheterization requires a physician's order in most cases.
- Urinary tract infection is the most common complication of being catheterized.
- Although catheterization is a "routine" procedure in health care, it is not routine to patients. They are often hesitant or reluctant about being catheterized. It often helps relieve the patient's anxiety to explain the purpose of the procedure, provide for privacy, and explain what is happening during the procedure.
- Remove no more than 800 to 1,000 cubic centimeters (cc) of urine at one time to prevent bladder collapse and electrolyte imbalance.
- If the catheter tip is accidentally inserted into the vagina, the catheter is contaminated and must be discarded. The caregiver will need to get a new kit and start over. Leave the first catheter in the vagina until you have successfully inserted the new sterile catheter in the urethral opening.

## Age-Specific Considerations

Patients of all ages may have concerns and fears about being catheterized. Children may fear where the tube will go inside their body. Elderly patients may fear a loss of mobility and independence. All patients may fear pain and the loss of privacy. To respond to these concerns, be certain to close the door or pull the curtain. Explain the procedure to the patient in terms that he or she can understand; use pictures if appropriate.

## Key Concept

The risk of infection increases with the length of time a catheter remains in place. Therefore, whenever appropriate, straight catheterization is preferred over indwelling catheterization because the catheter is removed at the end of the procedure.

## Steps for Inserting a Straight Urinary Catheter in a Female Patient

1. Wash hands.
2. Ask patient if she has allergies to latex or iodine. (If allergy exists, use latex-free gloves and catheter, and use hypoallergenic soap and water for cleaning.)
3. Explain the procedure to the patient.
4. Provide for privacy.
5. Position the patient in the dorsal recumbent position with knees flexed, exposing the labia.
6. Drape the patient so that only the perineum is exposed.
7. Assemble the equipment and put on gloves.
8. Prepare the items in the kit for use during insertion, maintaining clean technique.
9. With nondominant hand, separate the labia minora, and hold this position until the catheter is inserted.
10. Using cotton balls, cleanse the meatus with the iodine cleansing solution:
    a. Making one downward stroke with each cotton ball, begin at the labia on the side farthest from you, and move toward the labia nearest you.
    b. Afterward, wipe once down the center of the meatus.
    c. Wipe once with each cotton ball, and discard. (The forceps may be used to hold the cotton ball.)
11. Direct the open end of the catheter into the collection container. Lubricate and insert the tip of the catheter slowly through the urethral opening 3 to 4 inches or until urine returns.
12. Advance the catheter another 0.5 to 1.0 inches (Figure 1.7).
13. Allow urine to drain until it stops. Collect a sterile urine specimen if needed. Then remove the catheter slowly, allowing any additional urine to drain.
14. Cleanse the perineal area. Reposition the patient for comfort, and replace the linens.
15. Measure the amount of urine in the collection container, and record.
16. Remove and discard gloves; wash hands.
17. Document and report the results to the RN or preceptor.

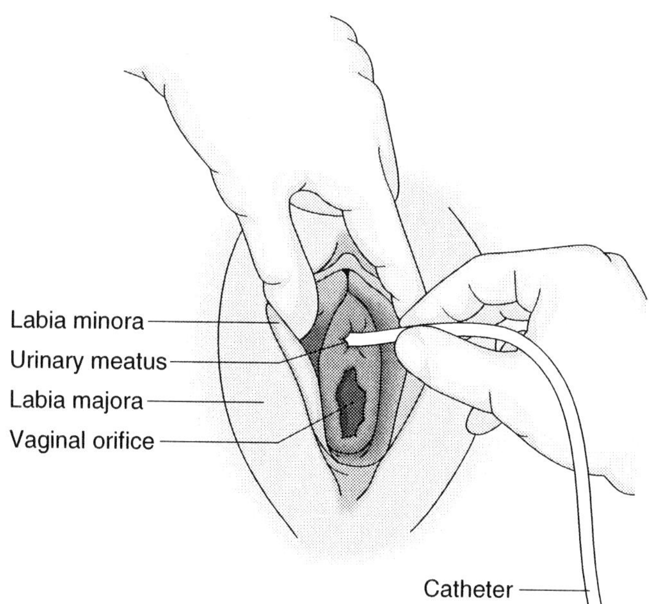


**Figure 1.7** Inserting a urinary catheter in a female patient.

## Steps for Inserting a Straight Urinary Catheter in a Male Patient

1. Wash hands.
2. Ask patient if he has allergies to latex or iodine. (If allergy exists, use latex-free gloves and catheter, and use hypoallergenic soap and water for cleaning.)
3. Explain the procedure to the patient.
4. Provide for privacy.
5. Drape the patient with bed linens so that only the penis is exposed.
6. Assemble the equipment and put on gloves.
7. Prepare the items in the kit for use during insertion, maintaining clean technique.
8. Remove the fenestrated drape from the kit, and using nondominant hand, place the penis through the hole in the drape. *Keep dominant hand sterile.*
9. Pull the penis up at a 90-degree angle to the patient's supine body.
10. With nondominant hand, gently grasp the glans (tip) of the penis; retract the foreskin if uncircumcised.
11. Using cotton balls, cleanse the meatus and the glans with the iodine cleansing solution, beginning at the urethral opening and moving toward the shaft of the penis; make one complete circle around the penis with each cotton ball. Direct the open end of the catheter into the collection container.
12. Lubricate and insert the tip of the catheter slowly through the urethral opening 7 to 9 inches or until urine returns (Figure 1.8).
13. Allow urine to drain until it stops. Collect a sterile urine specimen if needed. Then remove the catheter slowly, allowing any additional urine to drain.
14. Cleanse the perineal area, and replace the foreskin of the penis. Reposition the patient for comfort, and replace the linens.
15. Measure the amount of urine in the collection container, and record.
16. Remove and discard gloves; wash hands.
17. Document and report the results to the RN or preceptor.

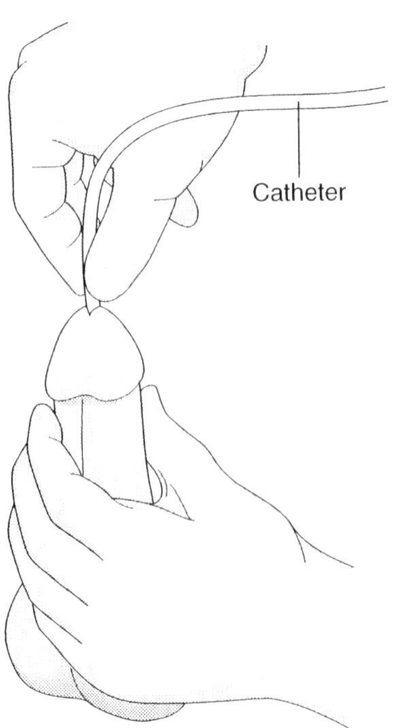


**Figure 1.8** Inserting a urinary catheter in a male patient.

# Clean Intermittent Catheterization—Home Use Only

This procedure is used for patients who are unable to empty their urinary bladder for several days and may use the procedure at home.

The procedure is performed almost the same as the procedure for inserting a straight urinary catheter, except for two differences:

**1.** Clean, not sterile, gloves are used.

**2.** The equipment is cleaned and reused.

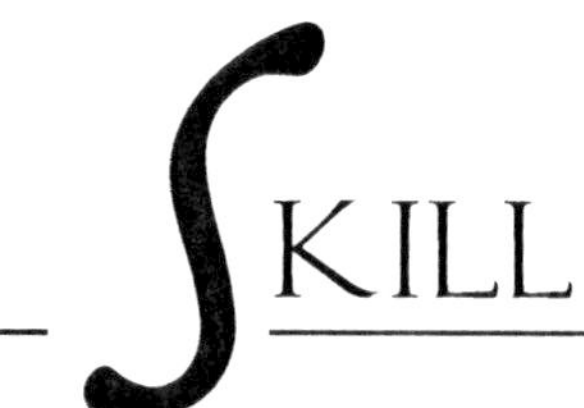

# SKILL

## Inserting an Indwelling Urinary Catheter

***Purpose*** Urinary catheterization, which involves inserting a hollow catheter up the urethra to the bladder under sterile conditions, is an ancient procedure. Some common reasons to use a catheter are to empty the urine from the bladder, to obtain a urine specimen, to keep the bladder empty (decompression) during certain procedures such as surgery, to instill medications, to bypass an obstruction, and to determine accurate urinary output.

### Objectives

**The caregiver demonstrates the ability to do the following:**

1. Gather the correct supplies.
2. Communicate using a style that reduces the patient's anxiety.
3. Ask the patient about any allergies (latex, rubber, iodine, paper, etc.).
4. Maintain sterile technique.
5. Check the balloon by inflating and deflating it.
6. Perform the catheterization.
7. Record the amount of urine obtained.
8. Report the results of the procedure to the RN or preceptor.

### Key Terms

**Bladder** A holding vessel for urine.

**Catheterization** The process of passing a tubular instrument into a body cavity to insert or remove fluids or gases.

**Kidneys** The organs that filter the blood to remove waste products and produce urine.

**Retention** A dangerous condition in which urine becomes trapped in the bladder. Retention can lead to loss of bladder tone, development of renal calculi, and urinary infection.

**Ureters** Connecting tubes that run between the kidneys and the bladder.

**Urethra** The normal outlet for urine from the body. The sphincter controls the elimination of urine.

### Supplies/Equipment

Solid drape • Fenestrated drape • Sterile gloves • Urinary catheter • Syringe • Lubricant • Cotton balls • Antiseptic solution • Urine collection tray • Specimen cup • Forceps

These items are usually contained within a kit.

### Pertinent Points

- Urinary catheterization requires a physician's order in most cases.
- Although catheterization is a "routine" procedure in health care, it is not routine to patients. They are often hesitant or reluctant about being catheterized. It often helps relieve the patient's anxiety to explain the purpose of the procedure, provide for privacy, and explain what is happening during the procedure.
- Remove no more than 800 to 1,000 cc of urine at one time to prevent bladder collapse and electrolyte imbalance.

- If the catheter tip is accidentally inserted into the vagina, the catheter is contaminated and must be discarded. The caregiver will need to get a new kit and start over. Leave the first catheter in the vagina until you have successfully inserted the new sterile catheter in the urethral opening.

### Age-Specific Considerations

Patients of all ages may have concerns and fears about being catheterized. Children may fear where the tube will go inside their body. Elderly patients may fear a loss of mobility and independence. All patients may fear pain and the loss of privacy. To respond to these concerns, be certain to close the door or pull the curtain. Explain the procedure to the patient in terms that he or she can understand; use pictures if appropriate.

### Key Concept

Infection is the most common complication of having an indwelling urinary catheter, and the risk of infection increases with the length of time the catheter remains in place. The caregiver's use of correct sterile technique significantly reduces the patient's risk for infection.

### Steps for Inserting an Indwelling Urinary Catheter in a Female Patient

1. Wash hands.
2. Ask patient if she has allergies to latex or iodine. (If allergy exists, use latex-free gloves and catheter, and use hypoallergenic soap and water for cleaning.)
3. Explain the procedure to the patient, emphasizing the need to maintain the sterile field.
4. Provide for privacy.
5. Position the patient in the dorsal recumbent position with knees flexed, exposing the labia.
6. Drape the patient so that only the perineum is exposed.
7. Remove the full drape from the kit with your fingertips, and place, plastic side down, just under the patient's buttocks (ask her to raise her hips).
8. Put on sterile gloves.
9. Prepare the items in the kit for use during insertion, maintaining sterile technique.
10. Test the balloon for defects. Deflate the balloon, and leave the syringe on the catheter (Figure 1.9). Liberally lubricate the catheter tip.

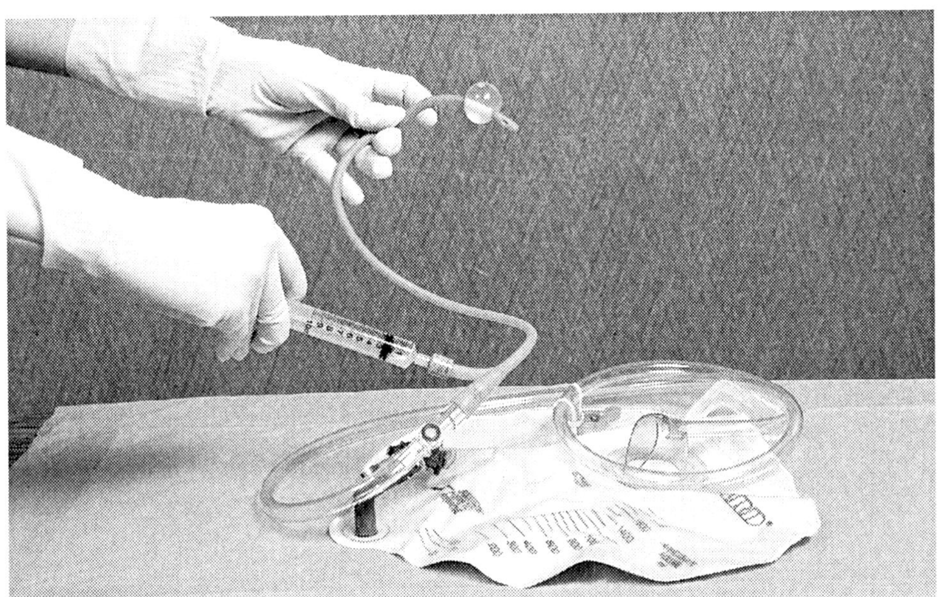

**Figure 1.9** Testing the retention balloon of a catheter with a syringe.

11. With nondominant hand, separate the labia minora and hold this position until the catheter is inserted. (Note: The dominant hand is the only sterile hand now; the contaminated hand continues to separate the labia.) Forceps may be used to hold the cotton ball.
12. Using cotton balls, cleanse the meatus with the iodine solution:
    a. Making one downward stroke with each cotton ball, begin at the labia on the side farthest from you, and move toward the labia nearest you.
    b. Afterward, wipe once down the center of the meatus.
    c. Wipe once with each cotton ball, and discard.
13. Insert the tip of the catheter slowly through the urethral opening 3 to 4 inches or until urine returns.
14. Advance the catheter another 0.5 to 1.0 inches.
15. Inflate the balloon with the attached syringe, and gently pull back on the catheter until it stops, or catches (Figure 1.10). Catch the urine in the collection tray or in the specimen cup (if needed).
16. Measure the amount of urine in the drainage bag, and record.
17. Position the collection bag lower than the bladder.
18. Remove and discard gloves; wash hands.
19. Document and report the results to the RN or preceptor.

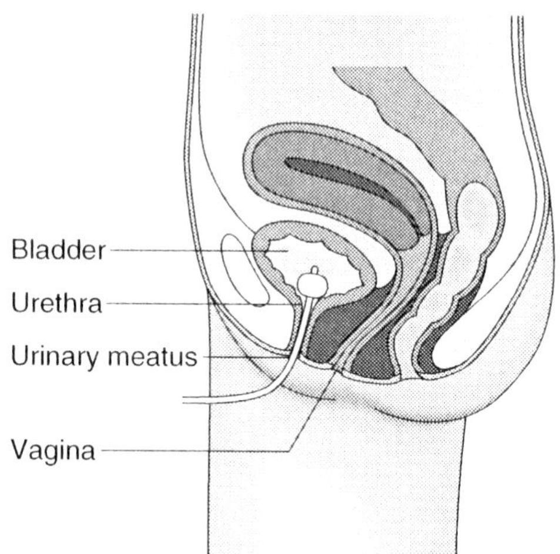


**Figure 1.10** Side view of female anatomy with indwelling urinary catheter in place.

## Steps for Inserting an Indwelling Urinary Catheter in a Male Patient

1. Wash hands.
2. Ask patient if he has allergies to latex or iodine. (If allergy exists, use latex-free gloves and catheter, and use hypoallergenic soap and water for cleaning.)
3. Explain the procedure to the patient.
4. Provide for privacy.
5. Assemble the equipment and put on gloves.
6. Prepare the items in the kit for use during insertion, maintaining sterile technique.
7. Test the balloon for defects. Deflate the balloon, and leave the syringe attached to the catheter (Figure 1.9). Liberally lubricate the catheter tip.
8. Remove the fenestrated drape from the kit, and using nondominant hand, place the penis through the hole in the drape. *Keep dominant hand sterile.*
9. Pull the penis up at a 90-degree angle to the patient's supine body.
10. With nondominant hand, gently grasp the glans (tip) of the penis; retract the foreskin if uncircumcised.
11. Using cotton balls, cleanse the meatus and the glans with iodine solution, beginning at the urethral opening and moving toward the shaft of the penis; make one complete circle around the penis with each cotton ball. Forceps may be used to hold the cotton ball.
12. Insert the tip of the catheter slowly through the urethral opening to the bifurcation (Y) of the catheter.
13. Inflate the balloon with the attached syringe, and gently pull back on the catheter until it stops, or catches (Figure 1.11).
14. Replace the foreskin of the penis on uncircumcised males.
15. Measure the amount of urine in the drainage bag, and record.
16. Position the collection bag lower than the bladder.
17. Remove and discard gloves; wash hands.
18. Document and report the results to the RN or preceptor.

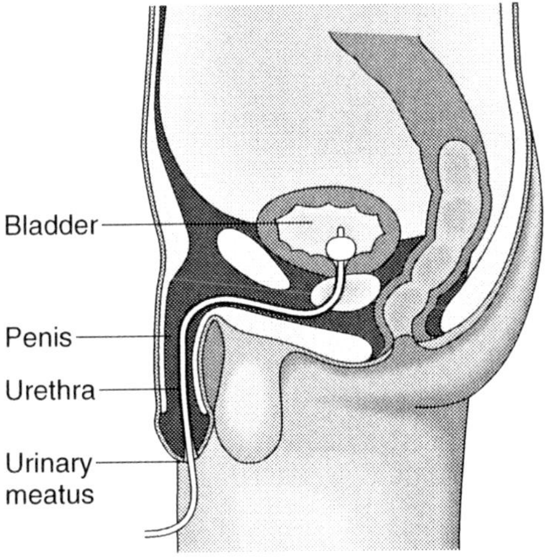


**Figure 1.11** Side view of male anatomy with indwelling urinary catheter in place.

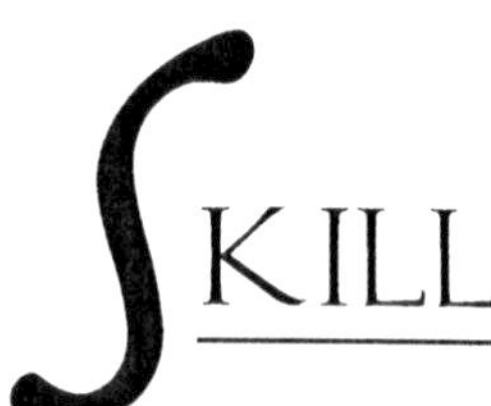

# SKILL

## Discontinuing an Indwelling Urinary Catheter

***Purpose*** The indwelling urinary catheter is removed when it is determined by the physician or by protocol that the patient is able to urinate on his or her own. It is also removed when the catheter needs to be changed for infection control or due to blockage.

### Objectives

**The caregiver demonstrates the ability to do the following:**

1. Gather the correct supplies.
2. Communicate using a style that reduces the patient's anxiety.
3. Correctly deflate the retention balloon before removing the catheter.
4. Record the amount of urine left in the drainage bag.
5. Report the results of the procedure to the RN or preceptor.

### Key Terms

**Drainage Bag** The bag that urine from the bladder drains into. It is attached to the indwelling catheter and collects the urine that drains from the bladder.

**Retention Balloon** The device that holds an indwelling urinary catheter in place in the bladder. It is filled with sterile saline solution. When the saline is removed, that section of the catheter collapses and becomes a narrow tube that can slide through the urethra.

### Supplies/Equipment

Protective pad or towel • Clean gloves • 10-cc syringe • Washcloth

### Pertinent Points

- Removing an indwelling urinary catheter requires a physician's order in most cases.
- Patients are often happy to have the tube removed but are hesitant that it will hurt. Be honest. Prepare the patient for a stinging sensation and then a feeling of relief when the catheter is out.
- Provide for privacy by closing the door or pulling the curtain.
- Provide for comfort by placing a pad under the patient to catch any urine that may drip during the procedure. Clean the patient's skin if needed.
- Note the condition of the tip of the catheter when you remove it. Be sure it is intact.
- If you note any white to green sediment, notify the RN or physician prior to removal. This may indicate an infection in progress and may require a culture collection of the catheter tip.
- If you notice a pungent odor, notify the RN or physician. Often, a culture of both the urine and the catheter tip will be ordered to determine whether an infection is the cause.

### Age-Specific Considerations

When removing a urinary catheter from a child, be honest and explain that the process might sting. Trust is a very important issue for children. If they cannot trust you, they will not feel secure in future interactions. Adolescents, adults, and the elderly may worry that they will not be able to urinate on their own once a catheter is removed. Reassure them that in the majority of cases, this is not a problem.

Key Concept

Care must be taken to properly deflate the retention balloon while holding the catheter. A catheter can be retracted accidentally into a male's urethra if the catheter is improperly cut to deflate the balloon. Should this occur, removal from the bladder requires cystoscopic surgery or radiological interventions. Remove the catheter using a slow, steady movement to minimize the patient's pain or discomfort.

Steps

1. Wash hands.
2. Explain the procedure to, and provide privacy for, the patient.
3. Gather the supplies.
4. Tuck a protective pad or towel under the patient's hips to catch any urine that may drip during the procedure.
5. Put on gloves.
6. Attach the syringe to the urinary catheter port, and draw back 10 cc of sterile saline solution (Figure 1.12). Be sure to remove all of the solution from the port to allow the balloon to collapse and the catheter to slip easily out of the urethra.
7. Tell the patient that you are ready to gently but firmly pull the catheter out. Encourage the patient to take a deep breath.
8. Clean up any urine that may have dripped.
9. Empty the drainage bag, and record the amount and characteristics of the urine.
10. Discard the catheter and the empty drainage bag in the trash.
11. Remove and discard gloves; wash hands.
12. Document and report the results to the RN or preceptor.

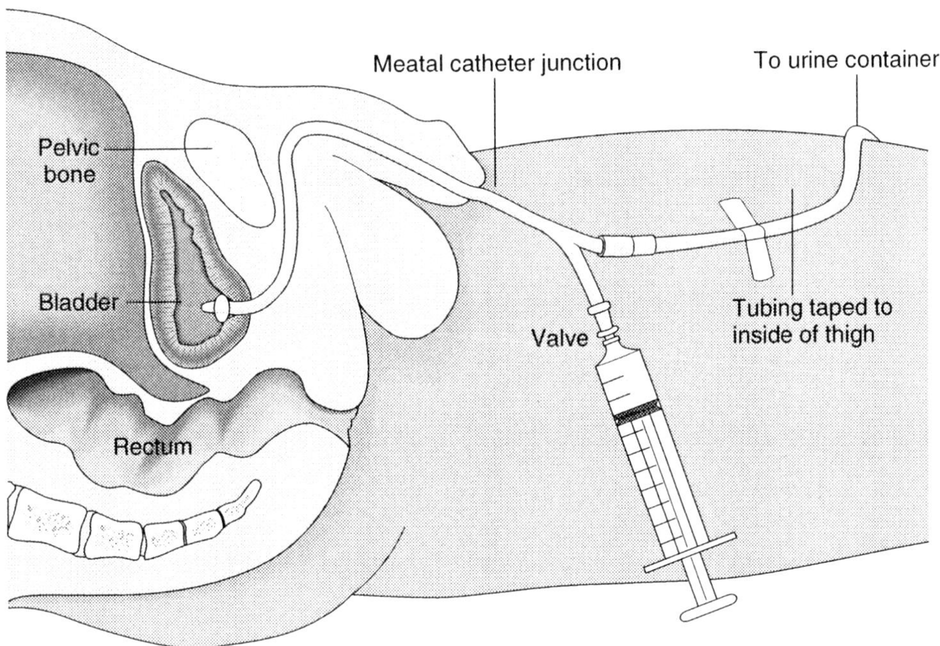


**Figure 1.12** Removing an indwelling urinary catheter. Always deflate the retention balloon before removing the catheter.

SECTION THREE

# Staple and Suture Removal

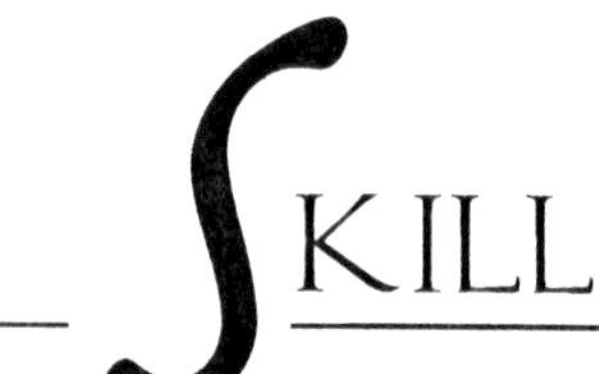

## SKILL

## Removing Staples

**Purpose** Staples are commonly used to hold the skin together after a surgical procedure. They allow the edges to come together as the healing process occurs (approximation and granulation). Once the physician has decided that sufficient healing has occurred, the staples are removed. Steri-Strips, a type of tape or bandage, are often applied to continue holding the skin together during the later stages of healing to minimize scarring.

### Objectives

**The caregiver demonstrates the ability to do the following:**

1. Gather the correct supplies.
2. Communicate using a style that reduces the patient's anxiety.
3. Maintain sterile technique.
4. Remove staples correctly.
5. Apply Steri-Strips correctly.
6. Report the results of the procedure to the RN or preceptor.

### Key Terms

**Approximation** A condition in which the edges of the incision or wound have new growth (granulation) and are sticking together.

**Dehiscence** A condition in which the edges of the incision, which were to have healed, come apart, revealing underlying levels of skin and tissue.

**Evisceration** A condition in which the underlying structures below the skin are revealed after dehiscence. Evisceration usually involves the bowel erupting out of the abdominal cavity onto the skin.

**Staple** A metal device that holds two edges of skin together so that healing can occur.

**Staple Extractor** A small metal device that slides under the staple in the patient's skin, lifts it up, and pinches it in the middle. Pinching the staple makes the ends rise up out of the skin.

### Supplies/Equipment

Sterile gloves • Steri-Strips • Scissors • Skin staple extractor • Skin prep swabs

### Pertinent Points

- Removing staples requires a physician's order in most cases.
- Patients are often happy to have the staples removed but are hesitant because they fear that it will hurt. Explain to the patient that there will be a slight, momentary discomfort as the staples are removed, but that it usually feels better to have them out.
- Provide for privacy and patient comfort before removing the staples. Close the door or curtain, and check to ensure that the patient is in a comfortable position.

## Age-Specific Considerations

Patients of all ages may be concerned about the appearance of the incision line. Others may focus primarily on getting the staples out. Give the patient time to look at the incision line if desired. Do not say that it looks good or bad, but do say that the wound is healing well if appropriate.

Children may fear mutilation or that the incision will pop open. Adolescents and adults may have body image issues, depending on the location of the incision line. The elderly may fear possible infection and the potential for longer healing times. Diabetic or extremely obese patients are likely to experience more difficulty or slower healing than are others.

## Key Concept

When taking the staples out, examine the incision line. If the edges are not approximated and it appears that the incision line is coming undone, **stop** removing the staples and call the RN or the preceptor to the room immediately with the call bell. Remain with the patient, and stay calm. Dehiscence does not happen often, but always check for it before removing all of the staples. A 2- by 2-inch or 2- by 3-inch gauze pad can be used to apply pressure to the dehisced area.

## Steps

1. Wash hands.
2. Explain the procedure to the patient.
3. Provide for privacy.
4. Assemble the equipment (Figure 1.13) and put on gloves.
5. Expose the incision line (remove the old dressing if necessary). Discard the dressing, and change gloves.
6. Open the supplies, and cut the Steri-Strips into 2- to 3-inch lengths.
7. Pull on sterile gloves. Remove every other staple. Slide the staple extractor under the staple to lift it, and then squeeze the handles of the extractor to crimp it (Figure 1.14). Gently lift the staple out of the skin. Note the healing progress.
8. Swab the skin with a prep swab (ask patient to determine whether they are allergic to prep); allow the area to dry thoroughly.
9. Apply a Steri-Strip to each place where a staple was removed (Figure 1.15).
10. Remove the remaining staples one at a time.
11. Apply the rest of the Steri-Strips to cover the incision line.
12. Remove and discard gloves; wash hands.
13. Document and report the results to the RN or preceptor.

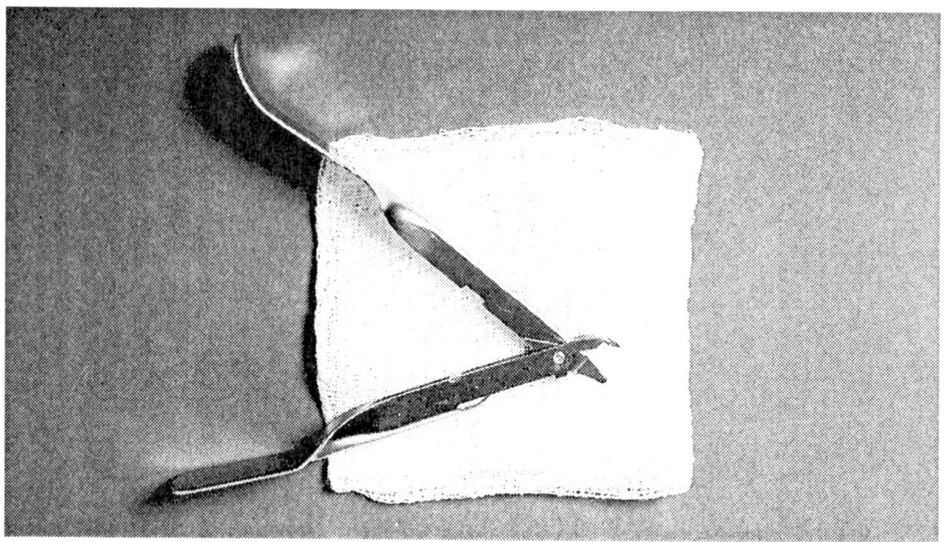

**Figure 1.13** Staple removal kit.

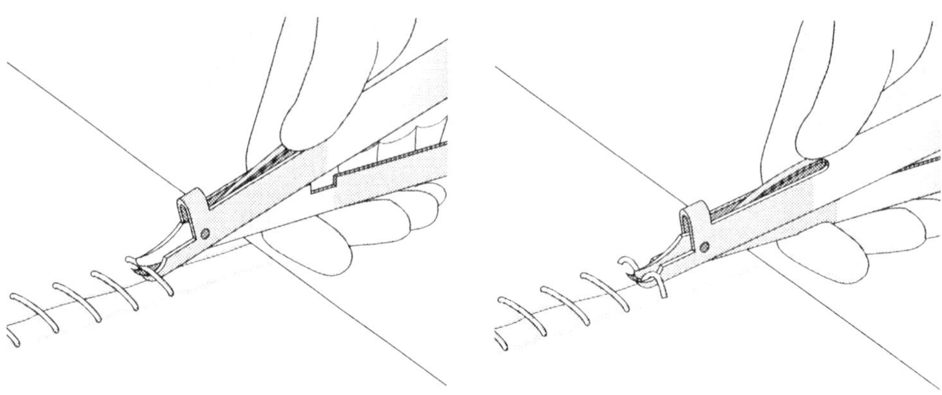

**Figure 1.14** Removing staples from an incision line.

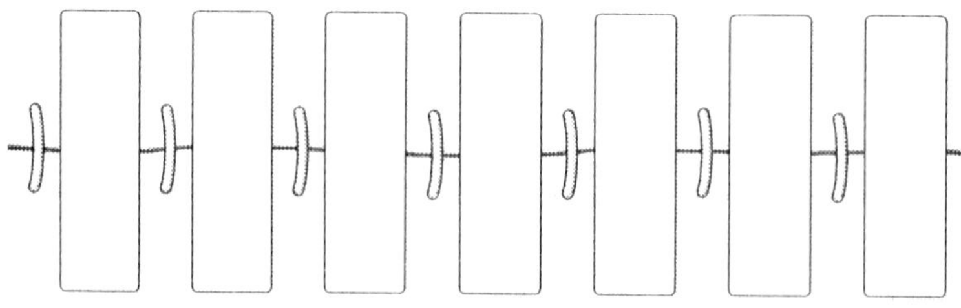

**Figure 1.15** Incision line with alternating staples and Steri-Strips. Apply a Steri-Strip immediately after removing each staple.

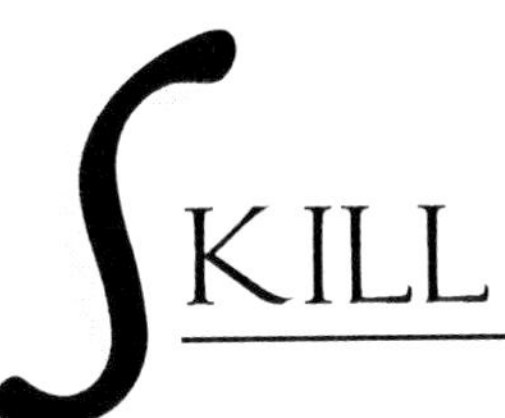

# SKILL

## Removing Sutures

***Purpose*** Sutures are commonly used to hold the skin together after a surgical procedure or injury to the body. They allow the edges to come together as the healing process occurs (approximation and granulation). Once the physician has decided that sufficient healing has occurred, the sutures are removed. Steri-Strips, a type of tape or bandage, are often applied to continue holding the skin together during the later stages of healing to minimize scarring.

### Objectives

**The caregiver demonstrates the ability to do the following:**

1. Gather the correct supplies.
2. Communicate using a style that reduces the patient's anxiety.
3. Maintain sterile technique.
4. Remove sutures correctly.
5. Apply Steri-Strips correctly.
6. Report the results of the procedure to the RN or preceptor.

### Key Terms

**Approximation** A condition in which the edges of the incision or wound have new growth (granulation) and are sticking together.

**Dehiscence** A condition in which the edges of the incision, which were to have healed, come apart, revealing underlying levels of skin and tissue.

**Evisceration** A condition in which the underlying structures below the skin are revealed after dehiscence. Evisceration usually involves the bowel erupting out of the abdominal cavity onto the skin.

**Forceps** A metal or plastic device that allows the user to pick up and lift small objects such as sutures.

**Sutures** A stitch put in place to close a wound or incision.

### Supplies/Equipment

Sterile gloves • Steri-Strips • Scissors • Forceps • Skin prep swabs

### Pertinent Points

- Removing sutures requires a physician's order in most cases.
- Patients are often happy to have the sutures removed but are hesitant because they fear that it will hurt. Explain to the patient that there will be a slight, momentary discomfort as the sutures are removed, but that it usually feels better to have them out.
- Provide for privacy and patient comfort before removing the sutures. Close the door or curtain, and check to ensure that the patient is in a comfortable position.

## Age-Specific Considerations

Patients of all ages may be concerned about the appearance of the incision line. Others may focus primarily on getting the sutures out. Give the patient time to look at the incision line if desired. Do not say that it looks good or bad, but do say that the wound is healing well, if appropriate.

Children may fear mutilation or that the incision will pop open. Adolescents and adults may have body image issues, depending on the location of the incision line. The elderly may fear possible infection and the potential for longer healing times. Diabetic or extremely obese patients are likely to experience more difficulty or slower healing than others.

## Key Concept

When taking the sutures out, examine the incision line. If the edges are not approximated and it appears that the incision line is coming undone, stop removing the sutures and call the RN or preceptor to the room immediately with the call bell. Remain with the patient and stay calm. Dehiscence does not happen often, but always check for it before removing all of the sutures. A 2- by 2-inch or 2- by 3-inch gauze pad can be used to apply pressure to the dehisced area.

## Steps

1. Wash hands.
2. Explain the procedure to the patient.
3. Provide for privacy.
4. Assemble the equipment (Figure 1.16) and put on gloves.
5. Expose the suture or the incision line (remove the old dressing if necessary). Discard the dressing and change gloves.
6. Open the supplies, and cut the Steri-Strips into 2- to 3-inch lengths.

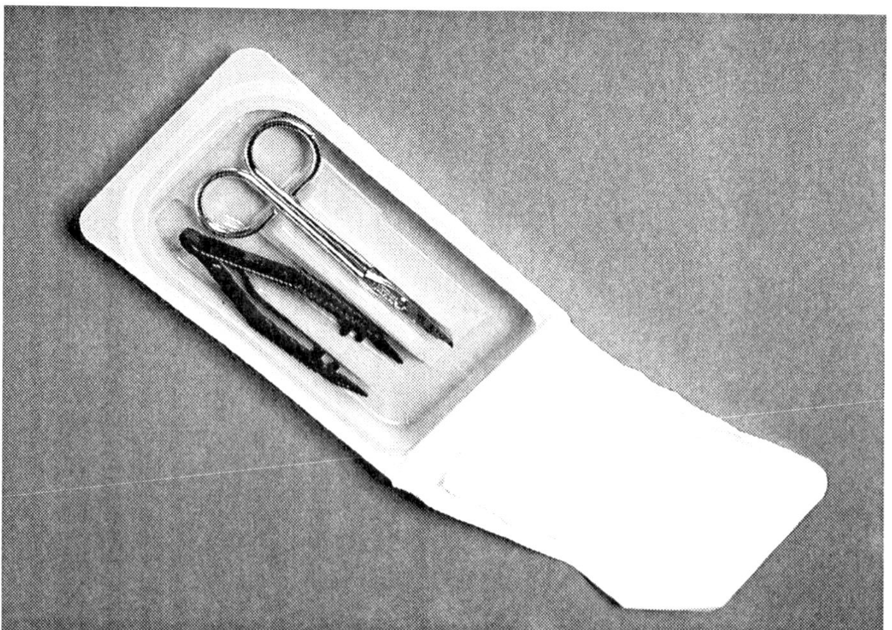

**Figure 1.16** Suture removal kit.

7. Put on sterile gloves. Remove every other suture (Figure 1.17). Lift the suture with the forceps, and then cut it with the scissors (Figure 1.18). Be sure to remove both/all pieces of suture with the forceps by gently lifting them out of the skin. Note the healing progress.
8. Swab the skin with a prep swab (ask patient to determine whether they are allergic to prep); allow the area to dry thoroughly.
9. Apply a Steri-Strip to each place where a suture was removed.
10. Remove the remaining sutures one at a time (Figure 1.18).
11. Apply the rest of the Steri-Strips to cover the incision line.
12. Remove and discard gloves; wash hands.
13. Document and report the results to the RN or preceptor.

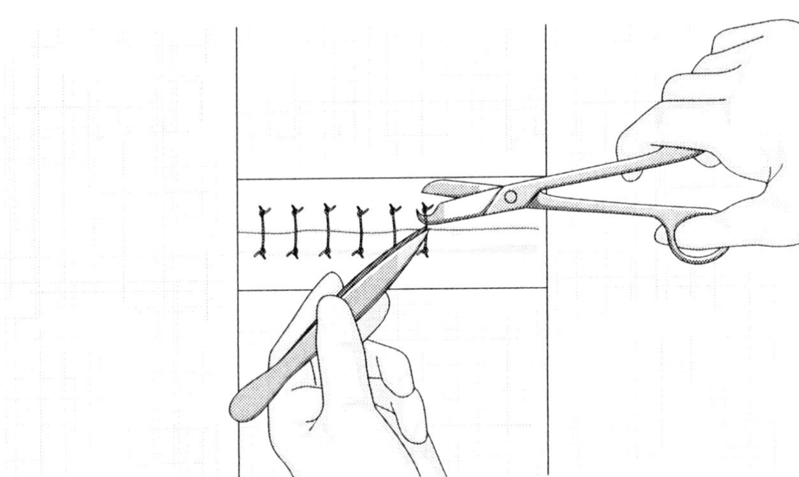

**Figure 1.17** Removing sutures from an incision line.

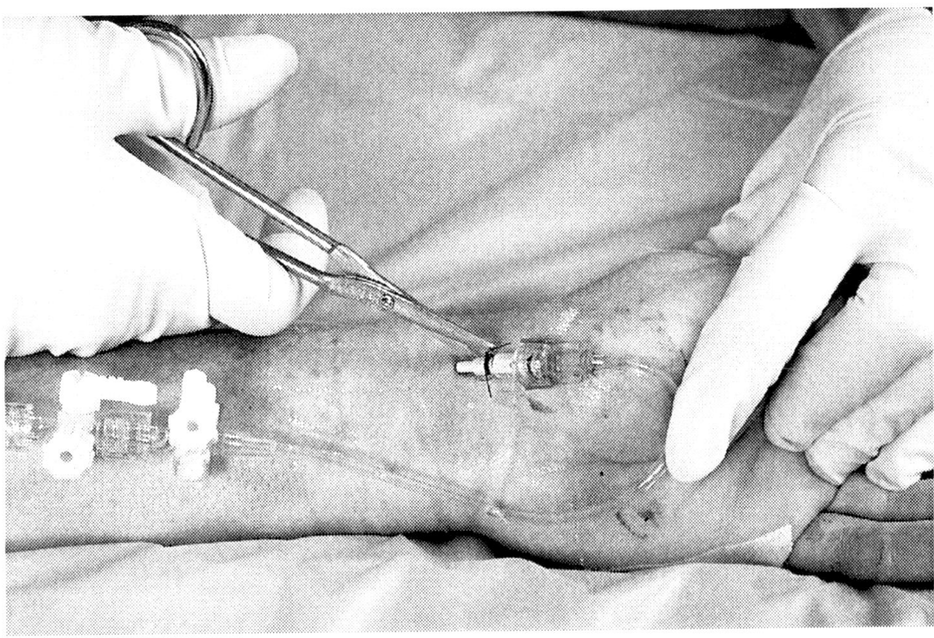

**Figure 1.18** Lifting and cutting a suture used to secure an IV line.

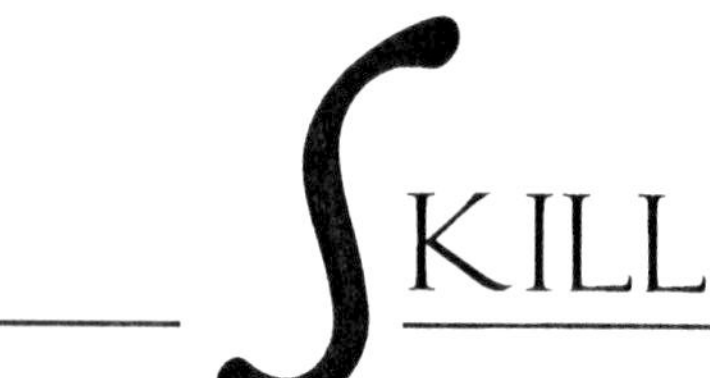

# SKILL

## Checking Blood Products

***Purpose*** Errors in matching the right blood to the right patient ***can result in death.*** Any blood given to a patient must be complementary and safe for the patient to receive. The collection, cross-matching, and typing process that blood administration requires are long and complex procedures. Every effort is made to ensure that the information related to the blood that is collected remains with that unit of blood. (Note: Some states restrict this skill to RNs and LPNs.)

### Objectives

**The caregiver demonstrates the ability to do the following:**

**1.** Identify the correct patient.

**2.** Verify the blood product to be administered to the patient.

**3.** Accurately complete the blood transfusion slip.

### Key Terms

**Blood Bank Identification Number** The number assigned to the blood product to use in matching it to the patient. The blood bank identification number helps prevent patients from receiving the wrong blood product, which could result in death for the patient.

**Blood Slip** A slip of paper that indicates the type of blood product, the patient's blood type, and the expiration date for the product. The blood slip is used to match the patient with the correct blood product.

**Blood Type** A unique characteristic of blood. Patients can have A, B, O, or AB type blood. Another characteristic is positive (+) or negative (−) factors. This represents the presence or absence of antigens in the blood.

**Expiration Date** The date after which a blood product is no longer safe to give.

**Patient Identification Number** The number assigned to the patient by the health care institution. This number is used on all paperwork or records associated with the patient. This process prevents patient records from being mixed up.

### Supplies/Equipment

Patient name or identification (ID) band • Blood slip • Blood product

### Pertinent Points

- Patients can only receive like-type blood or blood with fewer antigens than they possess. For example, a patient with AB+ blood can receive O− blood. O− blood is considered to be the universal donor, and AB+ blood is the most restrictive donor. In most cases, patients receive identically matching blood products to reduce the chance of error and potentially fatal complications for the patient. If you have any questions about whether the blood product is appropriate for a particular patient, contact the blood bank.
- Always check to make sure that the expiration dates on the blood slip and the unit of blood match. Also check to make sure that the blood product has not expired.

- Before beginning the procedure, determine which role you will play: checking the blood product or checking the blood slip. Both associates check the identity of the patient.
- Double-checking the blood assures both the caregivers and the patient that safety precautions are being followed. Explain to the patient that errors are very rare, and that the purpose of the procedure is to ensure safety.
- Use this time to educate the patient about the transfusion procedure used in your institution. Answer any questions that the patient and the family have.

## Age-Specific Considerations

Patients of all ages may have concerns, fears, and misconceptions about receiving blood. Address all issues with respect. Explain how the blood can help them, where it came from, and what they can expect to feel. Children as well as adults may fear that the transfusion will hurt.

## Key Concepts

- The blood slip contains all of the information regarding the characteristics of the blood and the type of blood that the patient needs. Double-checking the identification of the unit of blood, the patient, and the blood slip reduces the risk that the transfusion will harm the patient.
- It is important to relax and think clearly while checking blood products. If you rush through the procedure, you will not catch errors. Correctly identifying the patient who is to receive blood is crucial for patient safety.

## Steps

1. Ask the patient to spell his or her name as you check the spelling on the blood slip and on the patient's name band. (If the patient is unable to spell the name, ask another caregiver to read it aloud from the patient's ID band.)
2. Read aloud the patient identification number on the blood slip as a second caregiver (RN) checks it against the ID number on the patient's name band.
3. Read aloud the blood bank identification number, blood type, and expiration date from the blood slip as the second caregiver checks this information against the blood bag (Figure 1.19). Verify blood bank identification number, blood type, and expiration date as second caregiver reads aloud this information from the blood bag.
4. Immediately inform the RN of any discrepancy in the information.
5. Sign your name on the slip, indicating the double-check procedure, and give it to the RN to sign.

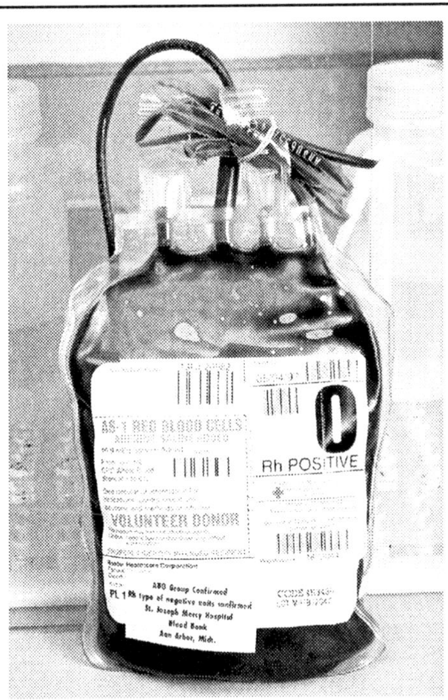


**Figure 1.19** Blood bag.

# Chapter 2
# Specimen Collection

## Introduction

Specimen collection is an important component of the caregiver's job. Patients receive treatment and are prescribed medications based on the findings of lab results. Specimens that are collected improperly or are contaminated in the process must frequently be obtained and analyzed again, resulting in unnecessary expense. Therefore, it is always important to acquire the desired specimen; record the correct information, including the patient's name, location, time, and date of collection, on the lab slip; and accurately document the results. The use of standard precautions prevents unnecessary risk and personal exposure of the caregiver involved in specimen collection or processing.

This chapter prepares caregivers to perform the following skills:

- Collecting a Sterile Urine Specimen
- Obtaining a Sputum Specimen
- Obtaining a Gastric Specimen
- Collecting Stool for Hemoccult Testing
- Checking Blood Glucose

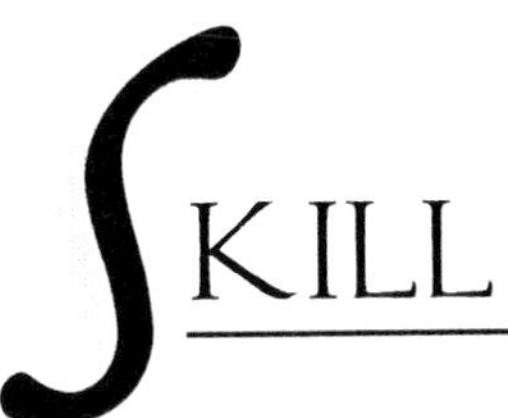

# SKILL

## Collecting a Sterile Urine Specimen

***Purpose*** A sterile urine specimen is needed to diagnose and treat many different diseases and disorders. The specimen must be sterile, or free of germs that are on the outside of the body, to get an accurate result. The specimen is obtained either by performing the straight catheterization procedure or by clamping an indwelling urinary catheter and withdrawing a sample of urine with a syringe from the tubing.

### Objectives

**The caregiver demonstrates the ability to do the following:**

1. Gather the correct supplies.
2. Communicate using a style that reduces the patient's anxiety.
3. Obtain a sterile urine specimen.
4. Apply the correct lab label.
5. Report the results of the procedure to the RN or preceptor.

### Key Term

**Specimen Identification** The process of ensuring that the correct patient's name is attached to each specimen. This includes identifying the correct patient from whom to obtain the specimen. If the specimen is obtained from the wrong patient, the result could be an inaccurate diagnosis or improper treatment.

### Supplies/Equipment

Gloves • Clamp • Alcohol swabs • 10-cc syringe • Sterile specimen cup • Lab label

### Pertinent Points

- Explain to the patient why the specimen is needed and how you will obtain it.
- When using the straight catheterization method, collect the urine in the sterile specimen cup as part of the procedure.
- When clamping an indwelling urinary catheter to collect a urine specimen, note the time the tubing is clamped. Remember to remove the clamp within 15 minutes.

### Age-Specific Considerations

Provide privacy, and avoid exposing the patient's genitals while collecting the sterile urine specimen. Ask visitors to step outside the room if that is the patient's preference.

Reassure all patients that collecting the specimen will not cause pain. A child who sees the needle may be fearful and require extra reassurance.

### Key Concept

An indwelling urinary catheter that is left clamped may cause pain, infection, or injury to the patient.

## Steps

1. Wash hands.
2. Identify the correct patient.
3. Explain the procedure to the patient.
4. Assemble the equipment and put on gloves.
5. Clamp the indwelling urinary catheter below the port by folding the plastic tubing in half and applying a metal or plastic clamp (Figure 2.1).
6. Wait no more than 15 minutes for a small amount of urine to collect in the tubing above the port.
7. Clean port with alcohol. Insert cannula (or needle, if cannula is not available) into the port, being careful not to poke all the way through the tubing.
8. Withdraw approximately 10 cc of urine (Figure 2.2).
9. Empty the urine from the syringe into the *sterile* specimen cup. Take care not to touch the rim or inside cover of the cap (this prevents contamination of the specimen).
10. Unclamp the catheter tubing and straighten it out. Be sure that the urine is now freely flowing.
11. Apply the correct lab label to the specimen cup and bag, according to institution policy.
12. Document the disposition of the specimen (e.g., sent/transported to lab) and report the results to the RN or preceptor.

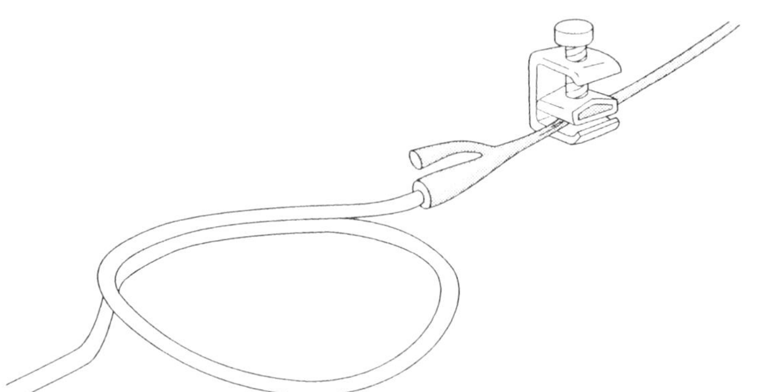

**Figure 2.1** Collecting a sterile urine specimen: clamping the catheter tubing.

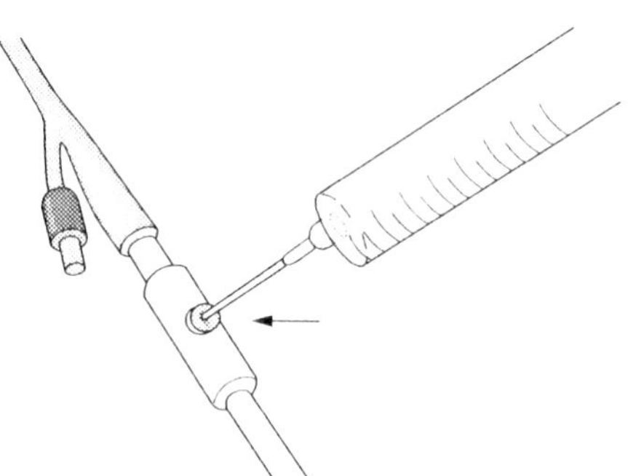

**Figure 2.2** Collecting a sterile urine specimen: withdrawing the urine.

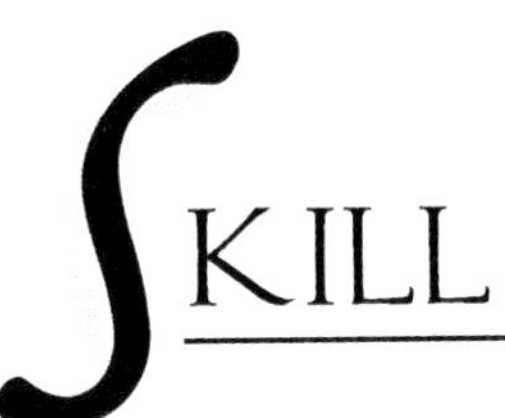

# SKILL

## Obtaining a Sputum Specimen

***Purpose*** The amount, color, and constituents of the sputum are important in the diagnosis of respiratory illnesses or infections. Sputum specimens are obtained from patients to determine whether they have respiratory infections or illnesses, including cancer of the lung, tuberculosis, or pneumonia. The best time to collect a sputum specimen is in the morning. After sleeping, the patient can often more easily expectorate accumulated secretions from the lungs and bronchial tubes.

### Objectives

**The caregiver demonstrates the ability to do the following:**

1. Gather the correct supplies.
2. Communicate using a style that reduces the patient's anxiety.
3. Obtain a sputum specimen.
4. Apply the correct lab label.
5. Report the results of the procedure to the RN or preceptor.

### Key Terms

**Expectorate** To cough up sputum from the lungs and spit it out of the mouth.

**Sputum** Secretions or materials coughed up from a patient's lungs. Sputum is thicker than saliva, the moist substance from the patient's mouth, and may contain mucus, pus, blood, or microorganisms.

### Supplies/Equipment

Gloves • Sputum cup • Tissues • Lab label

### Pertinent Points

- If the patient has eaten recently, it is a good idea to have her rinse her mouth with water before collecting the specimen. This will prevent food from mixing with the specimen when the patient spits out sputum.
- Have the patient take three or four deep breaths before expectorating. This will help ensure a good sample.

### Age-Specific Considerations

Older adults or young children may need extra assistance providing the sputum specimen. A demonstration of how to take deep breaths and cough up the sputum may be helpful. Some adults may be embarrassed or uncomfortable or may even find the process of obtaining the sputum to be nauseating. Provide reassurance and privacy to reduce their discomfort or embarrassment.

### Key Concepts

- Encourage the patient not to just spit into the cup. Explain that saliva and secretions from the nose are not the correct specimens.
- The best time of day to collect a sputum specimen is early morning before the patient brushes her teeth, uses mouthwash, or eats.

## Steps

1. Wash hands.
2. Identify the correct patient.
3. Explain the procedure to the patient.
4. Assemble the equipment and put on gloves.
5. Have the patient rinse out her mouth if she has eaten recently.
6. Ask the patient to take three or four deep breaths before coughing deeply from the lungs (Figure 2.3) and expectorating into the sputum cup.
7. Have the patient repeat step 6 until there is at least a tablespoon-size specimen. Provide the patient with tissues after she has produced the specimen.
8. Cover the specimen immediately, taking care not to touch the inside of the container.
9. Label the specimen immediately.
10. Document and report the results, or if specimen cannot be obtained, relay this information to the RN or preceptor.

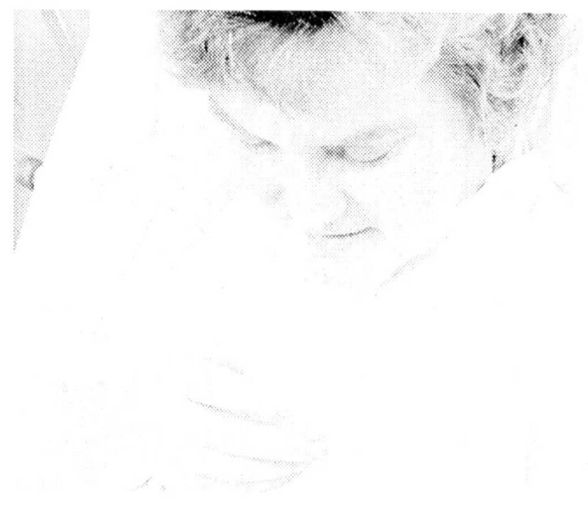

a

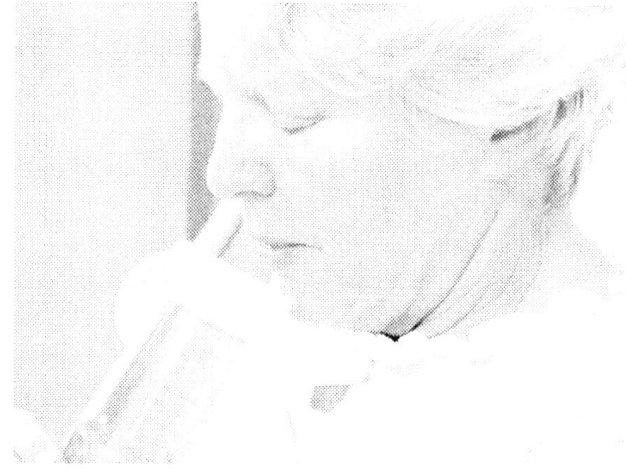

b

**Figure 2.3** **a** Collecting a sterile sputum specimen. **b** An acid-fast bacilli sputum specimen for tuberculosis.

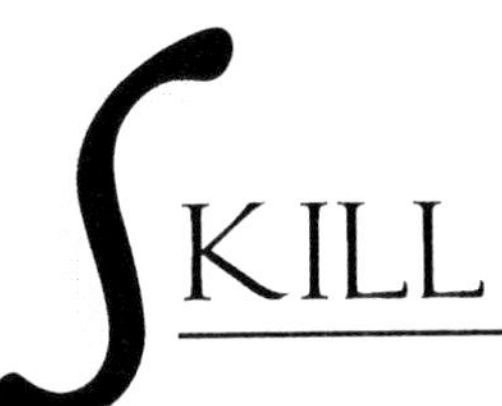

# SKILL

## Obtaining a Gastric Specimen

***Purpose*** A patient may have a nasogastric tube inserted for a number of reasons: to empty the stomach (decompression), to feed the patient (gavage), to wash the lining of the stomach (lavage), or to obtain a specimen for gastric analysis. One type of gastric analysis is the method of measuring the pH of the secretions. If the secretions are acidic, this may indicate the overproduction of acid by the stomach. A high level of acid may lead to discomfort for the patient and potential irritation of the stomach. A physician will often order an antacid to be administered when pH levels fall too low (often for 4 and below).

### Objectives

**The caregiver demonstrates the ability to do the following:**

1. Gather the correct supplies.
2. Communicate using a style that reduces the patient's anxiety.
3. Obtain a gastric specimen.
4. Apply the correct lab label.
5. Report the results of the procedure to the RN or preceptor.

### Key Terms

**Gastric Secretion** The type of fluid found in the stomach.

**Nasogastric Tube (NG Tube)** A tube that is inserted into one of the nares of the nose and passed down the esophagus into the stomach.

**pH** A measure of how acidic or alkaline a fluid is. Water has a pH of 7. A pH of less than 7 is considered to be acidic, and a pH of more than 7 is considered to be alkaline.

### Supplies/Equipment

Gloves • 60-cc syringe • Nitrazine paper • Specimen cup

### Pertinent Points

- Having a nasogastric tube in place is often uncomfortable for the patient.
- The patient may be alarmed at the thought of a caregiver doing something to the tube. Reassure the patient that the specimen collection process will not hurt.
- Explain all of your actions to the patient.

### Age-Specific Considerations

Older adults or young children may require extra reassurance that the procedure will not cause them additional discomfort. When obtaining the specimen, avoid moving the nasogastric tube more than necessary. The skin of elderly individuals or anyone with skin sensitivity can be easily irritated by the tape and pressure of the tube on the nostrils.

### Key Concept

Patients who have nasogastric tubes in place must remain with the head of the bed elevated at least 45 degrees. This prevents aspiration of gastric secretions into the lungs. Remember to maintain this positioning while obtaining the gastric specimen.

## Steps

1. Wash hands.
2. Identify the correct patient.
3. Explain the procedure to the patient.
4. Assemble the equipment, and apply gloves.
5. Disconnect from suction source or unclamp the nasogastric tube.
6. Insert the syringe into the unclamped port of the nasogastric tube.
7. Withdraw approximately 10 cc of gastric secretions into the syringe (Figure 2.4).
8. Reclamp the nasogastric tube, or reconnect it to the wall suction, as ordered.
9. Empty the contents of the syringe into the specimen cup.
10. Dip the end of the Nitrazine paper into the gastric secretion. If Gastrocult or another commercial product is used, follow the directions provided.
11. Note the color that the Nitrazine paper changes to. Compare the paper's color to the colors on the Nitrazine container and identify the closest color. This indicates the pH of the gastric secretions.
12. Document and report the level of the pH to the RN or preceptor, who will determine the need for any further action.

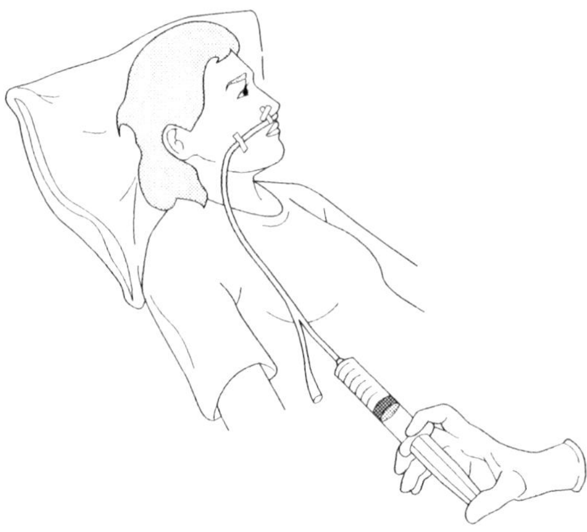

**Figure 2.4** Collecting a gastric specimen from a nasogastric tube.

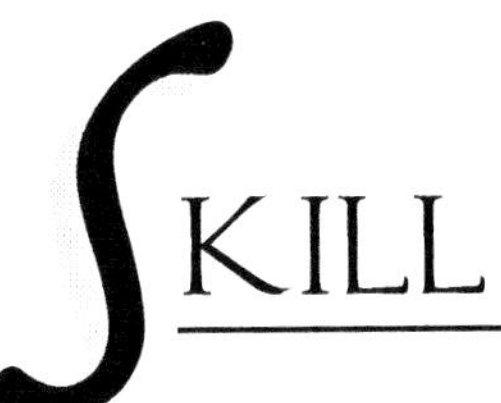

# SKILL

## Collecting Stool for Hemoccult Testing

***Purpose*** Hemoccult testing allows for the quick detection of blood in stool. It is a noninvasive test for the patient. The presence of blood in stool may indicate many diseases and disorders. Hemoccult testing is often used to detect bleeding due to polyps or cancer of the intestinal tract.

### Objectives

**The caregiver demonstrates the ability to do the following:**

1. Gather the correct supplies.
2. Communicate using a style that reduces the patient's anxiety.
3. Obtain an adequate stool sample for Hemoccult testing.
4. Apply the correct lab label.
5. Perform Hemoccult test and read the result.
6. Report the results of the procedure to the RN or preceptor.

### Key Terms

**Hemoccult Developer** The solution that generates or triggers the chemical reaction to indicate the presence of blood.

**Hemoccult Slide** The paper slide used to test for the presence of blood in stool.

### Supplies/Equipment

Gloves • Hemoccult slide • Applicator • Hemoccult developer • Lab label

### Pertinent Points

- Correct identification of the patient and the specimen is crucial for the correct results and diagnosis.
- Explain the test to the patient.
- Assist the patient to have a bowel movement by helping him to a commode chair or onto a bedpan.
- If the patient is using a toilet, a specimen can be collected using a new clean specimen hat placed in the back portion of the toilet.
- Provide for privacy to help the patient relax.

### Age-Specific Considerations

Some teenagers or adults may be embarrassed to be asked to give a stool specimen. Provide privacy, and encourage them to try to have a bowel movement at their usual time.

### Key Concepts

- The test results are most accurate when a clean bedpan is used to obtain the specimen.
- The patient should urinate before having a bowel movement to avoid mixing urine in the sample.
- Always wear vinyl or latex gloves when handling stool specimens.

## Steps

1. Wash hands.
2. Identify the correct patient.
3. Explain the procedure to the patient.
4. Assemble the equipment and put on gloves.
5. Label the Hemoccult slide with the patient's name, the date, and the address, if applicable (Figure 2.5a).
6. Collect a small amount of stool on the applicator.
7. Apply the stool to the box marked "Box A" on the slide (Figure 2.5b).
8. From a different area of the stool, collect another small sample and apply it to the box marked "Box B" on the slide.
9. Close the cover of the slide and secure.
10. Turn the slide over and open the other cover.
11. Wait 3 to 5 minutes before applying 2 drops of developer to each stool smear in "Box A" and "Box B" (Figure 2.5c).
12. Apply 1 drop of developer to the "performance monitor" section.
13. Wait 60 seconds to read the result. If the stool sample turns a light blue color like the "(+)" section of the performance monitor, it is a positive result. If there is no change, it is a negative result.
14. Document and report the results to the RN or preceptor.

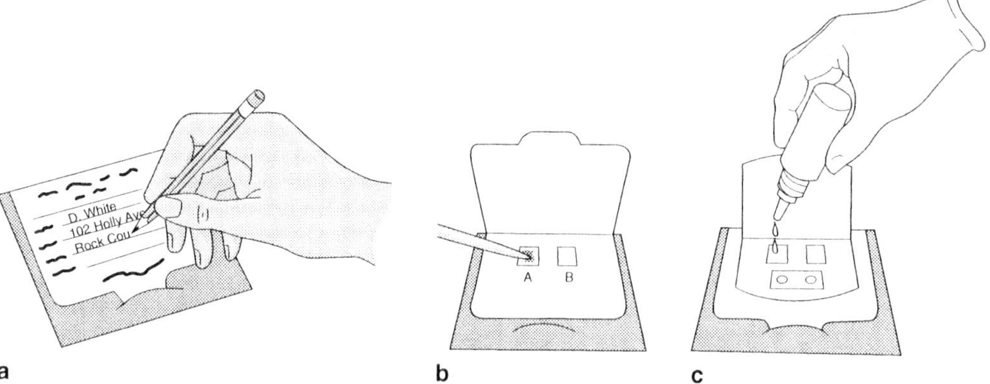


**Figure 2.5** Testing stool specimen for occult blood.

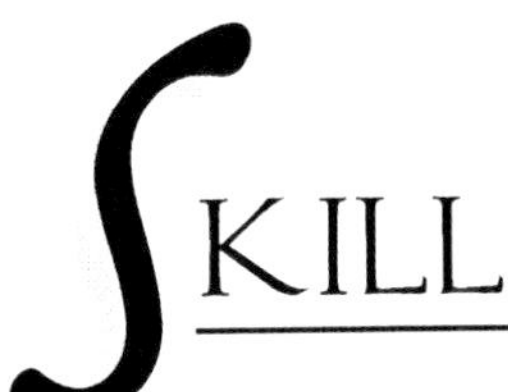

# SKILL

## Checking Blood Glucose

**Purpose** When a patient has diabetes or requires medications or treatments that may interfere with the body's ability to use insulin, it is important to monitor the level of the blood glucose. The most common method of testing blood glucose is with a blood glucose meter. Using a meter to determine when the blood glucose is high or low allows for early treatment with food or medication. There are many types of meters available. Learn about the type used by your institution or patient. New technology may eliminate or reduce the need for blood specimens.

### Objectives

**The caregiver demonstrates the ability to do the following:**

1. Gather the correct supplies.
2. Communicate using a style that reduces the patient's anxiety.
3. Prepare the blood glucose meter for a sample.
4. Obtain an adequate blood sample.
5. Record the results.
6. Report the results of the procedure to the RN or preceptor.

### Key Terms

**Diabetes Mellitus** A disorder caused by the body's inability to convert sugar into energy due to inadequate insulin production or inadequate insulin usage.

**Glucose** Sugar.

**Hyperglycemia** Abnormally high blood glucose.

**Hypoglycemia** Abnormally low blood glucose.

### Supplies/Equipment

Gloves • Blood glucose meter • Test strips • Lancet • Disposable pipet • Small bandage

### Pertinent Points

- Blood glucose monitoring allows for the early detection of hypoglycemia or hyperglycemia.
- The symptoms of hyperglycemia are air hunger (heavy, labored breathing), loss of appetite, nausea, vomiting, weakness, abdominal pain, increased thirst, sweet fruity breath, increased urination, and dulled senses.
- The symptoms of hypoglycemia are excessive sweating, faintness, hunger, irritability, numbness of the tongue and lips, headache, trembling, and blurred vision.
- If you note any of these symptoms or if the patient reports them to you, notify the nurse or preceptor immediately.
- Blood flow can be increased to the finger by (a) applying a warm, moist cloth 3 to 5 minutes prior to pricking the finger, (b) having the patient rub the fingers together, or (c) use of gravity by holding the hand so fingers point down.

### Age-Specific Considerations

Diabetes mellitus is a chronic disorder, and each patient adjusts to it in a unique way. Children may fear and dislike the intrusion of the needle pricks. Adolescents and adults may resent the intrusion as well as the lack of control that the disease creates. Adolescents may avoid following their treatment plans or diabetic diets because these things make them appear different from their friends. Adults and geriatric patients may fear potential complications or may be experiencing complications associated with diabetes.

### Key Concept

The primary use of blood glucose meters is to provide an accurate measure of the blood glucose, or blood sugar, level of diabetics. The goal is to keep the level as close to normal as possible. Medication and food requirements are influenced by the results of the test.

### Steps

1. Wash hands.
2. Identify the correct patient and explain the procedure.
3. Assemble the equipment (Figure 2.6) and put on gloves.
4. Match the code on the test strips to the number on the meter. Check the expiration date on the test strips. Discard them if they have expired. The code number may need to be reset. Follow the meter's instructions.
5. Remove a test strip from the container, and then close it. Do not touch the white area on the strip.
6. Use a disposable lancet or insert the lancet into the Penlet.
7. Place the end of the lancet firmly on the side of the patient's fingertip. Press the button on top of the Penlet.
8. Squeeze the finger gently to obtain a large drop of blood.
9. Slowly draw the blood up into the disposable pipet. Apply the blood sample to the test strip. This prevents cross-contamination of body fluids between patients. An alternative is to drop the blood directly onto the test strip if the machine is used for only one patient.
10. Wait the indicated amount of time for the results to appear on the meter.
11. Apply a bandage to the patient's finger.
12. Clean and dispose of the equipment as necessary.
13. Document and report the results to the RN or preceptor.

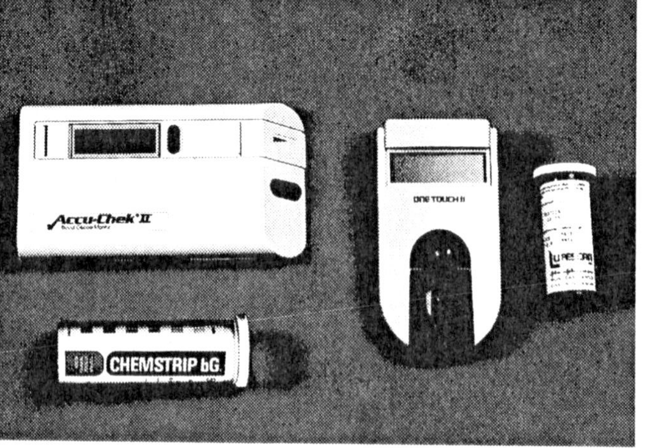


**Figure 2.6** One of the many different devices available for monitoring blood glucose.

# CHAPTER 3

# THE DIGESTIVE SYSTEM AND THE ADMINISTRATION OF ENTERAL NUTRITION

## INTRODUCTION

Adequate nutrition is vital for growth, tissue repair, energy, and resistance to infection. The foods we eat supply the nutrients and fluids for these processes. Caregivers use a variety of enteral feedings to provide nutrition for patients who are temporarily or permanently unable to feed themselves. Enteral feedings are tube feedings given to meet caloric and protein requirements when patients are unable to take adequate oral nutrition.

This chapter includes information on the basic anatomy and physiology of the digestive system. In addition, it prepares caregivers to perform the following skills:

- Inserting a Nasogastric Tube
- Administering a Nasogastric Tube Feeding
- Unclogging a Nasogastric Tube
- Discontinuing and Removing a Nasogastric Tube
- Administering an Enteral Feeding Using a Gastrostomy Tube
- Administering an Enteral Feeding Using a Gastrostomy Button
- Administering an Enteral Feeding Using a Jejunostomy Tube (J-Tube)

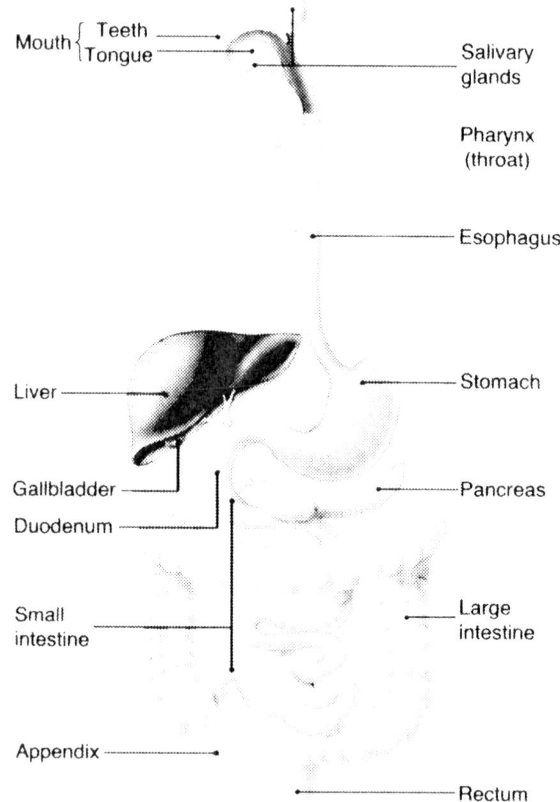


**Figure 3.1** Anatomy of the gastrointestinal system.

## Overview of the Digestive System

The digestive system breaks down food by mechanical and chemical means to a form that the body's cells can use. The digestive system consists of a hollow tube that begins at the mouth and extends to the rectum (anus) and is approximately 30 feet long. The portion of the digestive system from the stomach to the rectum is called the *gastrointestinal system*. It is here that the major part of the digestive process occurs (Figure 3.1).

The activities of the digestive system are complex. They include the secretion of enzymes, hormones, and electrolytes to assist chemically in the breakdown of food. The movement of food through the digestive system by a series of waves called *peristalsis* assists in the digestion of the food and enables the absorption of the end products of digestion into the bloodstream.

The process of digestion begins in the mouth with the mechanical act of chewing, which prepares the food for swallowing. During the process of chewing, the saliva secreted by the salivary glands softens the food mass, begins to dissolve it, and lubricates it for passage into the esophagus. In the esophagus, the food is carried by peristalsis to the stomach.

The main purpose of the stomach is to store, mix, and further break down the food into a semifluid mass called *chyme*. Various gastric juices secreted in the stomach cause the food to break down even further and liquefy. Other than alcohol, very little absorption occurs in the stomach. The food continues through the

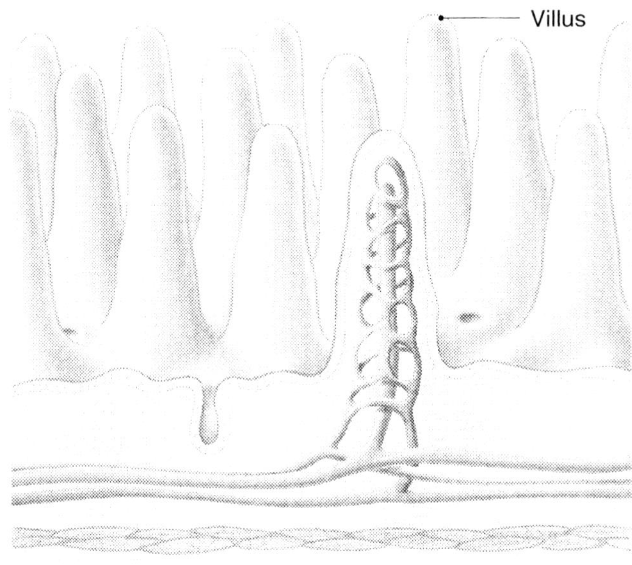


**Figure 3.2** Villi of the small intestine.

digestive system by slowly exiting the stomach through the duodenum, a portion of the small intestine. To aid in digestion, the small intestine also secretes several hormones that enter the bloodstream and stimulate the pancreas to release digestive secretions.

The lining of the duodenum is made up of thousands of tiny, finger-like projections called *villi* that are capable of absorbing the end products of digestion (Figure 3.2). Thus, the digestive process is completed in the small intestine, and the products of this process are absorbed over a 3- to 10-hour period. The products of digestion are moved into the bloodstream, where they are carried to individual cells.

Food that is not reabsorbed into the bloodstream continues on to the large intestine (colon). The major function of the proximal portion of the large intestine is to absorb water and electrolytes, such as sodium and chloride. The distal portion of the large intestine stores leftover products until defecation occurs.

In some patients, an abnormality or disease temporarily or permanently interferes with some portion of the digestive system. Therefore, to provide the body with required nutrients and fluids, the health care team explores and evaluates alternative methods. These methods may include intravenous (IV) feeding or some type of gastrointestinal (GI) feeding (nasogastric tube, gastrostomy tube, jejunostomy tube, etc.). Each method has its advantages and disadvantages and must be evaluated in terms of the treatment goals.

If the patient's health care team selects some form of gastrointestinal feeding, a dietitian or nutritionist collaborates with the physician to meet the patient's specific fluid, nutrient, and electrolyte needs. A formula or liquid feeding can be selected from a variety of commercially prepared products. The formula is then given to the patient by a nurse or multiskilled worker through a tube. Feedings are given either continuously around the clock or at regular times; the latter are called *bolus feedings*.

## Age-Specific Considerations

Infants and children might require alternative feeding methods to meet their nutritional needs due to respiratory distress, inability to tolerate oral feedings, physical abnormality, or illness. It is recommended that infants be given a pacifier to simulate regular feedings and to suck on to meet their oral gratification needs. Additionally, parents are encouraged to promote bonding by holding the infant during the feedings or at regular intervals. Physiologically, the infant is going through a rapid growth spurt that requires increased calories to meet metabolic requirements. Therefore, the dietitian must carefully calculate the caloric needs of infant patients.

Uncomfortable but not painful invasive procedures, such as GI feedings, might prompt an exaggerated avoidance response in toddlers. They are fearful of the loss of control, the separation from their parents or caregivers, and the restriction of their movement or activities that feedings might require. Toddlers are innately curious and energetic, which might lead them to pull on and potentially displace the tubes. Aspiration of nasogastric feedings can occur when the feeding tube is not inserted.

Throughout the preschool and school-age years, children are beginning to grow intellectually and are curious about the "why's" of procedures. Their questioning gives the caregiver an opportunity to provide simple explanations. Often caregivers use play or the use of dolls or puppets as a means to demonstrate key thoughts. Major fears of many children include mutilation, bodily injury, and the unknown. They might even perceive their feedings or medical condition as a punishment for something they did wrong.

Major issues for adolescents concern appearance, loss of control, separation from peers, and being different. Thus, hospitalization and the insertion of a feeding tube, even for a short time, often provoke much anxiety and sometimes behavior changes. Adolescents require complete explanations in private about what is happening to their body and why. Following the explanation, give the adolescent patient an opportunity to ask questions in a nonthreatening environment. Adolescents also need the chance to participate in some of the decision making regarding their care and daily routine (e.g., input into the time of their feedings).

Physiologically, middle-age adults begin to notice subtle changes in their basal metabolic rates that require changes in their caloric intake to avoid weight gain. Adult patients might have multiple stressors in their life that augment the anxiety of hospitalization. Examples of stressors include changes in their current lifestyle due to surgical procedures, feeding rituals, or preferences; the perceived loss of sexual appeal or desire due to the tubes; the perceived loss of youthfulness; and so on. Build on the adult's life experiences, and consider the various challenges facing adult patients when educating or teaching them. Assess the cognitive and developmental level of the patient before planning and implementing any educational activity. Remember to include the patient's primary caregiver, spouse, or significant other.

Patients of any age might have concerns and fears about having a tube placed. Young children might be fearful about where the tube will go inside their body. Adolescents and young adults are often concerned about their body image. Include the parents of children in your teaching. Pediatric patients and confused adult patients who are unable to understand the procedure might pose safety concerns. As people age, many changes occur in their nutritional requirements and their digestive systems. With increasing age, a gradual reduction in energy requirements takes place due to a lowering of the basal metabolism rate and decreased activity; therefore, fewer calories are required. This might be demonstrated in a smaller appetite. Chewing and swallowing difficulties might occur due to illness, inability to chew food effectively, or a diminished gag reflex. A variety of phenomena associated with aging might interfere with the absorption of nutrients from the intestine. Examples include atrophy of the salivary glands and decrease in enzymes in the stomach, pancreas, and small intestine. Diminished storage and utilization of nutrients from food might occur due to changes in the pancreas. Peristalsis, which moves food through the digestive system, slows down, perhaps leading to constipation. Beyond the basic physiological changes that occur with advanced age, other factors that influence the digestive system at this time include any other chronic illness or medical problem, psychological issues, physical pain, lack of teeth, and poorly fitted dentures. Food and eating are a significant part of everyday life. Therefore, it is important to provide the patient with other options for social involvement or recreation and oral gratification.

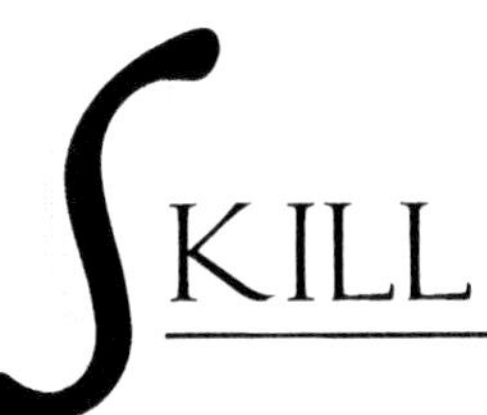

# SKILL

## Inserting a Nasogastric Tube

***Purpose*** A nasogastric tube is placed to meet the short-term nutrition and fluid needs of a patient who is unable to chew and swallow, as a postsurgical intervention, or to suction or decompress the stomach (Figure 3.3). If the nasogastric tube is used to decompress the stomach, a suction machine is attached after insertion of the tube.

Feedings may be given intermittently as a bolus (e.g., every 4 hours to simulate meals) or continuously. The type of formula used in the feeding is prescribed by the physician, frequently in collaboration with the dietitian, to meet the patient's nutritional needs.

### Objectives

**The caregiver demonstrates the ability to do the following:**

1. Gather the correct supplies.
2. Communicate using a style that reduces the patient's anxiety.
3. Ask the patient about any allergies (latex tape, etc.).
4. Follow Standard Precautions.

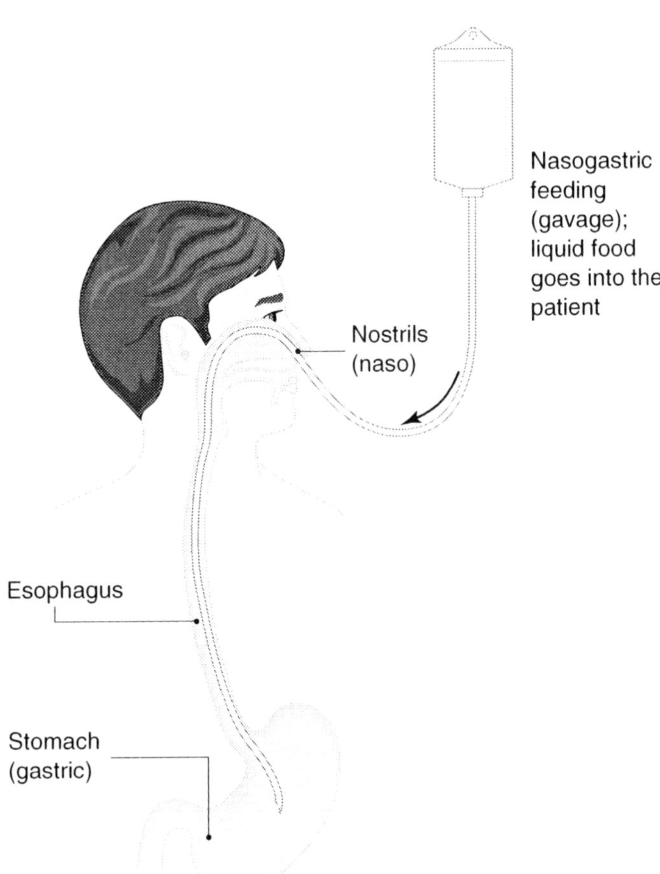


**Figure 3.3** Anatomic placement of the nasogastric tube.

5. Perform the procedure correctly.
6. Document the results of the procedure according to the institution's policy.
7. Report the results of the procedure to the RN or preceptor.

## Key Terms

**Aspiration** The inhalation of formula or fluid into the lungs.

**Auscultate** To listen for sounds from a particular part of the body, as with a stethoscope.

**Gastric** Pertaining to the stomach.

**Nasogastric Tube** A tube placed through one of the patient's nostrils, down the back of the throat, and through the esophagus into the stomach.

**Xiphoid Process** The pointed cartilage connected with the lower end of the sternum.

## Supplies/Equipment

Nonsterile gloves • Penlight or flashlight • Nasogastric tube (#8 to #16 French, red rubber or polyvinyl) • Water-soluble lubricant • Emesis basin • Glass of water and straw • Tape and scissors • Tongue blade • 50- to 60-cc catheter-tip syringe • Plug or clamp • Stethoscope • Safety pin • Tincture of benzoin (optional)

## Pertinent Points

- The insertion of a nasogastric (NG) tube requires a physician's order. This task may be delegated to a competent multiskilled worker.
- If using a red rubber tube, place it on ice before insertion to stiffen it. This is not necessary with polyvinyl tubes.
- To place an NG tube in an unconscious patient, elevate the head of the bed to a semi-Fowler's position, and stroke the patient's throat to stimulate reflex swallowing during insertion.
- Long-term complications of prolonged intubation include nasal erosion, sinusitis, esophagitis, gastric ulceration, and pulmonary aspiration.
- Documentation of the procedure should include the type and size of tube placed, the depth of insertion, the procedure used to verify correct placement, and the patient's response to the procedure.
- Oral hygiene should be provided and the lips moistened at least every 4 to 6 hours.

## Age-Specific Considerations

Infants and children might require alternative methods to meet their nutritional needs due to respiratory distress, inability to tolerate oral feedings, physical abnormality, or illness. It is recommended that infants be given a pacifier to simulate regular feedings and to suck on to meet their oral gratification needs.

Nasogastric tubes are available in various sizes. Be sure to choose the appropriate size for the patient.

Patients of any age might have concerns and fears about having a tube placed. Young children might be fearful about where the tube will go in the body. Adolescents and young adults are often concerned about their body image. Include the parents of children in your teaching. Pediatric patients and confused adult patients who are unable to understand the procedure might pose safety concerns.

## Key Concepts

- The insertion of an NG tube is an invasive procedure that might cause the patient to become anxious. It is important to explain the procedure and to offer the patient an opportunity to ask questions. In some cases, it might be necessary to premedicate the patient.
- When a nasogastric tube is placed, the patient is given nothing by mouth (NPO).

## Steps

1. Verify the physician's order.
2. Identify the correct patient.
3. Explain the procedure to the patient.
4. Wash hands.
5. Assemble the equipment (Figure 3.4).
6. Apply nonsterile gloves.
7. Inspect both nares for any obstructions using a penlight or flashlight.
8. Measure the distance from the tip of the nose to the xiphoid process, and mark it on the tube. (Note: The average length for an adult is 17 to 22 inches [45 to 55 cm].)
9. Ensure patency of the tube by flushing it with water.
10. Lubricate the first 6 to 8 inches (15 to 20 cm) of the tube with water-soluble lubricant.
11. Place the patient in a semi-Fowler's position.
12. Provide the patient with an emesis basin to use as needed.
13. Insert the tube into the naris, and gently advance it (Figure 3.5). (Note: Never force the tube. If you meet resistance, remove the tube and relubricate it, using the other naris if needed.)
14. If the patient is able, ask him to flex his head forward and take small sips of water to ease the

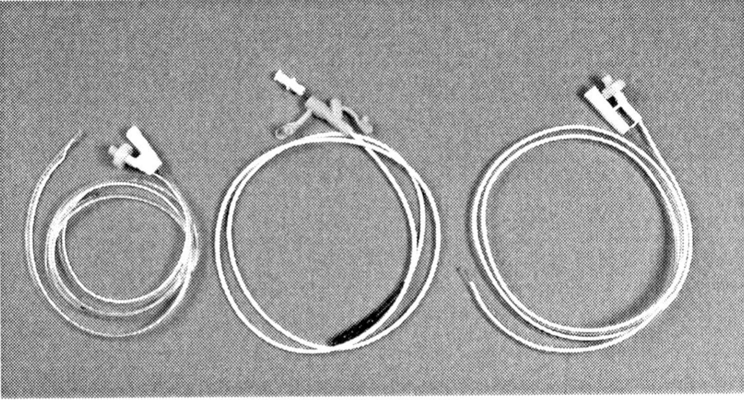

**Figure 3.4** Various types of feeding tubes.

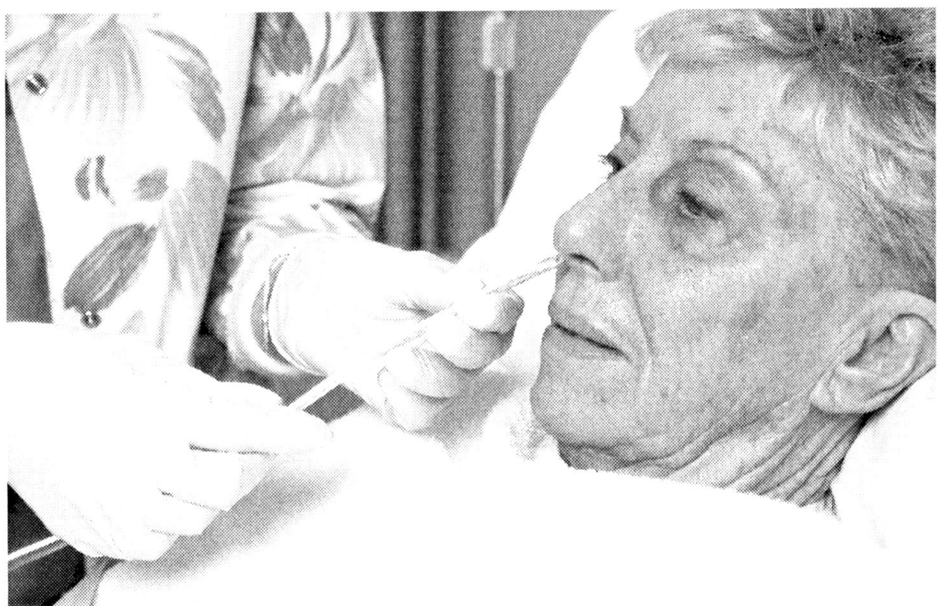

**Figure 3.5** Inserting a nasogastric tube in a patient.

tube's insertion. With each swallow, advance the tube 2 to 4 inches (5 to 10 cm).

15. When the tube has reached the mark you indicated earlier, secure the tube to the patient's nose by placing a 4- to 5-inch piece of tape under the nostrils with the sticky side up. Wrap the tape around the tube, and apply the sticky side of the tape to the opposite side of the nose. (Note: You may want to apply a small amount of tincture of benzoin to the nose to ensure that the tape will adhere.)

    An alternative way to secure the NG tube is to cut a 3-inch piece of 1-inch-wide adhesive tape in half lengthwise about two-thirds of the way up. Attach the uncut section to the adult's nose, and wrap the two tails around the NG tube to hold it in place.

16. Check to see if the tube was properly placed. Using the penlight, look at the back of the throat to see if the tube has curled at the oropharynx (back of the throat).

17. To ensure that the tube is in the stomach, attach the syringe to the tube, and aspirate for stomach contents. If the tube is placed correctly, you will be able to see pale yellow-green stomach contents. Reinstill the stomach contents by gravity flow to avoid electrolyte imbalance. To allow the contents to flow by gravity, remove the inside of the syringe, and hold the syringe barrel approximately 18 to 20 inches above the stomach.

    Another way to check for correct placement of the tube in the stomach is to inject approximately 10 cc of air into the open end of the tube and auscultate the epigastric area with a stethoscope. If the tube is correctly placed, you will hear a "whoosh" sound as the air passes through.

    Other tests for placement include asking the patient to hum. If the patient is unable to do so, the tube is in the trachea. If the patient burps when the tube is filled with air, it is in the esophagus.

18. Once correct placement has been verified, apply a plug or clamp to the tube, and connect the tube to the feeding apparatus or suction machine according to the physician's orders.

19. Attach the tube to the patient's gown by inserting a safety pin through a piece of tape that has been applied to the patient's tube.

20. Provide oral hygiene care and moisten the patient's lips after the procedure.

21. Wash hands and document and report the results of the procedure to the RN or preceptor.

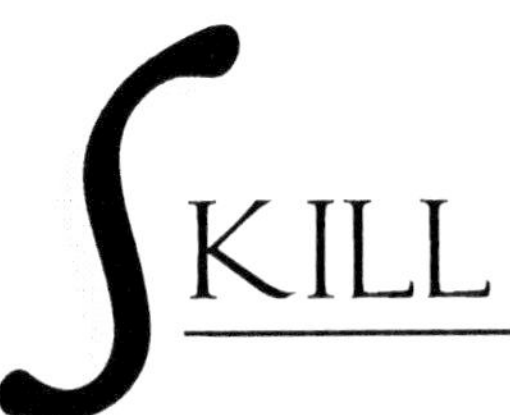

# SKILL

## Administering a Nasogastric Tube Feeding

***Purpose*** Enteral feedings are implemented to meet the nutrition and hydration needs of a patient by directly administering nutrients through the gastrointestinal tract. Indications for enteral feedings include patients who are comatose or on mechanical ventilation, patients who refuse to eat, and patients who are unable to maintain adequate oral nutrition (e.g., patients with cancer, stroke, head injury, or other trauma). Commercially prepared feedings are used.

### Objectives

**The caregiver demonstrates the ability to do the following:**

1. Gather the correct supplies.
2. Communicate using a style that reduces the patient's anxiety.
3. Ask the patient about any food allergies.
4. Perform the procedure while maintaining correct aseptic technique.
5. Document the patient's name, the amount of the feeding, and the patient's response.
6. Report the results of the procedure to the RN or preceptor.

### Key Terms

**Aspirate** To inhale formula or fluids into the lungs.

**Aspiration** The inhalation of formula or fluid into the lungs.

**Enteral Feeding** The process of administration of nutrition via the gastrointestinal tract (particularly tube feeding or oral supplements given to meet caloric and protein requirements when patients are unable to take adequate oral nutrition).

**Feeding** A commercially prepared formula designed to be a nutritional supplement.

**Nasogastric Tube** A tube of rubber or plastic that is inserted through the nostrils into the stomach.

**Peristalsis** Waves of involuntary muscle contraction within a hollow structure (e.g., the esophagus or intestines) that move the contents of the tube forward.

### Supplies/Equipment

Formula • Nonsterile gloves • 50-cc syringe • Emesis basin • Stethoscope • Tube feeding unit or bag • IV pole or hook • Feeding pump • Flush solution (usually water)

### Pertinent Points

- Nasogastric feedings require a physician's order. X-rays are often ordered and required to verify correct placement prior to the initiation of fluids.
- Feedings may be given continuously or intermittently as a bolus (e.g., every 4 hours).
- The schedule of tube feedings is planned to meet the patient's nutritional and fluid and electrolyte needs.
- The formula may be hung at room temperature for 8 to 12 hours.
- Baseline weight and laboratory values are often taken before enteral feedings are begun. Additionally, a patient may be placed on intake/output.

- As with all tube feedings, the patient's bowel status should be monitored. Observe for diarrhea for 30 to 60 minutes upon completion.
- The patient should remain in a semi-Fowler's position during the entire feeding.
- The patient should be observed frequently during the feeding for indications that the feeding tube has been dislodged (i.e., coughing, gagging, respiratory difficulties, change in skin coloration) or is causing discomfort (i.e., restlessness, abdominal tenderness).
- To facilitate digestion, the patient should be in an environment that promotes relaxation.
- Some institutions place a couple of drops of food coloring in the tube feeding to detect aspiration in high-risk patients.
- Some patients are allowed to have ice chips to reduce discomfort or irritation in the throat caused by the nasogastric tube. Offer these if ordered.

## Age-Specific Considerations

Patients of any age might have concerns about enteral feedings. Explain the procedure in words that the patient is able to understand.

School-age patients desire a more in-depth explanation with more detail than do younger patients. Older children want to become involved in decision making (e.g., the time scheduled for tube feedings).

Infants should be provided with a nipple to satisfy their sucking needs.

Normal age-related changes in the GI system include decreased peristalsis and delayed gastric emptying. These factors are important to bear in mind as you assess lab values and monitor residual volumes for older patients.

Diarrhea caused by feeding intolerance may lead to skin breakdown in all age groups.

## Key Concept

Correct verification of tube placement reduces the risk of aspiration. Check your agency's policy. Many institutions require that an RN administer the initial tube feeding to observe for any signs or symptoms of aspiration.

## Steps

1. Verify the physician's order for type of formula, rate, route, frequency, and amount of feeding.
2. Identify the correct patient.
3. Explain the procedure to the patient.
4. Assess the patient for any food allergies.
5. Wash hands.
6. Assemble the equipment.
7. Bring the formula to room temperature if it has been refrigerated.
8. Place the patient in at least a semi-Fowler's position for feeding. A high Fowler's position is preferred (Figure 3.6).
9. Apply nonsterile gloves.
10. Aspirate all of the stomach contents and measure the amount of residual to evaluate the absorption of the last feeding. Reinstill the stomach contents using the gravity method. (Remove the plunger of the syringe, and hold the syringe barrel approximately 18 to 20 inches above the abdomen.)
11. Evaluate the need to provide a feeding based on your institution's policy.
12. Fill the bag and tubing with formula, and hang the bag on the hook or IV pole.
13. If a bolus feeding is given, connect the feeding bag tubing to the patient's nasogastric tube.

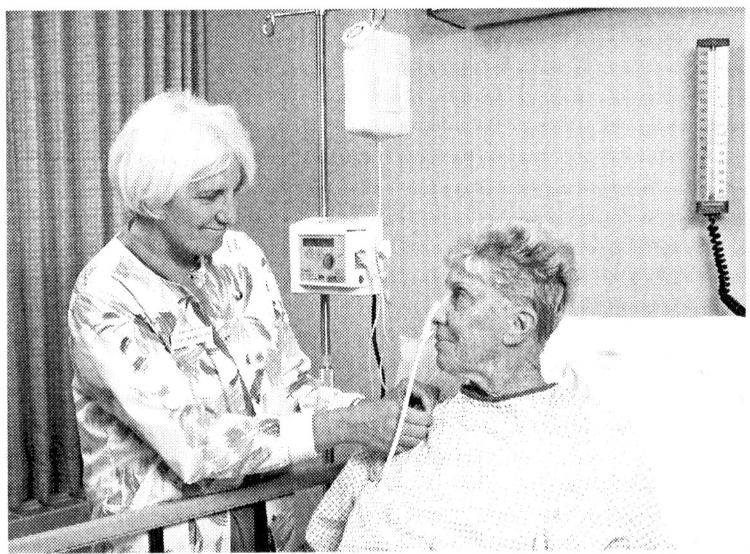

**Figure 3.6** Patient receiving a nasogastric feeding.

Note: Some institutions require a feeding pump to be used to regulate the feeding. Other institutions identify a drip factor (the number of cubic centimeters per hour) for running a feeding without a pump.

14. After the feeding is completed, flush the tubing with water according to your institution's policy. Normally, this is 30 to 50 cc water at room temperature. Follow the policy of your agency or institution regarding when to change the bag. In many places, they are changed once a day.
15. Reclamp the nasogastric tube.
16. Rinse the gastric feeding unit copiously with tap water only, and hang it to dry. Do not use soap.
17. Provide oral hygiene for the patient upon completion of the tube feeding.
18. Wash hands and document and report the results of the procedure to the RN or preceptor. Document the patient's name, the amount of the feeding provided, the patient's tolerance of the procedure, and his or her bowel status.

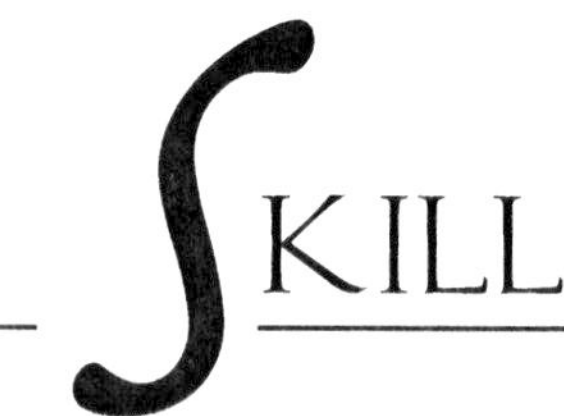

# SKILL

## Unclogging a Nasogastric Tube

**Purpose** A patient may have an obstructed feeding tube for several reasons, including solidified medications or feeding, thick secretions, solid stomach contents, and the use of a small-bore feeding tube. Several methods may be attempted to gently unclog the tube. The desired outcome is a patent feeding tube. If all efforts fail, the tube will have to be pulled and reinserted.

### Objectives

**The caregiver demonstrates the ability to do the following:**

1. Gather the correct supplies.
2. Communicate using a style that reduces the patient's anxiety.
3. Gently manipulate the feeding tube to facilitate patency.
4. Document the results of the procedure and the patient's response according to the institution's policy.
5. Report the results of the procedure to the RN or preceptor.
6. Notify the physician if the procedure is unsuccessful.

### Key Terms

**Enteral Feeding** The process of administration of nutrition via the gastrointestinal tract (particularly tube feeding or oral supplements given to meet caloric and protein requirements when patients are unable to take adequate oral nutrition).

**Patent** Open and unobstructed.

### Supplies/Equipment

Nonsterile gloves • Syringe: 5 to 20 ml for small-diameter feeding tube; 20 to 60 ml for feeding tubes larger than a #10 French • Liquid to unclog tube (e.g., warm water, carbonated beverage, acidic juice)

### Pertinent Points

- Attempts to unclog feeding tubes involve the risks of tube displacement, aspiration, tissue trauma, and patient injury. Therefore, it is important to minimize these risks by using the more conservative methods. Also, risks must be weighed against reinsertion of the feeding tube.
- All fluids used to flush tubes after feedings or medication administration should be counted as intake.

### Age-Specific Considerations

The volume of fluids used to unclog a tube should be proportional to the size of the individual. Very small children can have their tubes adequately flushed with 20 to 30 cc of water.

If unclogging an obstructed tube using cranberry juice, cola, or saline, consider whether the patient has diabetes or hypertension, which are seen most often in older adults.

### Key Concept

The optimal approach to maintaining patency of a feeding tube is to correctly follow procedures for administering medications and feedings.

## Steps

1. Identify the correct patient.
2. Explain the procedure to the patient.
3. Wash hands.
4. Assemble the equipment.
5. Apply nonsterile gloves.
6. Check the tube for placement.
7. Milk the tube from the point of insertion to the distal end, allowing gravity drainage.
8. If this does not unclog the tube, place warm water in a syringe. Gently inject a small amount of water into the tube, and pull back with a plunging action. You may want to leave the water in the tube for 10 to 15 minutes to dissolve a formula plug.
9. Milk the tube again, as described in step 7.
10. Other liquids, such as carbonated beverages or acidic juices, may be used as a solution (if recommended by the manufacturer of the tube) to unclog the tube following the method in step 8. Liquids may be left in the tube and clamped for 10 to 15 minutes.
11. Use the syringe to withdraw the liquid.
12. Monitor the patient for any symptoms of discomfort, abdominal distension, or distress.
13. If the tube becomes unclogged, flush it thoroughly with water and resume feeding.
14. If you are unable to unclog the tube, notify the nurse. The nurse will contact the appropriate physician for further intervention.
15. Wash hands and document and report the results of the procedure and the patient's response to the RN or preceptor.

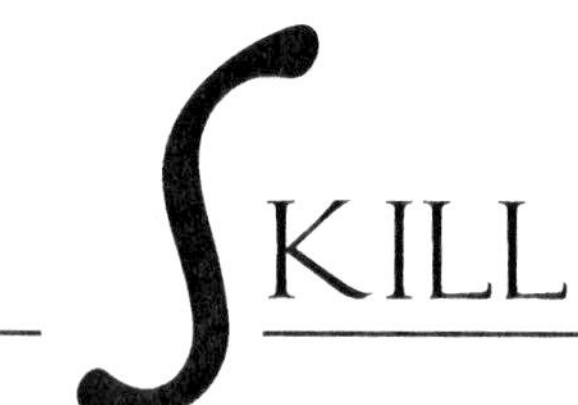

# SKILL

## Discontinuing and Removing a Nasogastric Tube

**Purpose** The nasogastric tube is discontinued and removed when the physician determines that the patient is able to eat, when protocol requires removal, or when another form of nutrition is supplied. It may also be removed secondary to a blockage in the tube.

### Objectives

**The caregiver demonstrates the ability to do the following:**

1. Gather the correct supplies.
2. Communicate using a style that reduces the patient's anxiety.
3. Perform the procedure while maintaining correct aseptic technique.
4. Document the results of the procedure according to the institution's policy.
5. Report the results of the procedure to the RN or preceptor.

### Key Term

**Nasogastric Tube** A tube placed through one of the patient's nostrils, down the back of the throat, and through the esophagus into the patient's stomach.

### Supplies/Equipment

Stethoscope • Towel or bed protector pad • Nonsterile gloves • Emesis basin (used in oral hygiene)

### Pertinent Points

- A physician's order is required for the discontinuation of a nasogastric feeding tube. Protocol may allow the removal and reinsertion of the tube secondary to a blockage without a separate physician's order.
- It is recommended that only a physician remove a nasogastric feeding tube placed for postoperative patients with gastric or esophageal resections. Hemorrhage could result from an injury to the suture line.

### Age-Specific Considerations

Patients of any age might have concerns about having a tube removed. Explain the procedure in words that the patient is able to understand.

School-age patients desire a more in-depth explanation with more detail than do younger patients. Older children want to become involved in decision making.

Explain to patients how they can help the removal process and decrease their discomfort or pain by staying as still as possible and exhaling slowly while the tube is removed.

### Key Concept

Prior to removal, assess the patient's abdomen for bowel sounds and distension.

Steps

1. Verify the physician's order.
2. Identify the correct patient.
3. Explain the procedure to the patient.
4. Wash hands.
5. Assemble the equipment.
6. Use stethoscope to assess the patient's abdomen for bowel sounds and any distension. Cover the patient's chest with a towel or bed protector pad.
7. Disconnect suction if used.
8. Apply nonsterile gloves.
9. Clamp the NG tube with your fingers and ask the patient to take a deep breath and to exhale slowly as you withdraw the tube.
10. Remove the tube in a slow, continuous motion (Figure 3.7).
11. Dispose of the tube and gloves appropriately.
12. Wash hands.
13. Provide oral and nasal hygiene.
14. Continue to monitor the patient for distension, alterations in nutrition, nausea, or vomiting.
15. Wash hands and document and report the results of the procedure and the patient's response to the RN or preceptor.

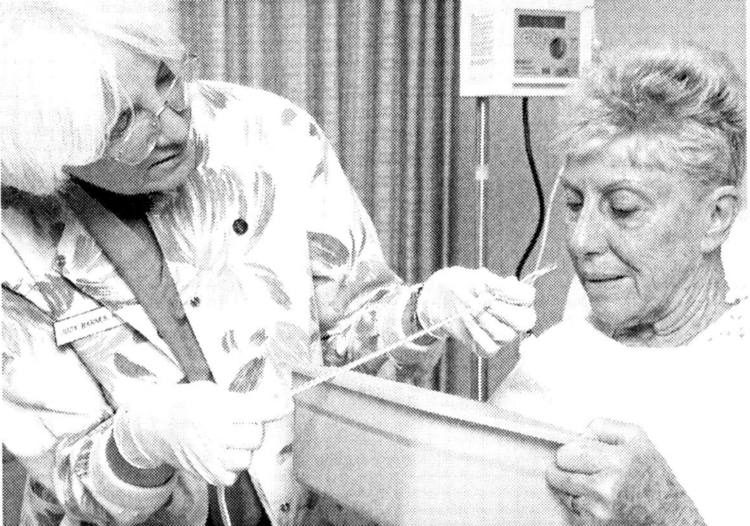

**Figure 3.7** Removing the nasogastric tube.

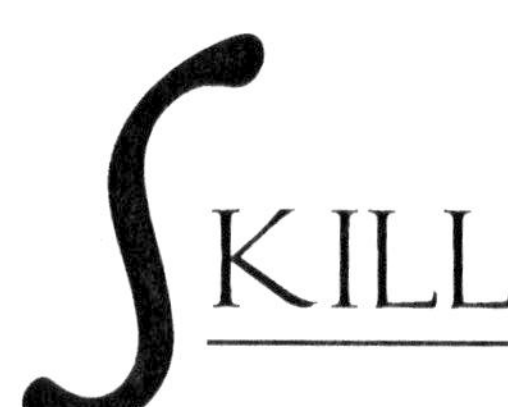

# SKILL

## Administering an Enteral Feeding Using a Gastrostomy Tube

***Purpose*** A gastrostomy tube provides an alternate route for gastric feedings. The tube is surgically placed into the stomach, which acts as a natural reservoir for the tube feedings. The tube can be visualized in the upper left quadrant of the abdomen. Commercially prepared feedings are used to meet the patient's nutrition and fluid needs.

### Objectives

**The caregiver demonstrates the ability to do the following:**

1. Gather the correct supplies.
2. Communicate using a style that reduces the patient's anxiety.
3. Ask the patient about any food allergies.
4. Perform the procedure while maintaining correct aseptic technique.
5. Document the results of the procedure according to the institution's policy.
6. Report the results of the procedure to the RN or preceptor.

### Key Terms

**Auscultate** To listen for sounds from a particular part of the body, as with a stethoscope.

**Enteral Feeding** The administration of nutrition via the gastrointestinal tract (particularly tube feeding or oral supplements).

**Gastrostomy Feeding Tube** A long, hollow, flexible feeding tube inserted into the stomach through a hole in the upper left quadrant of the abdomen.

**Proximal** Near the origin (e.g., the end of the feeding tube nearest the bag).

**Stoma** An opening in the skin created by a surgical procedure.

### Supplies/Equipment

Feeding tube and bag • Formula • 50- to 60-cc syringe with a catheter tip • Stethoscope • Nonsterile gloves • IV pole or hook • Flush solution (usually water) • Feeding pump (optional)

### Pertinent Points

- Tube feedings require a physician's order.
- Feedings may be given continuously or intermittently as a bolus (e.g., every 4 hours).
- The schedule of feedings is planned to meet the patient's nutritional and fluid and electrolyte needs.
- Baseline weight and laboratory values should be obtained before enteral feedings are begun. Additionally, a patient may be placed on intake/output.
- The formula may be hung at room temperature for 8 to 12 hours.
- Before the feeding, auscultate the abdomen. If bowel sounds are absent, hold the feedings and notify the physician.
- The patient should remain in a semi-Fowler's position during the entire feeding and for 30 to 60 minutes afterward. Other therapies and activities should be scheduled appropriately.
- As with all tube feedings, the patient's bowel status should be monitored. Diarrhea might occur due to feeding intolerance.

- Pressure from the gastrostomy tube or drainage of the gastric secretions might cause skin breakdown around the tube. Thus, it is important to monitor the skin around the tube daily.
- To facilitate digestion, the patient should be in an environment that promotes relaxation.
- Tube feedings may be held if aspiration of stomach contents equals more than 100 cc of fluid or exceeds two times the hourly rate. Check your procedure or policy.

## Age-Specific Considerations

Patients of any age might have concerns and fears about having a tube placed. Young children might be fearful about where the tube will go in the body. Adolescents and young adults are often concerned about their body image. Include the parents of children in your teaching. Pediatric patients and confused adult patients who are unable to understand the procedure might pose safety concerns. Infants should be provided with a nipple to meet their sucking needs. Intermittent feedings are preferred in infants because of the possible perforation of the stomach and irritation to the mucous membrane.

## Key Concept

It is important to verify tube placement to prevent aspiration and evaluate gastric residual before administering the feeding.

## Steps

1. Verify the physician's order for the type of formula, rate, route, frequency, and amount of feeding.
2. Identify the correct patient.
3. Explain the procedure to the patient.
4. Assess the patient for any food allergies.
5. Wash hands.
6. Assemble the equipment.
7. Bring the formula to room temperature if it has been refrigerated.
8. Auscultate for bowel sounds before administering the feeding.
9. Apply nonsterile gloves.
10. Aspirate the stomach contents and measure the amount of residual from the last feeding. Reinstill the stomach contents using a gravity method by removing the plunger of the syringe and holding it 18 to 20 inches above the abdomen.
11. Fill the bag and tubing with formula.
12. Place the patient in at least a semi-Fowler's position. A high Fowler's position is preferred.
13. Connect the feeding tube with the gastrostomy tube.
14. Initiate the feeding by placing the feeding bag approximately 18 to 20 inches above the abdomen on an IV pole or hook (Figure 3.8).
15. Monitor the patient during the feeding for any pain, abdominal swelling, nausea, vomiting, or respiratory distress.
16. After the feeding is completed, rinse the bag and feeding tube copiously with water. Clamp the proximal end of the feeding tube, and hang it to dry.
17. Inspect the gastrostomy dressing for any drainage or secretions. Change the dressing as needed.
18. Observe the stoma site for any skin breakdown.
19. Wash hands and document and report the results of the procedure to the RN or preceptor. Document the patient's response to the feeding, the name and amount of the feeding, and the patient's bowel status.

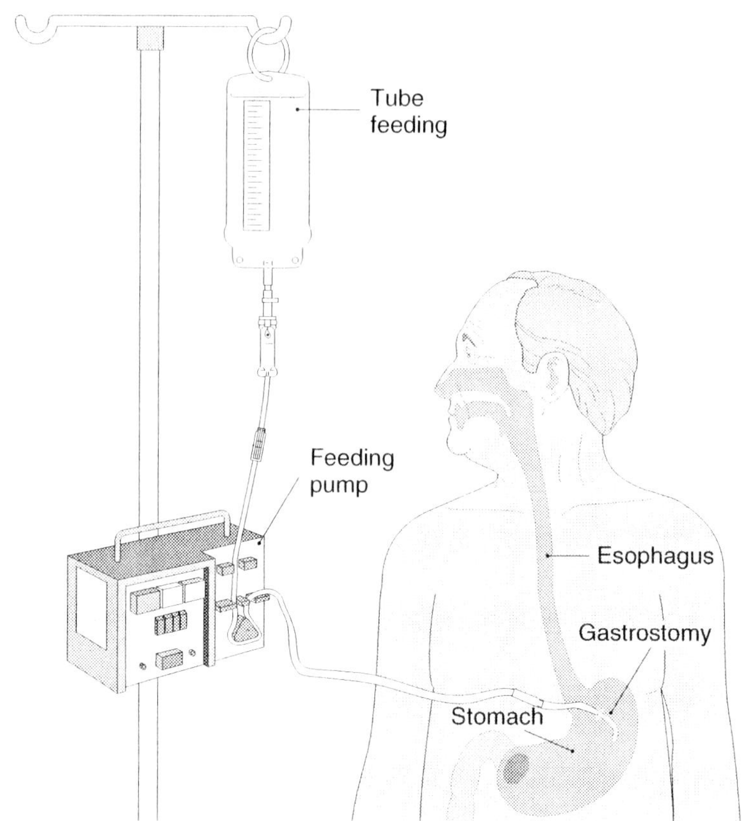


**Figure 3.8** Anatomic placement of the gastrostomy tube.

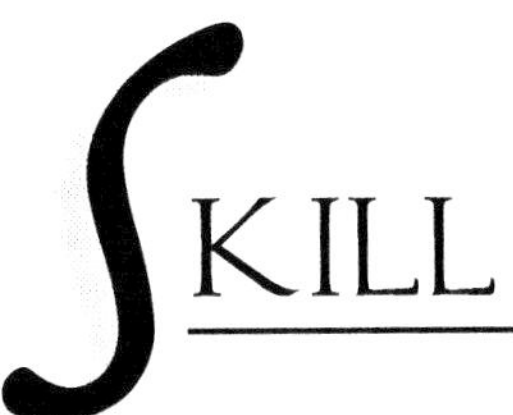

# SKILL

## Administering an Enteral Feeding Using a Gastrostomy Button

***Purpose*** Patients who are unable to maintain their nutritional status orally may be candidates for gastrostomy feeding. An opening, or stoma, to the stomach is surgically created in the left upper quadrant of the abdomen. A flexible silicone device called a button is placed in the stoma so that a tube can be inserted at regular intervals for feedings. This method may be more cosmetically pleasing than having a nasogastric tube in place to some patients for long-term therapy. Commercially prepared formulas are used.

### Objectives

**The caregiver demonstrates the ability to do the following:**

1. Gather the correct supplies.
2. Communicate using a style that reduces the patient's anxiety.
3. Ask the patient about any food allergies.
4. Perform the procedure while maintaining correct aseptic technique.
5. Report the results of the procedure to the RN or preceptor.
6. Document the amount and type of feeding and the patient's response to the feeding.

### Key Terms

**Aspiration** The inhalation of formula or fluid into the lungs.

**Auscultate** To listen for sounds from a particular part of the body, as with a stethoscope.

**Enteral Feeding** The administration of nutrition via the gastrointestinal tract (particularly tube feeding or oral supplements).

**Gastrostomy Feeding Tube** A long, hollow, flexible feeding tube inserted into the stomach through a hole in the upper left quadrant of the abdomen.

**Proximal** Near the origin (e.g., the opening of the gastrostomy button).

**Stoma** An opening in the skin created by a surgical procedure.

### Supplies/Equipment

Formula • Stethoscope • Nonsterile gloves • Feeding tube and bag • 50- to 60-cc syringe with a catheter tip • IV pole or hook • Feeding pump (optional) • Flush solution (usually water) • Gastrostomy button kit with obdurator

### Pertinent Points

- Tube feedings require a physician's order.
- The schedule of feedings is planned to meet the patient's nutritional and fluid and electrolyte needs.
- Baseline weight and laboratory values should be obtained before enteral feedings are begun. Additionally, a patient may be placed on intake/output.
- Insertion of a button requires a well-established gastrostomy site. This usually occurs 3 to 4 weeks after a surgical incision has been made. A Foley catheter is used to dilate the stoma gradually until the button size is reached.
- An antireflux valve at the distal end of the gastrostomy tube helps prevent backflow and the leakage of gastric contents.

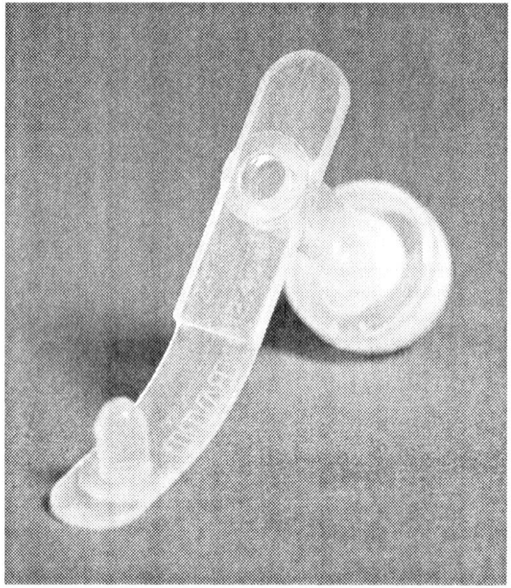

**Figure 3.9** Gastrostomy button.

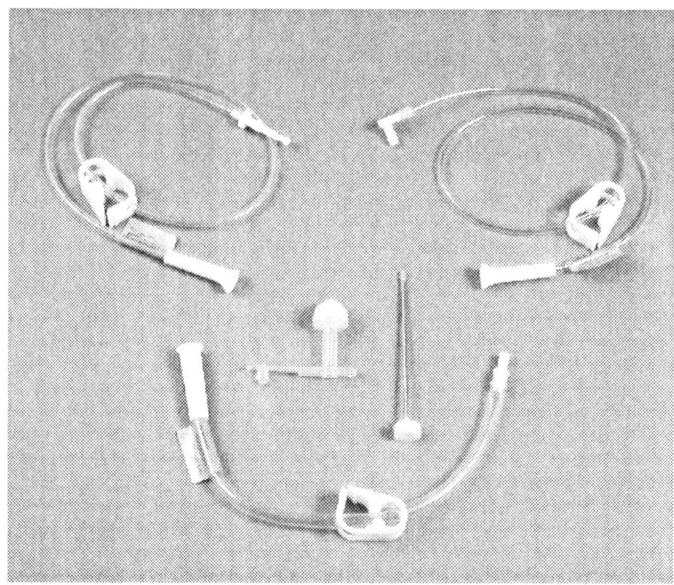

**Figure 3.10** Gastrostomy button and obdurator.

- A button kit includes an obdurator for ease of insertion, a stoma-measuring device, and a special feeding apparatus (Figures 3.9 and 3.10).
- To facilitate digestion, the patient should be in an environment that promotes relaxation.
- Elevate the patient's head for at least 30 to 60 minutes after a feeding is completed. If exercise or other activity is prescribed at regular intervals throughout the day, plan the feeding schedule to include the activity schedule.
- Drainage from gastric secretions or formula can cause skin breakdown. Monitor the skin integrity around the stoma. Be alert to the leakage of gastric contents, which can signal malfunction of the antireflux valve.
- The stoma should be cleaned one or two times a day with mild soap and water. It is suggested that it be allowed to air-dry approximately 20 minutes before any clothing is applied.
- As with all tube feedings, the patient's bowel status should be monitored. Diarrhea might occur due to a feeding intolerance.
- Feedings should be initiated with a weakened concentration of formula and advanced over a 24- to 48-hour period until maximal nutritional requirements are met. Initial feedings should start at 50 cc per hour.

## Age-Specific Considerations

Patients of any age might have concerns and fears about having a tube placed. Young children might be fearful about where the tube will go inside their body. Adolescents and young adults are often concerned about their body image. Include the parents of children in your teaching. Pediatric patients and confused adult patients who are unable to understand the procedure might pose safety concerns. Infants should be provided with a nipple to meet their sucking needs.

## Key Concept

When the gastrostomy button is used, the patient is given nothing by mouth.

## Steps

1. Verify the physician's order for type of formula, amount, route, frequency, and rate.
2. Identify the correct patient.
3. Explain the procedure to the patient.
4. Assess the patient for any food allergies.
5. Wash hands.
6. Assemble the equipment.
7. Bring the formula to room temperature if it has been refrigerated.
8. Use stethoscope to auscultate for bowel sounds.
9. Apply nonsterile gloves.
10. Attach the feeding tube to the proximal end of the button.
11. Use syringe to aspirate stomach contents to evaluate the amount of the gastric residual. Reinstill the stomach contents using the gravity method. (Remove the plunger of the syringe, and hold the syringe barrel approximately 18 to 20 inches above the abdomen.)
12. Fill the bag and tubing with formula.
13. Place the patient in at least a semi-Fowler's position. A high Fowler's position is preferred.
14. Initiate the feeding by placing the feeding bag approximately 18 to 20 inches above the abdomen on an IV pole or hook (Figures 3.11 and 3.12). (If using a pump, insert tubing and set rate.)
15. Monitor the patient during the feeding for any pain, abdominal swelling, nausea, vomiting, or respiratory distress.
16. Rinse the button with water (30 to 50 cc for an adult, 10 cc for a pediatric patient) after the feeding is completed and whenever medications are given.
17. Rinse the gastric feeding unit thoroughly with tap water only, and hang it to dry. Do not use soap. Change the bag and tubing per the institution's policy.
18. Observe the stoma site for any skin breakdown.
19. Wash hands and document and report the results of the procedure to the RN or preceptor. Document the name and amount of the feeding, the patient's bowel status, and the patient's response to the feeding.

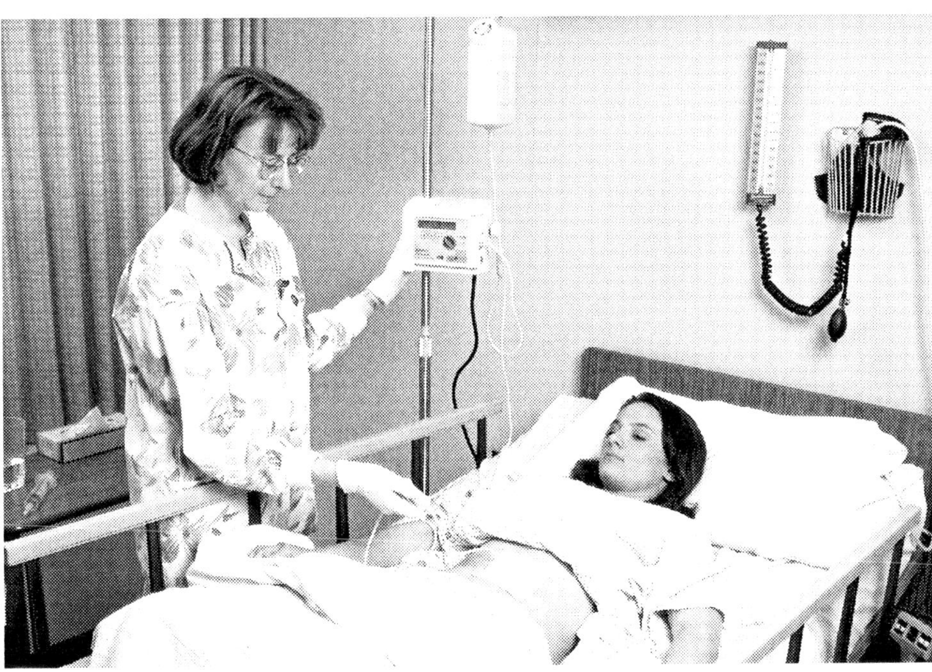

**Figure 3.11** Administering a gastrostomy tube feeding.

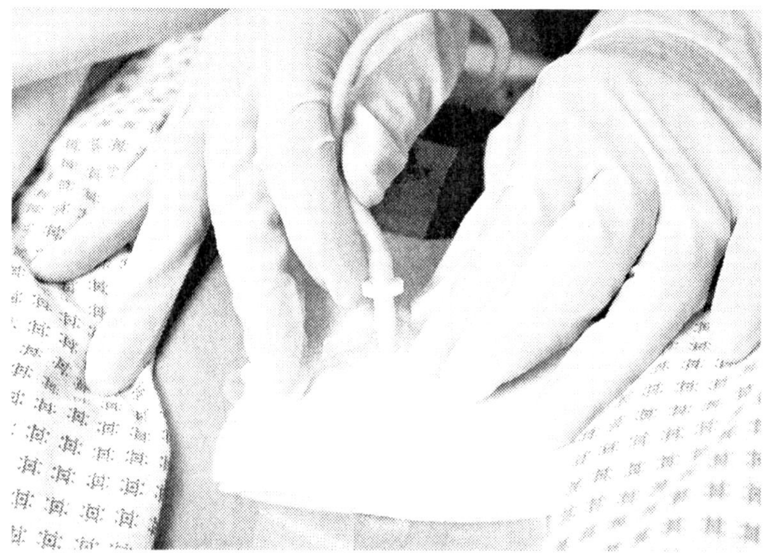

**Figure 3.12** Inserting the feeding tube in the gastrostomy button.

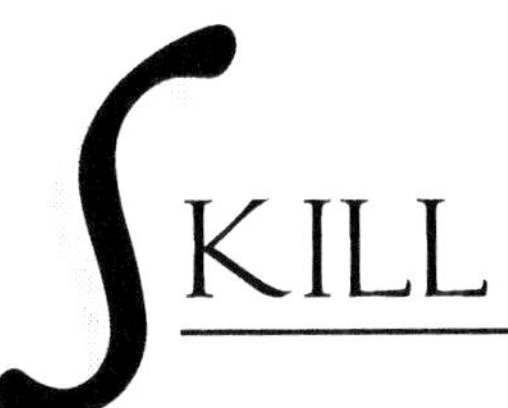

# Skill

## Administering an Enteral Feeding Using a Jejunostomy Tube (J-Tube)

**Purpose** Jejunostomy tubes are often used for gastric feedings for neurologically impaired patients who are at risk for aspiration, patients with stomach cancer, patients with extensive peptic ulcer disease, and those with chronic nausea and vomiting (Figure 3.13). The jejunostomy feeding tube is inserted surgically or via endoscopy. The tube exits the body through a puncture wound in the left lower quadrant of the abdomen (Figure 3.14). Commercially prepared formulas are used for the feeding to meet the nutritional needs of the patient.

### Objectives

**The caregiver demonstrates the ability to do the following:**

1. Gather the correct supplies.
2. Communicate using a style that reduces the patient's anxiety.
3. Ask the patient about any food allergies.
4. Perform the procedure while maintaining correct aseptic technique.
5. Report the results of the procedure to the RN or preceptor.
6. Document the results of the procedure according to the institution's policy.

### Key Terms

**Auscultate** To listen for sounds from a particular part of the body, as with a stethoscope.

**Endoscopy** A procedure in which an instrument is used to visualize or inspect the interior of the body.

**Enteral Feeding** The administration of nutrition via the gastrointestinal tract (particularly tube feeding or oral supplements).

**Gastric Reflux** The leakage of stomach contents back into the lower part of the esophagus.

### Supplies/Equipment

Formula • Stethoscope • Nonsterile gloves • 50- to 60-cc catheter syringe • Feeding tube and bag • IV pole or hook • Flush solution (usually water) • Feeding pump (if ordered)

### Pertinent Points

- Tube feedings require a physician's order.
- Baseline weight and lab values should be obtained before enteral feedings are begun. Additionally, a patient may be put on intake/output.

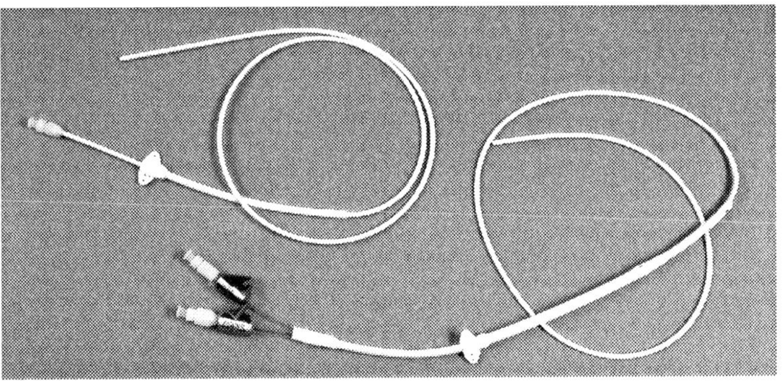

**Figure 3.13** Jejunostomy tube and jejunostomy–gastrostomy tube.

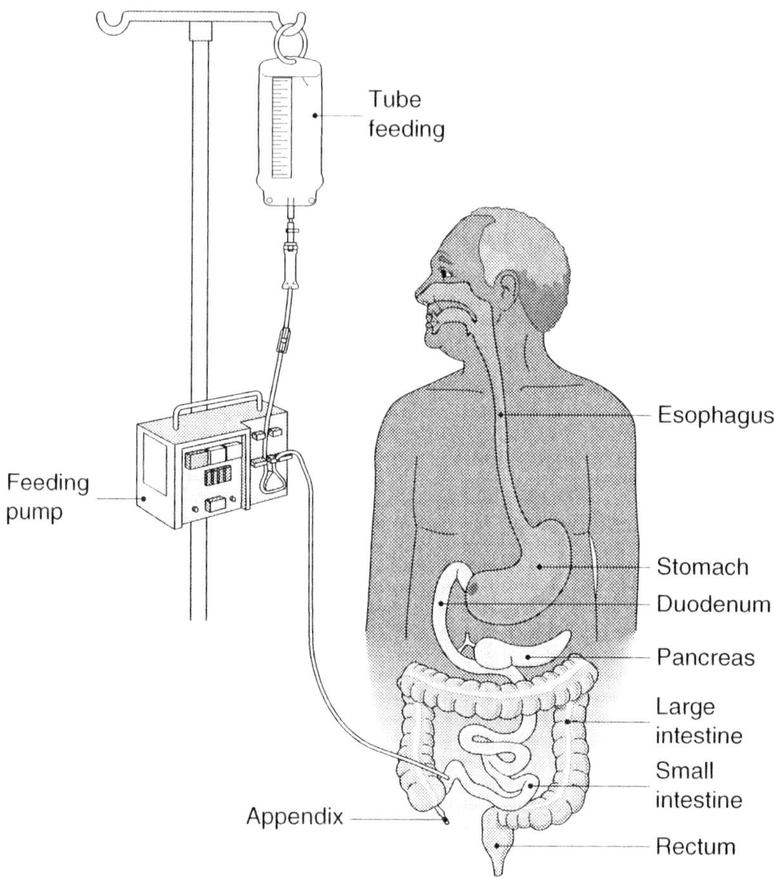


**Figure 3.14** Anatomic placement of the jejunostomy tube.

- Feedings must be continuous because the stomach is bypassed. This may cause diarrhea.
- Feeding pumps are usually used for continuous feedings.
- Formulas may be hung at room temperature for 8 to 12 hours.
- Auscultate for bowel sounds before each feeding. If none are present, notify the physician.
- The patient's bowel status must be monitored during the course of the feedings. (Usually, more than three loose stools in 24 hours is indicative of formula intolerance.)
- Skin integrity around the jejunostomy must be monitored regularly for breakdown secondary to the leakage of gastric secretions or other drainage.

## Age-Specific Considerations

Patients of any age might be concerned about the appearance of the tube in their abdomen. Adolescents and young adults especially might have body-image issues. Younger children might also express a fear of mutilation or of being hurt. Geriatric patients might have concerns about limited mobility due to the feedings. It is important to explain the tube, its function, and the feeding procedure in words appropriate to the patient's age and level of understanding.

## Key Concept

The primary purpose of enteral feedings is to provide adequate nutrition for the patient. The advantage of the jejunostomy tube is decreased gastric reflux. The patient is given nothing by mouth.

Steps

1. Verify the physician's order for type of formula, route, frequency, and rate.
2. Identify the correct patient.
3. Explain the procedure to the patient.
4. Assess the patient for food allergies.
5. Wash hands.
6. Assemble the equipment.
7. Bring the formula to room temperature if it has been refrigerated.
8. Use stethoscope to auscultate for bowel sounds.
9. Apply nonsterile gloves.
10. Use syringe to aspirate intestinal contents and check for a residual every 4 hours.
11. Measure the pH of the aspirated contents. Intestinal sites should be in the pH range of 6 to 7.
12. Place the patient in at least a semi-Fowler's position. A high Fowler's position is preferred.
13. Initiate and maintain continuous feeding by placing the feeding bag approximately 18 to 20 inches above the abdomen on an IV pole or hook (Figures 3.15 and 3.16).
14. Monitor the patient for any pain, discomfort, cramping, nausea, vomiting, or respiratory distress. Change the bag and tubing per the institution's policy.
15. After the feeding has infused, flush the tube with 30 to 50 cc of water for an adult or 10 cc of water for a child (Figure 3.17).
16. Wash hands and document and report the results of the procedure to the RN or preceptor. Document the amount and type of feeding and the patient's response to the feeding.

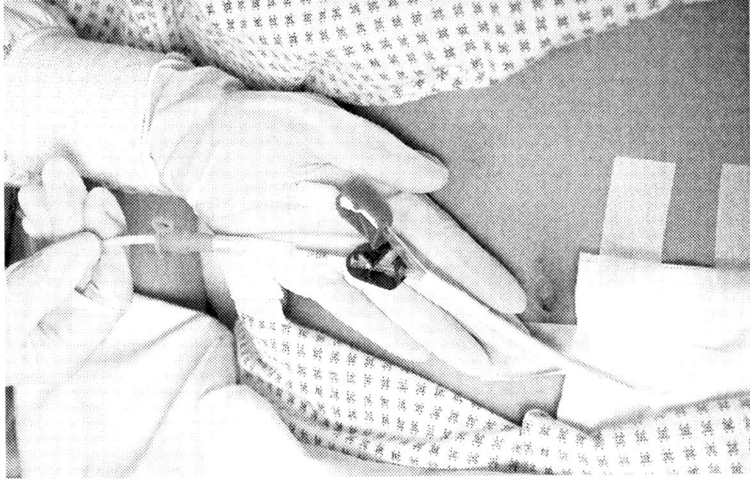

**Figure 3.15** Patient with a jejunostomy–gastrostomy tube.

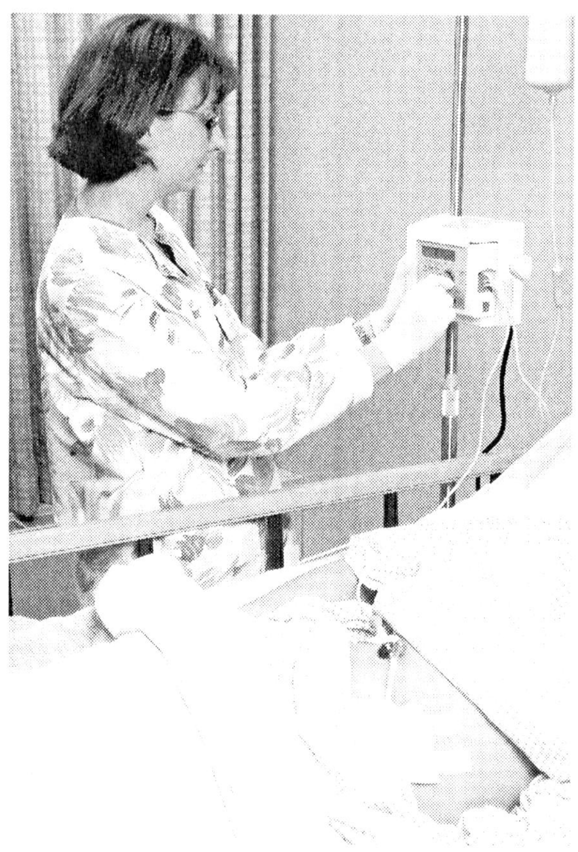

**Figure 3.16** Patient receiving a jejunostomy tube feeding.

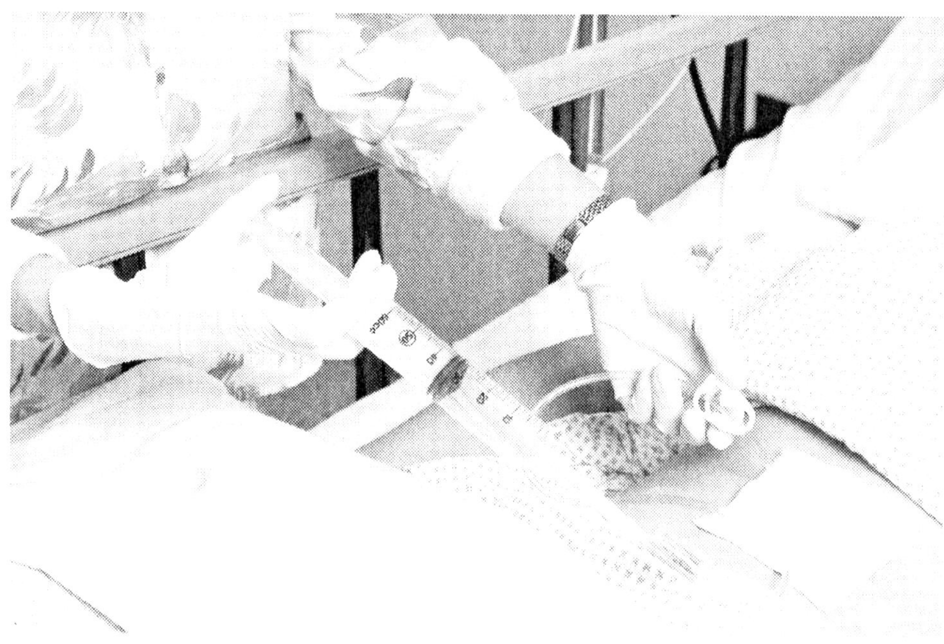

**Figure 3.17** Flushing the feeding tube.

# CHAPTER 4

# NEUROLOGICAL FUNCTION OBSERVATION

## INTRODUCTION

Caregivers often encounter patients with neurological problems. These patients have special needs due to conditions like cerebral vascular accidents (CVAs), brain tumors, spinal cord injuries, nerve conduction problems, dementias, and back pain. A good understanding of the anatomy and physiology of the human body and of specific neurological observation skills helps prepare caregivers to meet the special needs of these patients.

Caregivers must also know how to differentiate between delirium and dementia and how to care for a patient during a seizure. Patients with neurological impairments often experience sudden changes in their physical condition. They also face many psychosocial challenges, ranging from communication problems to sudden changes in body image. Having solid knowledge of the neurologically impaired patient allows the caregiver to respond rapidly, confidently, and with greater empathy.

This chapter describes neurological functions and explains how to perform neurological observations and care for a patient during a seizure.

# Neurological Function

The brain is the master control of the body and the most prominent component of the central nervous system. The brain controls the many conscious and unconscious movements we perform every day. There are twelve cranial nerves in the body. These major nerves of the brain send messages to other parts of the body to help coordinate major functions, such as seeing, hearing, feeling, walking, talking, and thinking. The spinal cord relays messages from the brain to the rest of the body to coordinate movement, sensation, and temperature control.

## Objectives

**This section prepares caregivers to do the following:**

1. Describe the basic anatomy and physiology of the central nervous system.
2. Acquire a basic understanding of the cranial nerves.
3. Describe the function of the spinal cord.

## Key Terms

**Aneurysm** A bulging and weakening in a portion of a blood vessel wall.

**Babinski Reflex** The reflexive movement observed when the bottom of the foot is stimulated from the heel up to the toes and the toes fan out. This is an abnormal reflex in anyone over 18 months old.

**Basal Ganglia** A brain structure that provides for basic and subconscious body movement.

**Bilateral** Pertaining to or affecting both sides of the body (e.g., both arms or both eyes).

**Brain Stem** The portion of the brain that controls motor, sensory, and reflex functions. Most of the cranial nerves begin in the brain stem. It consists of the midbrain, the medulla, and the pons.

**Central Nervous System** Consists of the brain (cerebrum and cerebellum) and the spinal cord. One of the two main divisions of the nervous system that serves to coordinate and control the body.

**Cerebral Cortex** The outer layer of the brain.

**Cerebrospinal Fluid** A clear, colorless, odorless fluid that acts as a cushion protecting the central nervous system. Cerebrospinal fluid is produced at a rate of 25 to 35 cubic centimeters (cc) per hour by the choroid plexus, which is located in the ventricles and spinal cord.

**Cerebellum** The part of the brain, located behind the brain stem, that controls the coordination of voluntary movement.

**Cerebrum** The largest and uppermost portion of the brain. It is divided into the right and left hemispheres. Memory, speech, writing, and emotional response are controlled by the cerebrum.

**Coma** A decreased level of consciousness in which the person cannot be aroused even when exposed to unpleasant stimuli.

**Contralateral** Pertaining to or affecting the opposite side of the body.

**Corpus Callosum** The major connecting pathway between the right and left hemispheres of the brain.

**Decerebrate** A rigid body position in which the arms and legs are extended. The body assumes decerebrate posturing when intracranial pressure is intense. It indicates that the cerebrum is being affected and is a more severe sign than decorticate posturing.

**Decorticate** A rigid body position in which the arms and legs are flexed. The body assumes decorticate posturing when intracranial pressure is intense. It indicates that the cortex is being affected and is a slightly less severe sign than decerebrate posturing.

**Diencephalon** The portion of the brain that consists of the thalamus and the hypothalamus.

**Dilation** The widening of the pupils.

**Flaccid** Lacking muscle tone or resistance in a limb or in the entire body. Flaccidity is a very late sign of intense intracranial pressure.

**Frontal Lobe** A lobe of the cerebrum that controls movement, short-term memory, emotional responsiveness, behavior, and speech.

**Hemiplegia** The paralysis of one side of the body.

**Infarction** An area of tissue death related to the loss of blood circulation.

**Ipsilateral** Pertaining to or affecting the same side of the body.

**Lesion** A defect or injury to the body.

**Lethargy** Drowsiness.

**Meninges** The outer lining of the central nervous system. The meninges include the pia, the arachnoid, and the dura.

**Motor Function** The ability to move any part of the body. These movements can be either voluntary or involuntary.

**Neuron** A nerve cell.

**Occipital Lobe** The lobe of the cerebrum that controls sight.

**Parietal Lobe** The lobe of the cerebrum that interprets sensations and proprioception.

**Proprioception** The ability to sense the position of one's limbs with one's eyes closed.

**Sensory** Pertaining to any of the senses (hearing, sight, etc.).

**Skull** The hard, protective, outer covering of the brain.

**Spinal Cord** The spinal cord is one of the main components of the central nervous system. It conducts both sensory and motor impulses to and from the brain, controls many reflexes, and allows for movement and sensation in the body.

**Stroke** A brain attack; a prolonged or permanent loss of brain function due to loss of blood supply.

**Temporal Lobe** The lobe of the cerebrum that controls hearing, speech, and long-term memory.

**Ventricles** Fluid-filled cavities within the brain stem and brain. There are four ventricles: the right and left lateral ventricles, the third ventricle, and the fourth ventricle.

## The Central Nervous System

The central nervous system (CNS) is made up of the brain (the cerebrum and the cerebellum) and the spinal cord (Figure 4.1). The CNS is a vital system for the human body. It is amazing in its complexity and function, and much is still unknown about exactly how this system works. The following discussion of the anatomy and physiology of the CNS is intended to provide a basic understanding of the structures of the CNS and their function.

### The Skull

The skull is the bony framework that protects the brain. It is composed of eight cranial bones and fourteen facial bones (Figure 4.2). The brain, which lies in the closed "box" formed by the skull, is actually many distinct structures. Just beneath the skull are the three layers, or membranes, of the meninges. The pia mater is the innermost covering. Then comes the arachnoid layer, and then the outermost layer, the dura mater. The meninges, along with the cerebrospinal fluid produced in the ventricles, protect or pad the brain from injury inside the skull.

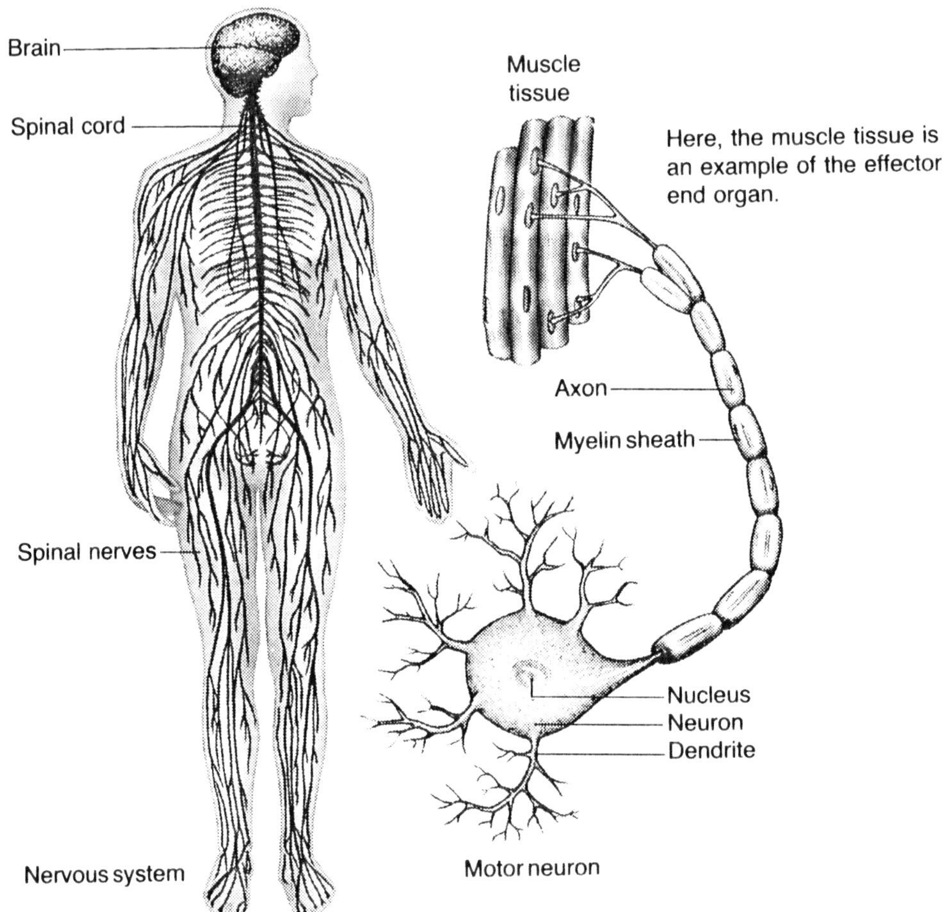


**Figure 4.1** Anatomy of the nervous system.

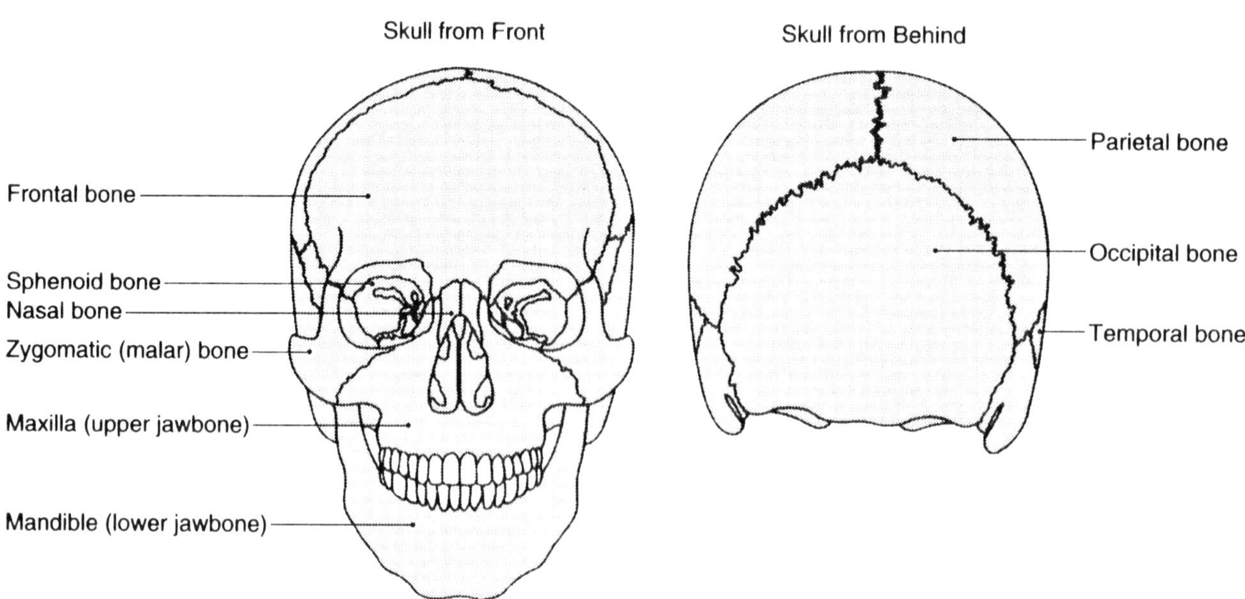


**Figure 4.2** The major bones of the skull.

## The Cerebrum

One of the largest structures of the brain is the cerebrum. This structure is known for the numerous wrinkles, or convolutions, that can be seen on its surface. The convolutions increase the surface area of the brain. The cerebrum is divided into two halves called hemispheres. The right hemisphere controls the left side of the body, and the left hemisphere controls the right side of the body.

Each hemisphere of the cerebrum is composed of four lobes, each of which has its own distinct function. The frontal lobe controls many processes. One of the most important is motor function. The other functions are often related to what is thought of as personality. These include emotional responsiveness, short-term memory, behavior, and portions of speech. Located in the parietal lobe is the primary sensory control area. The parietal lobe also controls the functions of body awareness and object perception. The third lobe, the temporal lobe, is responsible for the sense of hearing, long-term memory, and much of the ability to speak. The fourth lobe is the occipital lobe, which is located in the back of the skull. It is primarily involved in controlling the sense of vision.

## The Cerebellum

The cerebellum is located behind the brain stem. It controls the coordination of voluntary movement. The ability to walk and move in a coordinated fashion is a result of the role of the cerebellum. This structure is also responsible for the refinement of muscle movement, the coordination of muscles, and balance.

## The Brain Stem

The brain stem is located deep within the center of the hemispheres of the brain. Brain stem components are involved in making connections with the spinal cord through the medulla. The brain stem contains all of the nerve fibers that pass between the hemispheres of the brain and the spinal cord, and all of the cranial nerves except the olfactory nerve (CN I) arise from the brain stem. There are twelve pairs of cranial nerves. They carry impulses for bodily functions, such as smell, vision, ocular movement, pupil contraction, muscular sensation, chewing, facial expression, glandular secretion, taste, hearing, skin sensation, equilibrium, swallowing, and movement of the tongue, head, and shoulders. Other structures in the brain stem include the midbrain, the pons, and the medulla oblongata. These structures work together to relay information back and forth from the spinal cord.

## The Diencephalon and the Basal Ganglia

Between the brain stem and the cerebellum are two structures that are very important to brain function. The first is the diencephalon. This small structure serves as a regulator for the body. It controls appetite, temperature, emotions, and hormone secretions. It also serves as the "executive secretary" for the body as it relays information from the body to the cerebrum. It is where the sense of instinct and the urge for self-preservation are located. The second structure is the basal ganglia. This structure serves to control basic, subconscious body movements, such as muscle tone, and the automatic movements involved in walking and balance.

## The Spinal Cord

The spinal cord is the third major component of the CNS (Figure 4.3). It arises from the medulla oblongata and extends to the second lumbar vertebra. It is made up of the spinal cord, which is covered by the three layers of the meninges. It carries both motor and sensory impulses to and from the brain and controls many reflexes in the body. Thirty-one nerves originate from the spinal cord: eight cervical, twelve thoracic, five lumbar, five sacral, and one coccygeal. Compression of any of

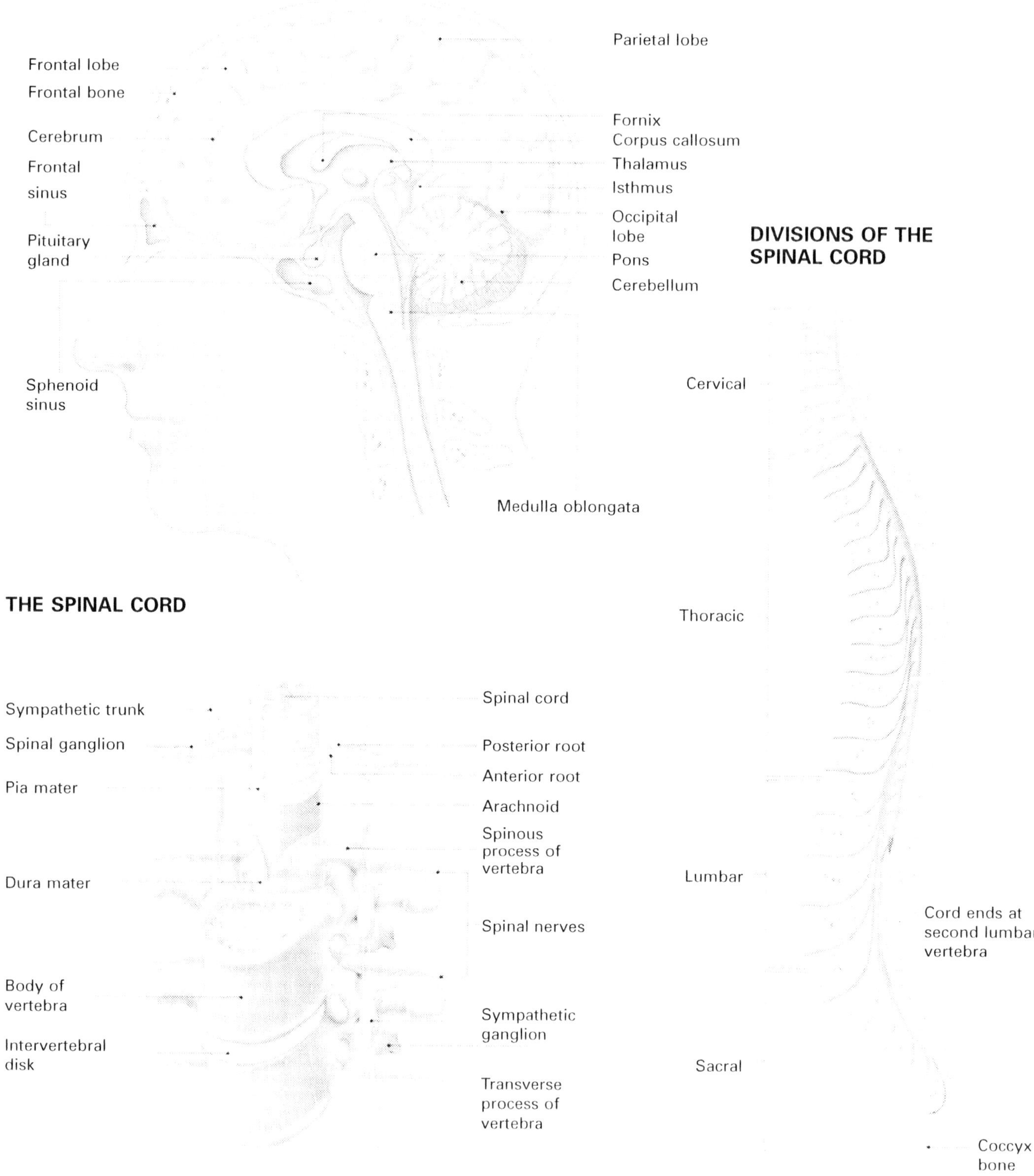


**Figure 4.3** The brain and spinal cord.

the nerves results in severe pain, and injury to the nerves or to the cord might result in paralysis. The extent of paralysis is related to the level of injury: The more serious the injury, the more extensive the paralysis.

### Cerebrospinal Fluid

Cerebrospinal fluid flows around the brain and the spinal cord and serves to cushion and protect these structures. It is made in the ventricles, which are located near the center of the brain. Because the brain is contained in the skull, a hard, fixed container, only so much cerebrospinal fluid can be managed by the brain before pressure is applied to the lobes and structures of the brain. When swelling occurs, the caregiver will see loss of function from the structures involved. The brain cannot tolerate much swelling before loss of function appears. It is for this reason that caregivers need excellent observation skills.

### Cerebral Blood Flow

The circulation of the brain is unique in the body. Systemically, the brain is given priority over other structures of the body to ensure a constant supply of nutrients to its tissues. The brain has a unique ability to assist in maintaining a constant blood flow. This is called autoregulation. The blood vessels have the ability to respond to changes in pressure within the lumen of the vessels. When the vessels experience increased blood pressure, they constrict to avoid decreased blood flow and tissue damage. When the blood vessels experience decreased blood pressure, they dilate to increase the blood flow to the brain. The brain can only autoregulate up to a certain point. When intracranial pressure increases, the astute caregiver will see several signs and symptoms in the patient. These include headache, nausea and vomiting, memory alterations, changes in speech and judgment, and decreased respirations. Late signs and symptoms appear when intense pressure is being applied to the brain. These include Cushing's triad (wide pulse pressure, decreased heart rate, and abnormal respirations), pupil dilation, and posturing (decorticate, decerebrate, and flaccid).

## Neurological Observation

### Introduction

Performing a neurological observation provides valuable insight into the baseline and subsequent neurological functioning levels of the patient. Many factors can influence a patient's neurological functioning, including medications and their side effects, many disease processes, lack of sleep, infections, and trauma, to name a few. Learning to accurately check the patient's pupils and perform a Glasgow Coma Scale assessment and a Rancho Los Amigos Scale assessment will allow the caregiver to provide more expert care.

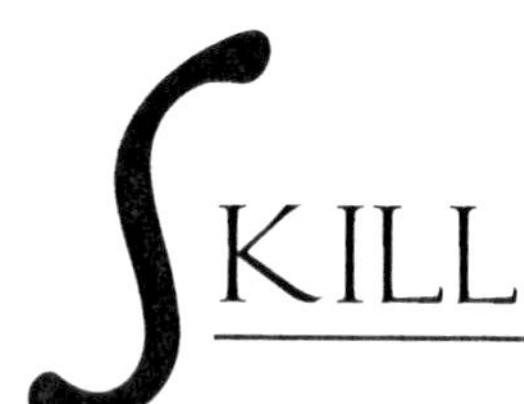

# SKILL

## Performing a Pupil Check

***Purpose*** Checking the patient's pupils is an important aspect of the neurological observation. Their size, shape, and reaction to light are the areas that are most frequently evaluated. This information is important because the findings are directly related to the functioning of the central nervous system (CNS). The pupil observation is unlike other aspects of the neurological check because it can be performed and provide valuable information regardless of the patient's level of consciousness.

Not unlike observation of the other systems, it is extremely important to establish baseline data so that subsequent pupil checks can be compared to the initial observation. It is important to use the appropriate technique when evaluating the pupils and to recognize and communicate any changes noted.

The acronym *PERRLA* (pupils equal, round, reactive to light, accommodating) is used to document the normal finding of a pupil observation. The size of the pupil and its reaction to light (brisk, sluggish, or no reaction) are also documented. The size of the pupil should be recorded before and after constriction (Figure 4.4).

### Objectives

**The caregiver demonstrates the ability to do the following:**

1. Gather the correct supplies.
2. Communicate using a style that reduces the patient's anxiety.
3. Describe the components of a pupil check.
4. Perform a pupil check correctly.
5. Document the results of the procedure according to the institution's policy.
6. Report the results of the procedure to the RN or preceptor.

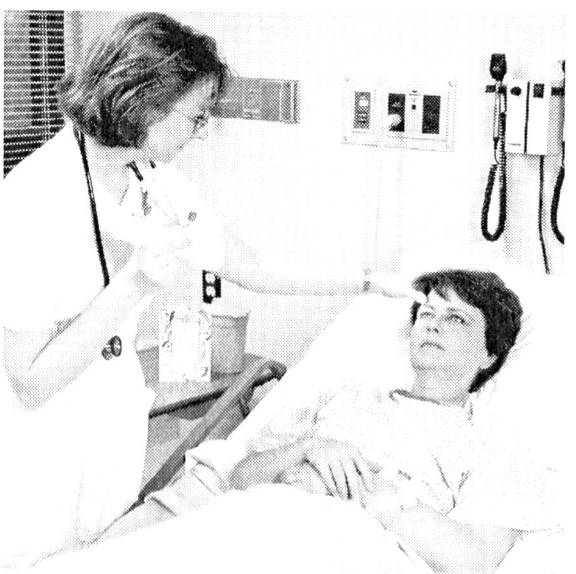

**Figure 4.4** Checking a patient's pupils.

## Key Terms

**Accommodation** Pupillary constriction that occurs when the patient changes the focus from a distant object to a close one.

**Anisocoria** The finding of a difference in the size of the right and left pupils.

**"Blown" Pupils** Pupils that are dilated and fixed.

**Dyscoria** Irregular pupil shape.

**Pupil** The central opening in the iris that permits light to enter the eye.

**Reactive** Responsive to a stimulus.

## Supplies/ Equipment

Pupil size chart • Penlight

## Pertinent Points

- It is important to obtain a health history from the patient or family to establish any preexisting conditions, such as cataracts, cataract surgery, iridectomy, glaucoma, and medications, that might affect the pupils' shape, size, or reaction.
- Pupils that are unequal usually indicate a CNS dysfunction. However, it has been noted that about one person in four with intact functioning of the CNS will present with asymmetrical pupils.
- It might be impossible to assess the pupils of patients who have extremely swollen eyes.

## Age-Specific Considerations

The size of the pupil changes throughout the life span. At birth, the pupil is small, but it enlarges during childhood. As we age, the pupil decreases in size. In older adults, the pupils show a decrease in the reactivity to light and might have cataracts, glaucoma, or visual deficits. This should be taken into consideration when checking pupils.

## Key Concept

Although a change in the level of consciousness is usually the first sign of increased intracranial pressure, changes in the shape, size, and reactivity of the pupils are also extremely important findings. All changes, including changes in the level of consciousness, sluggish reaction, unequal pupils, and ovoid-shaped pupils, must be reported immediately.

## Steps

1. Identify the correct patient.
2. Explain the procedure to the patient, regardless of their level of consciousness.
3. Wash hands.
4. Assemble the equipment.
5. If necessary, help the patient open his or her eyes for the pupil observation.
6. Check the size of the pupils by measuring them with the pupil size chart or ruler. Measure the right and left pupils individually. Normal pupil size ranges from 2 to 6 millimeters (mm) in diameter.
7. Look at the shape of the pupil on the right and then at the one on the left. Both should be round.
8. Check the pupils for reaction to light:
   a. Turn off the lights or darken the patient's room.
   b. Ask the patient to look straight ahead at an object.
   c. Hold the penlight approximately 6 inches in front of the patient's right eye.
   d. Observe the size of the pupil when it constricts and the dilation of the pupil when the

light source is removed (direct light reflex).

e. Note whether the reaction time is brisk or sluggish or whether the pupil is nonreactive.

f. Repeat steps c, d, and e on the patient's left pupil.

g. Observe the opposite pupil when checking the pupillary constriction to light (direct light reflex). The opposite pupil should constrict at the same time and dilate when the light is removed (consensual light reaction).

9. Check for accommodation if the patient is able to follow instructions:

   a. Place your finger approximately 8 inches in front of the bridge of the patient's nose.

   b. Instruct the patient to look at an object in the distance and then directly at your finger.

   c. The pupils should constrict and converge as the patient focuses on your finger.

10. Wash hands, and document and report the results of the procedure to the RN or preceptor. Document these findings:

    a. PERRLA (pupils equal, round, reactive to light, accommodating) for normal findings

    b. Size of pupils

    c. Reactivity—brisk, sluggish, or nonreactive

11. Immediately report any changes from the previous check.

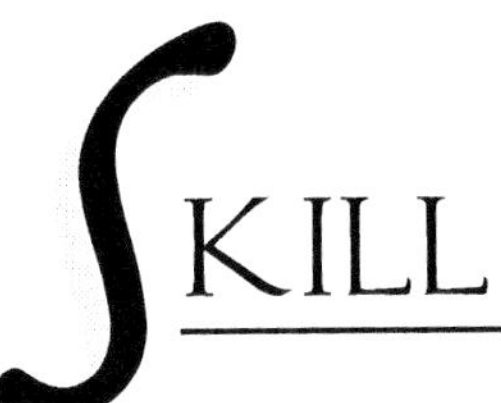

# SKILL

## Performing a Neurological Check Using the Glasgow Coma Scale

***Purpose*** Neurological checks are performed for many reasons. The most obvious reason is to assess the level of functioning of the central nervous system. Other reasons to perform a neurological check are to detect a dysfunction of some part of the nervous system, to monitor the patient's response to a medical intervention, and to gain information to make decisions for patient management both within the health care system and at home. These checks are performed as part of the initial patient assessment and at timed intervals afterward. The initial assessment allows caregivers to learn the baseline, or "normal," level of functioning before planned procedures or other medical interventions. The neurological check is performed after medical interventions to monitor for changes in intracranial circulation and intracranial pressure. These conditions will impair the functioning of the various structures of the brain, depending on where the pressure or loss of blood circulation has occurred.

Many factors influence the type and frequency of the neurological check performed for a patient. One of these factors is the setting in which the patient is receiving care (e.g., the scene of an injury, an emergency room, an intensive care unit, a rehabilitation unit, an outpatient clinic). Another factor is the purpose for care (life-threatening emergency, identifying the cause of a problem or complaint, monitoring after intervention, or planning for ongoing care). Another factor is the condition of the patient. The patient might be unconscious, semiconscious, or conscious. Other factors that influence the neurological check include the presence of a spinal cord injury, the age and developmental level of the patient, the intellect of the patient, and social and cultural factors.

The Glasgow Coma Scale (GCS) is commonly used to assess the neurological function of patients based on behavioral responses. It is used in a wide range of settings to get a quick idea of the level of functioning of the central nervous system. The scale assesses the patient's ability in the areas of eye opening, motor response, and verbal response. Verbal response to the questions of the GCS might be decreased as a result of the use of alcohol, drugs, or medications. The patient's score is based on the best patient response in each area (Table 4.1). The GCS is one component of a neurological check. Depending on the depth of the assessment, other factors will be tested to establish the functioning of a component of the neurological system.

### Objectives

**The caregiver demonstrates the ability to do the following:**

1. Communicate using a style that reduces the patient's anxiety.
2. Explain the purpose of the Glasgow Coma Scale.
3. Describe the components of the Glasgow Coma Scale.
4. Perform a neurological check correctly.
5. Document the results of the procedure according to the institution's policy.
6. Report the results of the procedure to the RN or preceptor.

### Key Terms

**Command** An instruction to do something.

**Deficit** A condition that is less than normal. A deficit exists when a patient receives a less than optimal score on the Glasgow Coma Scale.

**Noxious** Unpleasant.

**Oriented** Having the ability to correctly state one's name, the time, where one is, and what is happening.

## Supplies/Equipment

None

## Pertinent Points

- It is very important to use the scale consistently to generate both a baseline assessment and an ongoing record of assessments. When neurological checks are ordered for a patient, it is important to perform them on time and not to miss one. Patients might have to be awakened in order to assess their level of functioning.
- The Glasgow Coma Scale is used at different intervals depending on the intensity of the neurological status at risk. For example, critically ill patients with neurological issues are often monitored every 15 minutes. Postoperative neurological checks might start at once every 15 minutes and progress to every hour, then every 4 hours, and then to every shift when a stable status has been established.
- Always give patients the score that reflects their best attempt. For example, if they were asleep but are able to wake up in a minute or two and tell you clearly who they are, where they are, and what time it is, they should get credit for a 4 on the alertness scale. If they are only able to open their eyes and look at you when you talk or shout to them, then they should get a score of 3 on this portion of the scale.
- Other types of neurological tests are often performed with the Glasgow Coma Scale. Some of these include tests of pupil functioning, tests of muscle strength (having the patient press down on the tester's hands or pull away from the tester), and other tests for item recollection, memory, and so on that indicate how well the brain and CNS are functioning.

## Age-Specific Considerations

As people age, they experience biological changes to the CNS. The most frustrating changes for patients are often noted in the sensory areas: sight, hearing, taste, touch, and reaction time. Assess whether an older patient can hear and see you. Many older individuals find it embarrassing to admit that they have impaired hearing or eyesight and might pretend to have a higher level of functioning than they actually have. Allow time for the patient to respond to questions. It is always important to refer to the baseline assessment of the patient, as increased delays in response are an early sign of impaired neurological function. Older patients often have less strength and slower response than younger patients.

For pediatric patients, different scales are often used to assess neurological abilities. Young children are just beginning to develop their cognitive, verbal, and motor abilities.

## Key Concept

Neurological function deteriorates rapidly. Pupil dilation and posturing are critical signs of neurological impairment. It is important to notice subtle differences in patient response and to report any changes in neurological function immediately to a physician.

## Table 4.1 Sample Neurological Exam for ICU Patients

| | |
|---|---|
| I. Level of consciousness | Alertness (e.g., awake, arouses to voice, arouses to pain)<br>Orientation to time, place, others, self (verbal or written response)<br>Motor response to command or pain or spontaneous<br>Response to simple commands (if none, check response to pain—nail bed pressure)<br>Response to painful stimuli (order correlates with Glasgow Coma Scale) |
| II. Respiration | Regular without distress<br>Difficulty keeping airway clear (tongue/sections blocking)<br>Irregular or Cheyne Stokes respirations (due to increased intracranial pressure [ICP]) |
| III. Vital signs | Watch for raised blood pressure (BP) and lowered pulse (due to increased ICP). |
| IV. Motor | Look for difference in strength between right and left sides.<br>-Hand grips<br>-Arm drift<br>-Leg lifts<br><br>Look for difference in muscle tone between right and left sides.<br>(Look for abnormal muscle tone—spastic or flaccid.)<br><br>If differences in tone or strength between sides of body are present, then check once/shift for<br>-Presence of Babinski (abnormal finding)<br>-Deep tendon reflexes (only significant if there is a difference between sides)<br><br>Watch for tremors, seizure activity, and primitive reflexes.<br>-Sucking<br>-Yawning<br>-Chewing |
| V. Pupils | In assessments below, look for differences between right and left.<br>-Size<br>-Reaction to light (direct and consensual—both eyes)<br>-Shape (describe irregularities)<br>-Briskness of reaction |
| **Beginning of Each Shift**<br>Cranial Nerve Exam:<br>**On Alert Patient** | **On Unresponsive Patient** |
| I. Olfactory (smell—don't usually test) | Don't test |
| II. Optic—test one eye at a time; ask patient to correctly identify the number of fingers held up. | Normal response =<br>-Blink to threat (open hand coming toward opened eyes, test eyes together<br>-Pupils react to light |
| III. Oculomotor—Have patient look to one side, then up, then down.<br>IV. Trochlear<br>V. Abducens | III, IV, V may be indirectly checked by the Doll's Eyes reflex—which also indicates intactness of brain stem (Doll's Eyes reflex present—turn head to side and eyes should conjugately move in opposite direction).<br>Doll's Eyes present = normal<br>Doll's Eyes absent = abnormal<br>Expect Doll's Eyes to be absent with Nembutal coma. |

(continued)

| | |
|---|---|
| (Normal if able to move both eyes in all directions equally).<br>↑ ↑<br>← →<br>↓ ↓<br>If patient is alert and c/o double vision—check for disconjugate gaze. Look for position of reflection on each eye and compare | |
| VI. Trigeminal: ciliary reflex (blink when eyelashes stroked). | Ciliary—same<br>Corneal reflex—check only if ciliary is absent.<br>(Normal = blink when cornea is lightly stroked with cotton.)<br>Pin prick in nose—check only if corneas absent<br>(Normal = blink from pain.) |
| Check facial sensation on forehead, cheek, and jaw.<br>Test jaw strength (have patient clench teeth—try to move jaw back and forth). | |
| **On Alert Patient** | **On Unresponsive Patient** |
| VII. Facial: Test facial strength. (Have patient wrinkle forehead, smile, puff out cheeks with air. Look for differences between right and left.) | Look for flattened nasal labial fold and widened palpebral fold on weak side. |
| VIII. Vestibulocochlear: hearing. (Don't usually test in ICU.) | Don't test hearing. |
| Watch for nystagmus (eye jerks in one direction and drifts back slowly). Can only check for nystagmus on alert patient (represents vestibular and/or cerebellar lesion). | Caloric testing done by MD (cold saline in ear if VIII is intact, will see nystagmus opposite side of the saline infusion. Using warm saline—will see nystagmus toward same side of the infusion). (caloric oculovestibular water [COW]) |
| IX. Glossopharyngeal: Compression results in hoarseness and decreased ability to swallow | Check for normal presence of gag (both sides of palate) and swallow |
| X. Vagus | |
| XI. Accessory: Have patient turn head and shrug shoulders against resistance. | Don't test |
| XII. Hypoglossal: Stick out tongue (will deviate to weak side). | Don't test |

Adapted from sample Neurological Exam for I.C.U. patients, St. Joseph Mercy Hospital, Ann Arbor, Michigan. Used with permission.

## Observing for Signs of Increased Intracranial Pressure

A patient often deteriorates in a stepwise fashion:

1. Decreased level of consciousness on RAS
2. Respiration—blocked airway
   —irregular rate/depth
3. BP up, pulse down (pressure on vital sign center in medulla)
4. Weakness on one or both sides (compression of motor tracts—cortex and midbrain)
5. Dilation of one pupil and decreased reaction to light (CN III)
6. Both pupils fixed and dilated—cerebral anoxia (CN III)

Report any signs of increased intracranial pressure (ICP) to the RN or your supervisor.

---

### Steps

1. Identify the correct patient.
2. Wash hands.
3. Note the patient's level of wakefulness as you approach. Note whether the sleeping patient arouses when you call or whether you must gently tap him or her. Some patients only awaken when given a noxious stimulus, such as being rubbed on the sternum. Unconscious patients are unarousable. Record the patient's best level of alertness.
4. For the test of verbal ability, it is important to give patients who have been sleeping a bit of time to orient themselves before you ask them the neurological assessment questions.
5. Explain the procedure to the patient. Explain that you need to ask some questions to see how the patient's neurological system is working. Ask the following questions in a clear voice to assess the patient's verbal response:
   - **a.** What is your name?
   - **b.** Where are you right now?
   - **c.** What's today's date? What year is it?
   - **d.** Why are you here?

   Record the patient's best level of alertness. Note that in patients who have tracheostomies, if they can mouth the correct response or write it, they should be given credit for this and not given a low score because they cannot vocalize.
6. Test the patient's motor response. Give the patient a simple command, such as "Please squeeze my hands or fingers" (Figure 4.5). This part of the assessment tests the patient's ability to follow commands as well as the patient's symmetry in the strength of the hands. Have the patient shut her eyes and extend her arms out straight. Check for drift (Figure 4.6). Record the score that reflects the patient's best attempt on the motor section of the scale.
7. Wash hands and document and report the results of the procedure to the RN or preceptor. Report any changes in scores from the previous check.

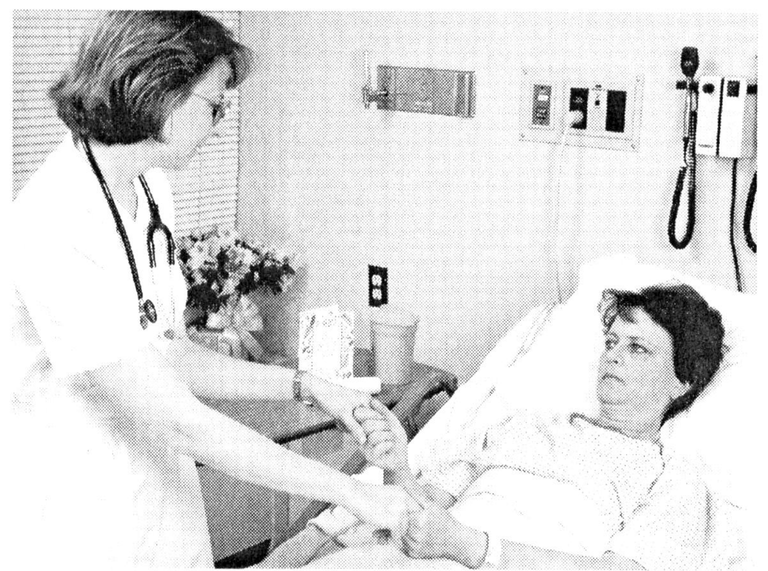

**Figure 4.5** Having the patient squeeze the caregiver's hands or fingers to check strength.

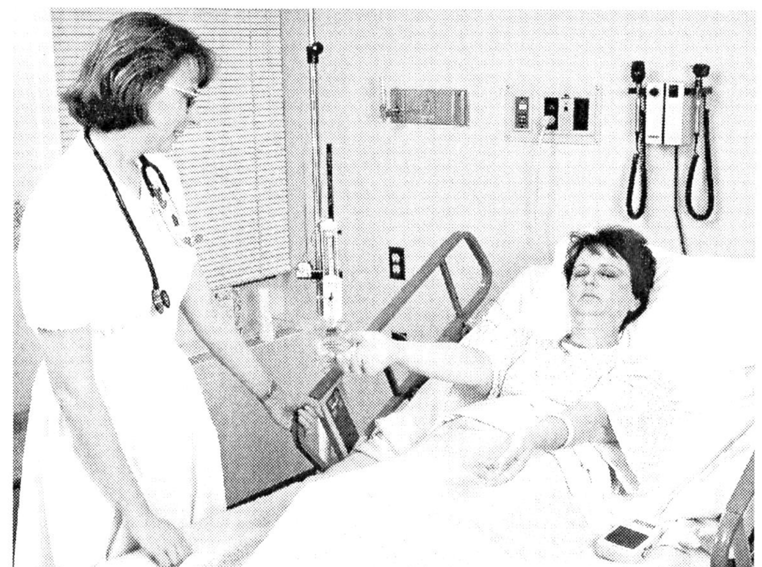

**Figure 4.6** Drift.

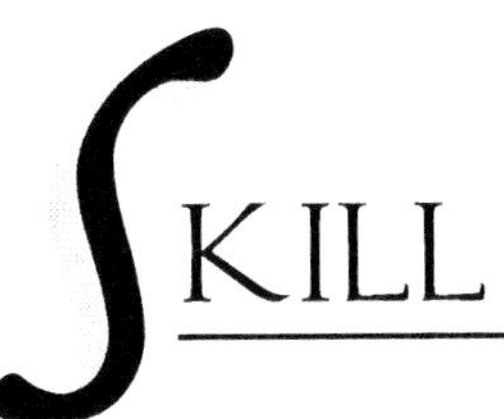

# SKILL

## Giving Rancho Los Amigos Cognitive Level Care

***Purpose*** The Rancho Los Amigos Cognitive Scale is used to evaluate the behavior of the head-injured patient in relation to cognitive functions as the patient progresses through the rehabilitation process. The scale is divided into eight levels of functioning. The cognitive abilities assigned to the levels range from no response to purposeful and appropriate response. The purpose of the evaluation is to systematically organize an individualized plan of care with appropriate nursing interventions.

Management of the head-injured patient is challenging and frustrating for the patient, the family, and the caregiver. As the patient moves through the different levels on the Rancho scale, the behavior observed might include loss of inhibition, agitation, aggressiveness, and impulsiveness. Generally accepted social behavior sometimes does not seem to exist for the head-injury patient. The patient's use of profanity, his or her confabulation of stories, and the sexual overtone of the patient's behavior and conversation are disturbing for the family. Other deficits include decreased reaction time; increased information-processing time; short- and long-term memory issues; difficulty concentrating, learning, and relearning tasks; and decreased ability to solve problems. Depending on the injury, the patient might also suffer from a motor impairment. Head-injured patients need to be independent, but their lack of self-awareness of their deficits makes patient safety a major concern.

Although each head-injured patient's recovery is unique, the Rancho scale sets goals for each level. Nursing intervention to achieve optimum functioning for the patient can be planned based on the patient's level of cognitive ability. Improvement in cognitive functioning can continue to occur for years after a head injury. Health care providers who deliver appropriate stimulation and care management can make a difference in the patient's long-term outcome.

### Objectives

**The caregiver demonstrates the ability to do the following:**

1. Communicate using a style that is appropriate to the patient's cognitive level.
2. Plan care activities based on the patient's cognitive level.

### Key Terms

**Cognition** Awareness; the mental processes by which knowledge is acquired.

**Deficit** A condition that is less than normal.

**Head Injury** One of a variety of conditions, including intracerebral bleeding; skull fracture; and concussion, contusion, or laceration of the brain.

**Rehabilitation** The process of assisting the patient to attain his or her highest level of physical, psychosocial, and cognitive functioning.

### Supplies/Equipment

None

### Pertinent Points

- The patient's previous educational level, personality, adjustment patterns to everyday stressors, and past experiences are key factors in the rehabilitation process.
- A good understanding of the different levels of the recovery process helps the family and the caregiver avoid personalizing the patient's inappropriate behavior.

- Complete recovery and return to the patient's pre-illness state are not always feasible.
- The Rancho scale should only be used during the first few weeks or months after a head injury to evaluate the patient's progress.

## Age-Specific Considerations

Head injury occurs in all age groups. The severity of the injury determines the patient's level of independence and the number of tasks that he or she must relearn during the recovery phase. The relearning of tasks such as speaking, walking, dressing, and other basic activities of daily living (ADLs) can be an overwhelming and lengthy journey for the patient and the family. The patient's role, responsibilities, vocation, and family relationships sometimes change drastically immediately after a head injury and possibly for the duration of the patient's life.

Nursing interventions should be based on the Rancho scale and not on the patient's chronological age. Older adult patients might experience biological changes related to the aging process in addition to the cognitive changes resulting from the head injury. Age-related changes include decreased visual acuity and hearing and decreased reaction time. Older adults usually have more residual neurological deficits than do younger patients. The Rancho level is a general guideline for planning care; nursing interventions must then be modified to meet the patient's individual and age-specific needs (Table 4.2).

## Key Concept

- The brain-injured patient might experience visual problems, such as the loss of peripheral vision or double vision.
- Restraints usually increase the patient's agitation and aggression.
- Communicate with comatose patients as if they could hear and respond appropriately. Talking to comatose patients might improve their outcome.
- Changes you observe in neurological function should be documented and reported.

## TABLE 4.2 Rancho Los Amigos Cognitive Scale

| Level | Behavior |
|---|---|
| Level I: no response | Is unresponsive to any stimulus. |
| Level II: generalized response | Gives limited, inconsistent, nonpurposeful responses. Responds to pain, but response might be delayed. |
| Level III: localized general response | Gives purposeful responses. Might follow simple commands, focus on presented object, and respond to discomfort. |
| Level IV: confused, agitated response | Exhibits heightened state of activity, confusion, disorientation, aggressive and bizarre behavior. Is unable to do self-care and is unaware of present events. Attention span is short. |
| Level V: confused, inappropriate response | Appears alert, responds to commands, is distractable, does not concentrate on task, gives agitated responses to external stimuli, is verbally inappropriate, performs previously learned tasks, but is unable to learn new ones. |
| Level VI: confused, appropriate response | Exhibits goal-directed behavior, but needs cuing; can relearn old skills, such as ADLs; has serious memory problems and some awareness of self and others. |
| Level VII: automatic, appropriate response | Exhibits robot-like appropriate behavior, minimal confusion, slow recall, poor insight into condition. Initiates tasks but needs structure. Has poor judgment and problem-solving and planning skills. |
| Level VIII: purposeful, appropriate response | Is alert and oriented, recalls and integrates past events, learns new activities, and can continue without supervision; is independent in home and living skills, is capable of driving. Defects in stress tolerance, judgment, and abstract reasoning persist. May function at reduced level in society. |

Adapted from the original scale co-authored by Chris Hagen, Ph.D.; Danese Malkmus, M.A.; Patricia Durham, M.A. Communication Disorders Service, Rancho Los Amigos Hospital, 1972. Revised 11/15/74 by Danese Malkmus, M.A., and Kathryn Stenderup, O.T.R. Revised scale 1997 by Chris Hagen. Used with permission.

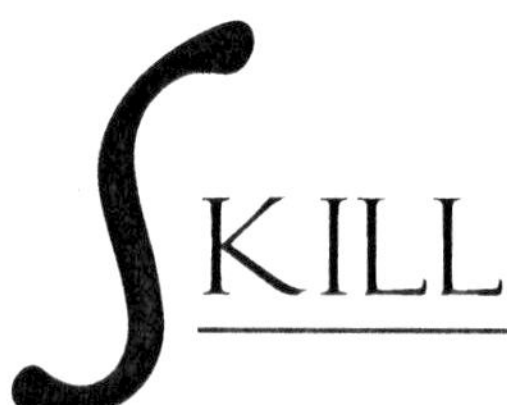

# SKILL

## Caring for a Patient During a Seizure

***Purpose*** Many conditions can lead to seizure activity, including cerebral neoplasm, cerebrovascular disturbance, infectious disorders, and cerebral trauma. Other causes of seizure activity are drug overdose, electrolyte imbalance, vitamin deficiency, diabetes mellitus, and nontherapeutic anticonvulsant drug levels. It is always important to establish the cause for the seizure so that appropriate interventions can be implemented to prevent another seizure. The caregiver's keen observation and documentation of the patient before, during, and after a seizure can directly affect the patient's outcome.

In the International Classification of Seizures system, all seizures are classified as either partial or generalized, based on clinical data and electroencephalographic findings. Partial seizures usually do not result in loss of consciousness and involve only a part of the brain. Generalized seizures result in loss of consciousness and involve the whole brain. In the generalized tonic–clonic seizure, more commonly known as a grand mal seizure, the patient progresses through the tonic phase, the clonic phase, and the postictal period (the time period immediately after a seizure).

Status epilepticus is a condition in which seizures occur in succession for a period of at least 30 minutes, during which the patient does not regain consciousness. It is usually a result of brain lesion, encephalitis, stroke, head trauma, metabolic disorder, or nontherapeutic anticonvulsant drug levels in a patient who has been diagnosed with epilepsy. Inappropriate care for this patient can result in respiratory arrest, brain damage, and even death. Therefore, this type of seizure activity is always considered to be a medical emergency.

### Objectives

**The caregiver demonstrates the ability to do the following:**

1. Gather the correct supplies.
2. Communicate using a style that reduces the patient's anxiety.
3. Describe the differences among seizure classifications.
4. Describe the care of a patient during a seizure.
5. Document appropriate observations made during a seizure.
6. Report the results of the procedure to the RN or preceptor.

### Key Terms

**Aura** A peculiar sensation that precedes a seizure, such as a visual disturbance, numbness, or a premonition. The sensation is specific to the patient.

**Clonus** A type of spasm in which muscle contraction and relaxation cause the body to jerk.

**Seizure** A sudden change in brain activity that causes motor or sensory activity.

**Seizure Disorder** A condition that describes a patient who has had a history of seizures.

**Tonus** A contraction of all of the skeletal muscles.

### Supplies/Equipment

Padding for the side rails • Suction setup • Oxygen • Intravenous (IV) setup

## Pertinent Points

- A partial seizure might indicate the onset of a generalized seizure.
- A padded tongue blade should never be used to force the patient's mouth open.
- During a generalized tonic–clonic seizure, the patient might become very cyanotic and might stop breathing for 30 to 60 seconds.
- The blood pressure during the postictal state could be high because of the physical activity of the seizure or low because of the diversion of blood to the central circulation.
- Children in status epilepticus are more likely to suffer brain damage than are adults.
- Observation and documentation of pre-, during, and postseizure activities can help determine the cause and necessary treatment for the seizures.

## Age-Specific Considerations

Seizures can occur in patients of any age. All patients will be concerned that a seizure will occur at school, at work, or in public and will cause them embarrassment. They will need reassurance and education about compliance with a medication schedule. When the seizure activity is related to trauma or a bad prognosis is related to a brain tumor, adults of all ages will need time to grieve their loss. Parents of infants will need reassurance of the cause of seizure and the likelihood of its recurrence.

## Key Concept

Stay with the patient during the seizure. Call for help or put on the bathroom nurse call light. Do not leave the patient alone.

## Steps

1. Note the time of onset.
2. Protect the patient:
   a. Do not restrain the patient.
   b. Loosen tight clothing or restraints.
   c. Cushion the area around the patient to avoid the patient's hitting anything hard.
   d. Place a pillow under the patient's head.
   e. Do not leave the patient alone. Call for help or turn on the bathroom nurse call light.
   f. Do not attempt to place an airway or padded tongue blade in the patient's mouth while the jaw is clenched.
3. Speak calmly, and let the patient know you are there and are going to help.
4. Provide for privacy.
5. Turn the patient to the side as the seizure begins to cease.
6. Suction the patient.
7. Comfort the patient and offer reassurance.
8. Provide care during the postictal state:
   a. Maintain an adequate airway.
   b. Check the patient's vital signs.
   c. Check the patient's neurological status, including muscle strength, level of consciousness, and pupils.
9. The RN should notify the physician of the patient's status. The following orders might be given:
   a. Set up an intravenous line for the administration of fluids and medications. Normal saline 0.9 percent will be needed if Dilantin is administered.
   b. Prepare to draw blood to test for glucose, electrolytes, anticonvulsant drug level (if the patient is currently on medication), toxic substances, and drugs.
   c. Obtain a pulse oximetry. (see page 192).

10. Call for immediate medical assistance if another seizure occurs. Subsequent or multiple seizures increase the risk for status epilepticus.
11. Wash hands and document and report the following observations to the RN or preceptor:
    a. Time of onset and duration
    b. Activity at onset and aura
    c. Seizure activity, type of movements (tonic, clonic), tremors, body parts involved, head–eye deviation
    d. Unilateral or bilateral movements and any sequencing
    e. Presence of cyanosis or incontinence
    f. Observations during the postictal state: speech impairment, weakness in the extremities, confusion, lethargy, headache.

# CHAPTER 5

# PHLEBOTOMY AND IV THERAPY

## INTRODUCTION

Caregivers often encounter patients who must have their blood drawn for various tests. Collecting blood specimens for laboratory testing allows physicians and caregivers to identify the patient's status, confirm a diagnosis, and assess the extent of the patient's disease. Physicians determine treatment plans or order medications based on the test results. Intravenous (IV) lines have become so commonplace that most hospitalized patients have one in place. Health care has evolved to the point that some patients are discharged with an IV in place so they can continue to receive IV antibiotics, chemotherapy, or pain medications in their home. Caregivers must frequently assess the IV site as complications may occur that require interventions.

This chapter includes information on selecting veins and recognizing problems in IV therapy as well as preparing caregivers to perform necessary skills. There is variation throughout the United States in who may start IVs or infuse fluids. Check with your employer or instructor.

SECTION ONE

# Phlebotomy

## Selecting a Vein

Determining which vein to use is one of the primary considerations to be taken into account before starting an IV. In a young, healthy adult, there is often an abundance of peripheral hand and arm veins to choose from. Unfortunately, this is not usually the case. Age, illness, previous therapies, and other factors frequently limit the number of veins from which a caregiver will have to choose.

### Adult

In reviewing the hand and arm veins from distal to proximal (from the fingers toward the shoulder), first the veins of the fingers, or the *digital* veins, are found (Figure 5.1). These veins are located along the lateral (side) and dorsal (top) portions of the fingers. The catheter of choice for use in these veins is a small-gauge (22-gauge) catheter that can be anchored securely in this area. A padded tongue blade can be used to splint the finger and prevent dislodging. The veins of the fingers are usually not the best choice when starting an IV. They are generally smaller than the veins of the forearm and therefore provide less hemodilution and a greater likelihood that phlebitis will occur.

Next are the three *metacarpal* veins, which are located on the back of each hand and begin at the junction of the digital veins (Figure 5.1). The catheter of choice for these veins is usually a 22- or 20-gauge catheter. Use a short catheter, $\frac{3}{4}$ or 1 inch in length, to prevent catheter flexion as the joints of the hand and wrist are moved. A flexible catheter should be used instead of a metal needle, if possible, when using the finger or hand veins for IV therapy. This area has many joints, and a metal needle could easily become dislodged from the vein if not immobilized

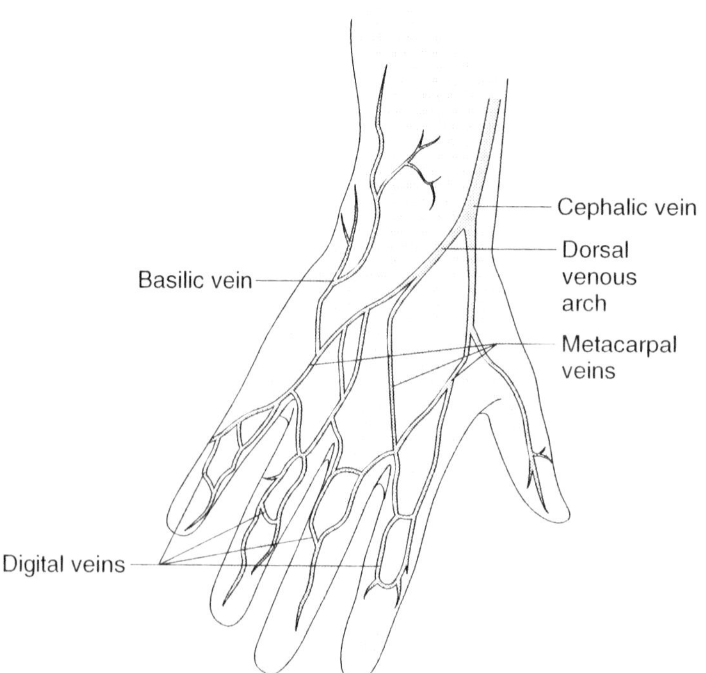


**Figure 5.1** Superficial veins of the fingers and hand.

by an arm board. Because of restriction of movement and limited size, the veins of the fingers and hand are not normally the first choice for long-term or irritating therapies.

The veins of the forearm are usually the veins of choice in selecting a site for IV placement in an adult. These veins are usually larger, straighter, and more easily secured than are the veins of the fingers and hands. The long bones of the arm serve as natural arm boards, and the flat surfaces of the forearm allow the IV to be more easily secured with less loss of mobility for the patient (Figure 5.2).

The *cephalic* vein originates from the metacarpal veins near the base of the thumb and travels along the radial bone of the forearm. This vein is often referred to as the intern's friend because of its prominence and relative ease of accessibility. The *basilic* vein originates from the metacarpal veins on the opposite side of the hand. It follows the course of the ulnar bone up to the elbow and then travels along the inner aspect of the upper arm, where it joins the cephalic vein at the axillary vein near the shoulder.

Both the cephalic and basilic veins of the forearm, along with the median basilic and accessory cephalic veins, are good choices for IV therapy. Catheters or needles from 22- to 18-gauge are normally used. Because these veins have a tendency to roll, secure traction is required to increase the success of the IV start.

Begin IV therapy at the most distal vein that can be palpated. Subsequent venipunctures should be proximal to the last venipuncture site. Remember, if a vein has chemical phlebitis (an irritation from medications infused) and you start an IV distal to that site, the irritating substance may continue to flow through that vein toward the heart, thereby worsening the phlebitis.

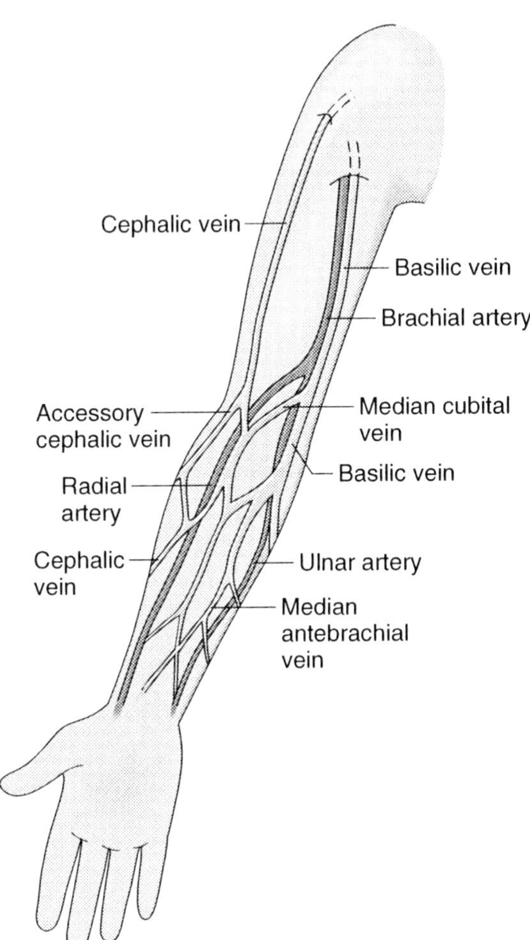


**Figure 5.2** Superficial veins of the forearm.

The *antecubital* veins, located at the inner aspect of the elbow, are a good choice in emergency situations and are the veins of choice for blood drawing. All sizes of catheter are acceptable, especially large 18- or 16-gauge catheters for rapid infusion of fluids or blood products. This site is usually uncomfortable for the patient because flexion of the elbow must be prevented in order for the IV to flow properly. If this site is used in an emergency, it is preferable to change the site within 24 hours if possible.

## Infant and Child

Depending on the child's age, it is usually more difficult to find an appropriate site for IV therapy in a pediatric patient than in an adult. IVs are frequently started in the hand, forearm, antecubital fossa, and upper arm. As these are considered to be the preferred sites, they should be used or evaluated first. The foot and lower leg are normally reserved for children below walking age.

The veins of the hand include the digital and metacarpal veins. The forearm veins commonly used are the supplementary cephalic, the basilic, and the median antecubital. The upper arm contains the basilic and the cephalic veins. The main veins of the foot and leg are the greater and lesser *saphenous* veins.

Less optimal sites for IVs in children include the wrist, abdomen, axilla, and knee. These are usually only considered in infants or very small children. These sites should be considered only when the preferred sites are not available. Infiltration in any of these sites may cause nerve or tissue damage.

The scalp is another site that is often used in infants up to 12 to 18 months of age. The scalp has many superficial veins, including the *frontal* or *metopic*, the *superior temporal*, the *occipital*, and the *posterior auricular* veins. Care must be taken to distinguish these veins from arteries in the scalp (Figure 5.3).

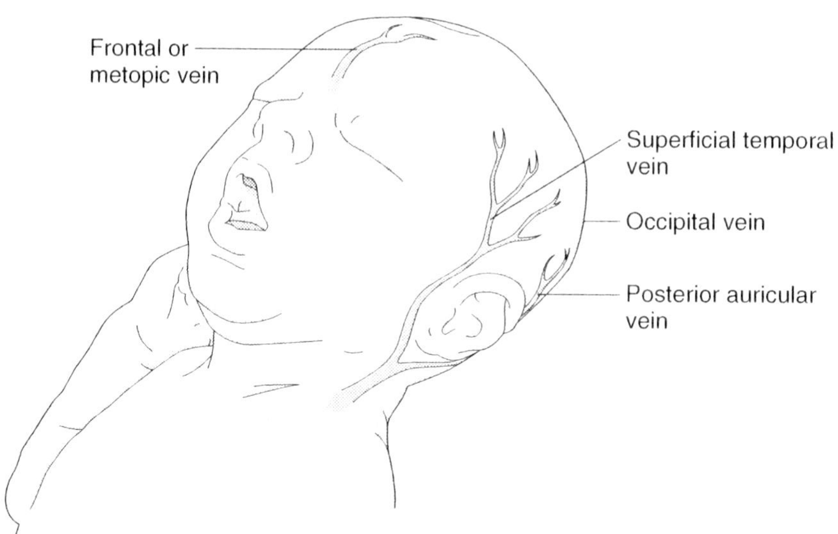


**Figure 5.3** Sites for infant scalp vein infusions.

## Key Information

If an artery is accidentally used—as indicated by bright red, pulsating blood return—the IV should be removed immediately and pressure held on the site until the bleeding stops. A pressure bandage should be applied and kept in place for 30 minutes. When an artery is accidentally punctured, many facilities require that an incident report be completed and a supervisor, physician, or pathologist notified.

Care must be taken to prepare the infant's parents before they see the child; the sight of an IV placed in an infant's head can be distressing. The child's hair might need to be shaved or clipped. Remove the smallest amount of hair necessary to achieve a clear site and to affix the IV securely. Figure 5.4 shows how a rubber band may be used as a tourniquet on the baby's scalp.

Small-gauge, thin-walled over-the-needle catheters are usually preferred to winged, metal needles in children and infants. Usually, 24- to 22-gauge catheters are used in infants and children. Catheters as small as 26-gauge may be used for therapy in neonates.

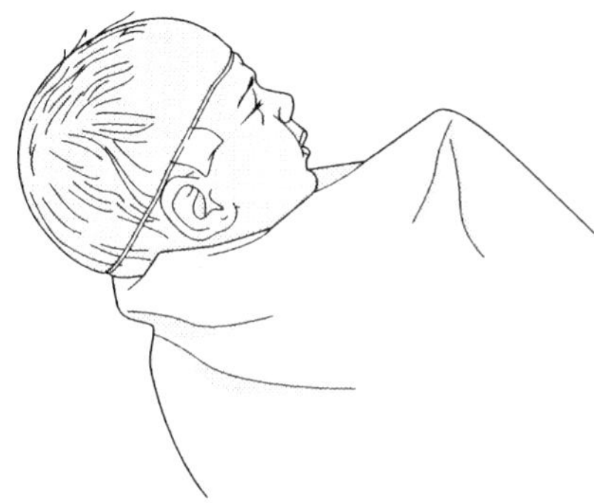

**Figure 5.4** Applying a tourniquet on an infant head.

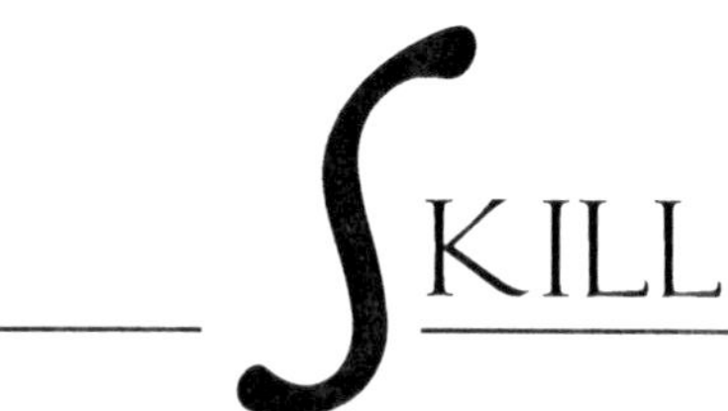

# SKILL

## Blood Specimen Collection

***Purpose*** Blood, which flows through the patient's arteries and veins, is usually drawn from peripheral veins in the patient's arms or hands to be tested for many things. Physicians order blood tests to measure electrolyte balance, abnormal functioning of body organs, blood counts, bacterial invasion, and other things that assist them in diagnosing and treating illness.

### Objectives

**The caregiver demonstrates the ability to do the following:**

1. Gather the correct supplies.
2. Communicate using a style that reduces the patient's anxiety.
3. Maintain sterile technique and use standard precautions.
4. Identify the correct colored tubes to be used for each test that the doctor has ordered.
5. Correctly perform the venipuncture.
6. Draw blood in the appropriate order related to the color of the blood tube.
7. Apply pressure and place a sterile bandage over the venipuncture site.
8. Dispose of the needle in a sharps container.
9. Correctly label the blood tubes.
10. Arrange for the blood to be taken to the laboratory.
11. Report the results of the procedure to the RN or preceptor.

### Key Terms

**Uncoagulated Blood** Blood that is collected in a tube and mixed with an anticoagulant so it does not clot. This allows the blood specimen to be tested in a liquid form with the cells in suspension.

**Coagulated Blood** Blood that is collected in a tube and allowed to clot. As the blood stands, a clear liquid, called serum, separates from the clotted blood cells.

**Hematoma** An accumulation of blood beneath the skin that results in a discoloration of the skin. Also called a bruise.

**Peripheral Vein** Surface vein that can be used as a site for venipuncture.

### Supplies/Equipment

Vacutainer system with appropriate tubes, needle, and holder • Tourniquet • Clean disposable gloves • Alcohol swabs • Sterile gauze • Sterile adhesive bandage

### Pertinent Points

- A physician's order is required for obtaining a blood specimen.
- Patients are often anxious about being stuck by a needle and about the amount of blood to be taken.
- A confident attitude and a reassuring manner will serve to calm patients and gain their cooperation. If the patient expresses concern, explain that relatively little blood will be taken. Explain also that there will be some discomfort during the procedure, but that if the patient holds very still, the discomfort will be minimized.

- Blood alcohol levels are drawn with dark blue top tubes. These are a time sensitive, high priority when the individual is accompanied to the emergency, urgent care, or ambulatory center by law enforcement personnel.
- The order used when drawing several specimens:
  1. Red top or SST tubes—used for general tests, especially electrolytes (contain no anticoagulants—clear empty tubes)
  2. Blue top—contain anticoagulants (heparin levels)
  3. Lavender top—contain anticoagulants (used for cell counts, complete blood cell [CBCs], hematocrits [HCTs])
- Check your lab manual or ask your supervisor, for any special test tube requirements. No one wants to have blood redrawn because the wrong tube was used.
- Observe the puncture site for swelling or hematoma during and after the venipuncture. Discontinue venipuncture if a hematoma forms. Apply gentle pressure over the venipuncture site for 2 to 3 minutes. If the patient is on anticoagulant therapy, apply gentle pressure for up to 5 minutes to prevent bleeding.
- If you cannot obtain the sample within two venipunctures or if you cannot find an appropriate vein to stick, notify the RN immediately. Do not stick a patient more than twice.
- Unacceptable sites for blood collection include arteries, heparin locks, fistulas, shunts, bovine or Gortex grafts, foot and leg veins, hematomas, mastectomy sites, above an IV site, scarred or burned areas, and edematous areas.

## Age-Specific Considerations

Patients of any age might have a fear of needles. Explain what you are going to do before beginning the procedure. Assess the patient's ability to immobilize the limb that you are sticking. Children and confused individuals of any age might need to be physically restrained to prevent movement when the needle is in the skin.

One of the most important things for improving success in venipuncture in children is to prevent movement of the selected site. Always try to have another caregiver assist with immobilization. Parents are usually not ideal for this purpose because they are not always able to continue to hold their children as they become upset or cry in pain.

## Key Concepts

- Check the patient's name or armband for positive identification.
- Do not attempt to stick a patient more than twice. Have another caregiver attempt the draw.
- Never attempt a venipuncture without feeling or seeing a vein.
- Do not keep the tourniquet on the patient's arm for more than 2 minutes.
- Do not prelabel tubes. Initial requisition slips only after the specimen has been collected.
- Use standard precautions and follow all agency policies and procedures.
- Discard needles only in the appropriate boxes or containers.
- Never draw a blood speciman above an IV site.
- Blood specimen tubes without anticoagulants are always filled before those with anticoagulants. Verify which tube is required any time you are unsure.

## Steps

1. Wash hands.
2. Assemble the equipment (Figure 5.5a).
3. Identify the correct patient.
4. Explain the procedure to the patient, emphasizing the need to hold the selected arm as still as possible.
5. Put on gloves.
6. Attach the needle to the Vacutainer holder (Figure 5.5b).
7. Select the correct tubes for the blood samples you are going to draw.
8. Insert one tube into the holder, and push the tube stopper partway into the needle. (Tubes without anticoagulants are always filled before those with anticoagulants.)
9. Apply the tourniquet 3 to 4 inches above the elbow.
10. Select a site for venipuncture. Assess the antecubital space of both arms to locate the best site (Figures 5.5c and d).
11. Clean the venipuncture site with an alcohol swab (Figure 5.5e). Allow to dry for several seconds. Do not touch the site after cleaning.
12. Remove the needle cover.
13. Use nondominant hand to secure and stretch the skin below the site. This stabilizes the vein and prevents it from rolling.
14. Carefully insert the needle through the skin, bevel up, in one fluid motion (Figure 5.5f).
15. Secure the Vacutainer holder with one hand while firmly pushing the tube into the holder with the thumb of the other hand (Figure 5.5g). When the tube is full, withdraw it (Figure 5.5h). If the blood specimen tube has additives, gently invert it eight to ten times to mix the additive with the blood. Insert the next tube into the holder, and repeat the process until all of the required samples have been drawn.
16. Release the tourniquet.
17. Place sterile gauze over the venipuncture site, and withdraw the needle from the skin (Figure 5.5i).
18. Apply pressure to the site for 2 to 3 minutes. (More time might be needed for patients who are on anticoagulant therapy.)
19. Discard the needle in a sharps container (Figure 5.5j).
20. Apply a sterile adhesive bandage to the site (Figure 5.5k).
21. Label the tubes with the patient's name, the date and time, and your initials.
22. Finish filling out the requisitions (Figure 5.5l).
23. Remove and discard gloves; wash hands.
24. Ensure that the blood samples and requisitions are delivered to the proper laboratory for testing.
25. Document and report the results to the RN or preceptor.

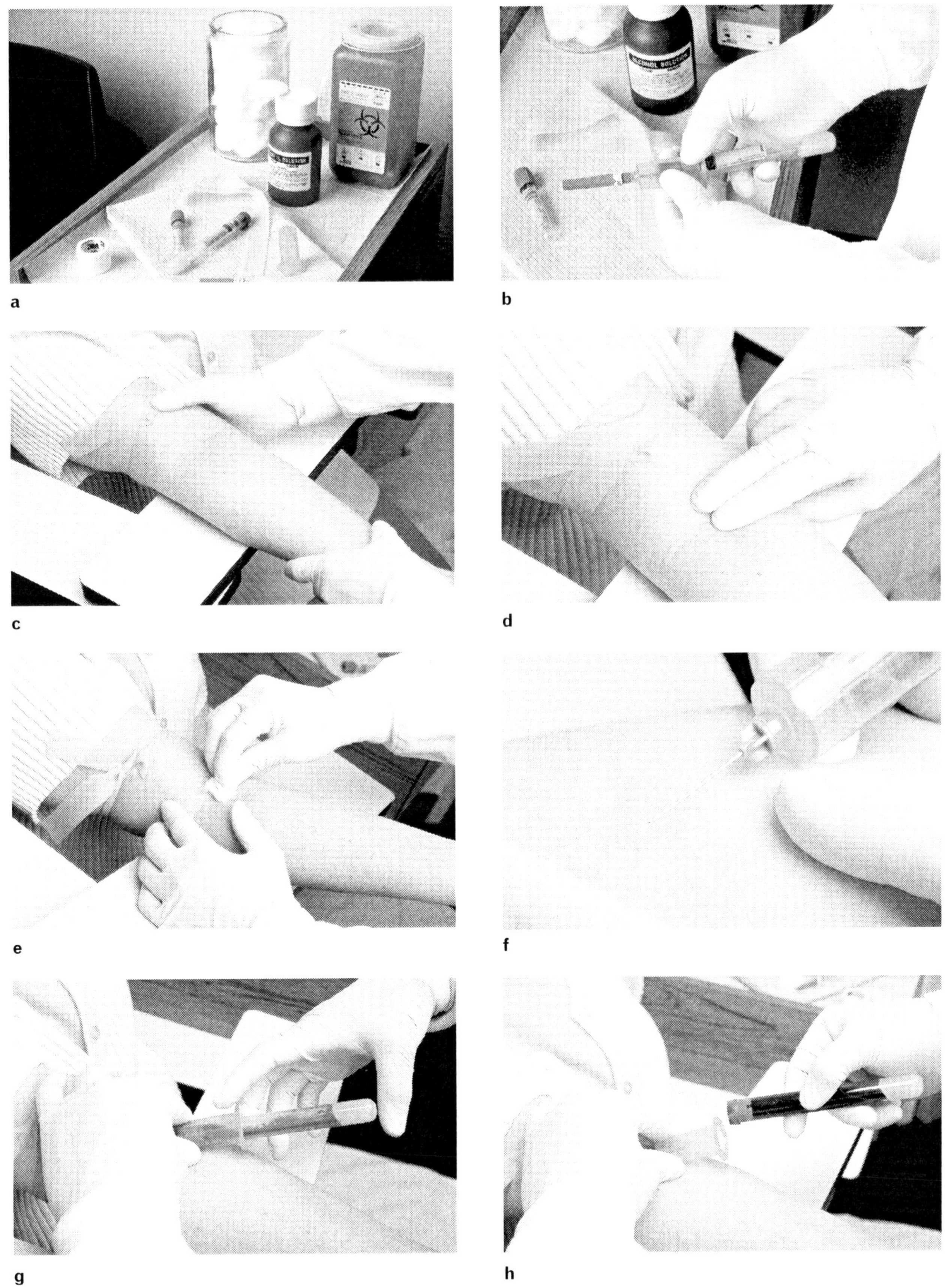

Figure 5.5 Using a Vacutainer to draw blood.

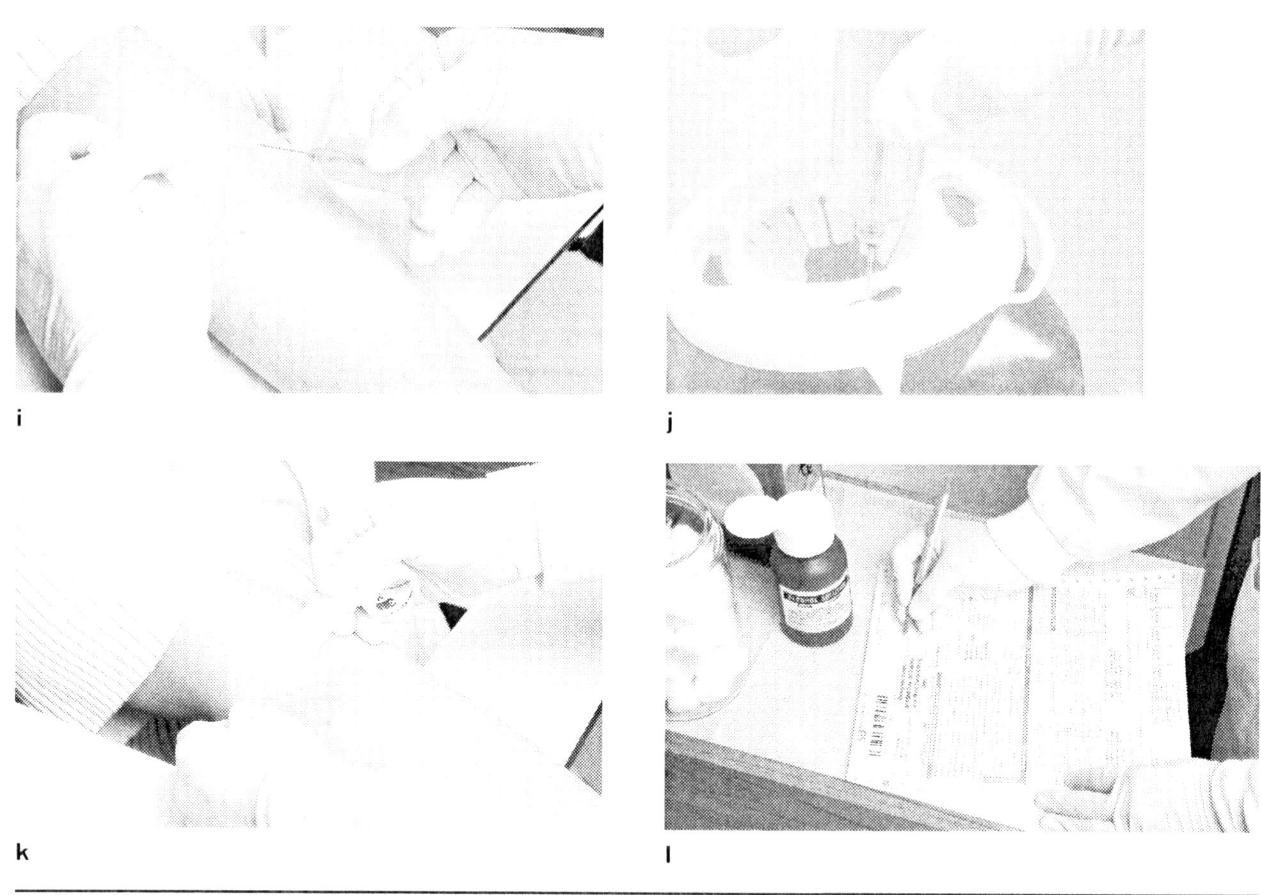

i

j

k

l

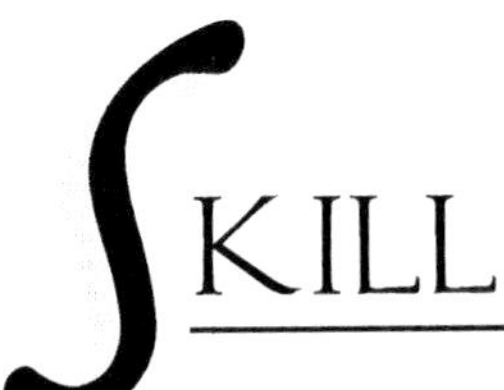

# SKILL

## Obtaining Blood Cultures

***Purpose*** When a patient is suspected to have a septicemia, blood cultures are obtained to identify the causative microorganisms. Blood cultures are drawn when a patient is feverish or having chills with a spiking fever. Blood cultures are usually ordered in sets (one aerobic and one anaerobic), which are usually drawn from more than one venipuncture site, often spaced over a period of time.

### Objectives

**The caregiver demonstrates the ability to do the following:**

1. Gather the correct supplies.
2. Communicate using a style that reduces the patient's anxiety.
3. Maintain sterile technique and use standard precautions.
4. Correctly identify aerobic and anaerobic blood culture bottles.
5. Correctly prep the venipuncture site and the blood culture bottle tops.
6. Correctly perform the venipuncture.
7. Inject the blood into the blood culture bottles using sterile technique.
8. Apply pressure and place a sterile bandage over the venipuncture site.
9. Dispose of the needle in a sharps container.
10. Correctly label the blood culture bottles.
11. Arrange for the blood to be taken to the laboratory.
12. Report the results of the procedure to the RN or preceptor.

### Key Terms

**Aerobic** Able to live only in the presence of free oxygen.

**Anaerobic** Able to live without air, like some microbes.

**Septicemia** An infection in the blood; the absorption of pathologic organisms into the blood, where they multiply rapidly.

### Supplies/Equipment

2 needles • 20-cc syringe • Blood culture bottles • Povidone–iodine swabs • Sterile gauze • Tourniquet • Sterile disposable gloves • Sterile adhesive bandage • Alcohol pad or wipe

### Pertinent Points

- A physician's order is required for obtaining a blood culture.
- Patients are often anxious about being stuck by a needle. A confident attitude and a reassuring manner will serve to calm patients and gain their cooperation. Explain that there will be some discomfort during the procedure, but that if the patient holds very still, the discomfort will be minimized.
- Observe the puncture site for swelling or hematoma during and after the venipuncture. Apply gentle pressure over the venipuncture site for 2 to 3 minutes.

### Age-Specific Considerations

Patients of any age might have a fear of needles. Explain what you are going to do before beginning the procedure. Assess the patient's ability to immobilize the limb that you are sticking. Children and confused individuals of any age might need to be physically restrained to prevent movement when the needle is in the skin. This is especially important in drawing blood cultures because of the necessity for strict asepsis in getting the blood into the culture bottle.

## Key Concepts

- Extreme care must be taken in preparing the skin and in preventing contamination during the procedure. Contamination of the blood culture by bacteria on the skin can cause an incorrect diagnosis of infection or a delay in treatment while the blood culture is repeated to verify the results.
- If you cannot obtain the sample within two venipunctures or if you cannot find an appropriate vein to stick, notify the RN immediately. Do not stick a patient more than twice.
- Never draw blood cultures above an IV site.

## Steps

1. Wash hands.
2. Assemble the equipment.
3. Identify the correct patient. Ask if patient is allergic to iodine. If yes, use alcohol only.
4. Explain the procedure to the patient, emphasizing the need to hold the selected arm as still as possible to prevent failed venipuncture or contamination.
5. Attach a needle to the 20-cc syringe (Figure 5.6b) or use a butterfly needle (Figure 5.6a).
6. Prepare the blood culture bottles by removing the cap from the rubber diaphragm, being careful not to touch the rubber stopper.
7. Apply the tourniquet 3 to 4 inches above the elbow.
8. Select a site for venipuncture. Assess the antecubital space of both arms to locate the best site.
9. Put on gloves.
10. Clean the venipuncture site with an alcohol pad and povidone–iodine swab. Using a circular motion, start from the venipuncture site and continue outward approximately 3 inches. Repeat twice. Allow to dry. Do not touch the site after cleaning.
11. Remove the needle cover.
12. Use nondominant hand to secure and stretch the skin below the site. This stabilizes the vein and prevents it from rolling.
13. Carefully insert the needle through the skin, bevel up.
14. When the vein has been entered and blood return is obtained, slowly pull back the plunger and withdraw 20-cc of blood or use a blood culture adaptor (Figure 5.6a).
15. Release the tourniquet.
16. Place sterile gauze over the venipuncture site and withdraw the needle from the skin.
17. Apply pressure to the site for 2 to 3 minutes. (More time might be needed for patients who are on anticoagulant therapy.)
18. Change the needle, and inject 10 cc of blood through the diaphragm of the anaerobic bottle. Next, place 10 cc of blood in the aerobic bottle. Try not to inject air into either bottle; this is especially important in the anaerobic bottle (Figure 5.6b).

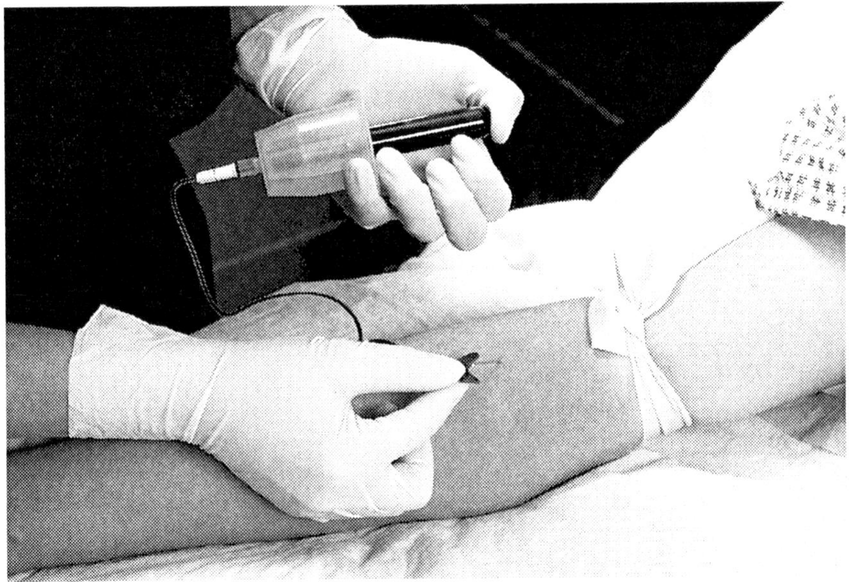

a

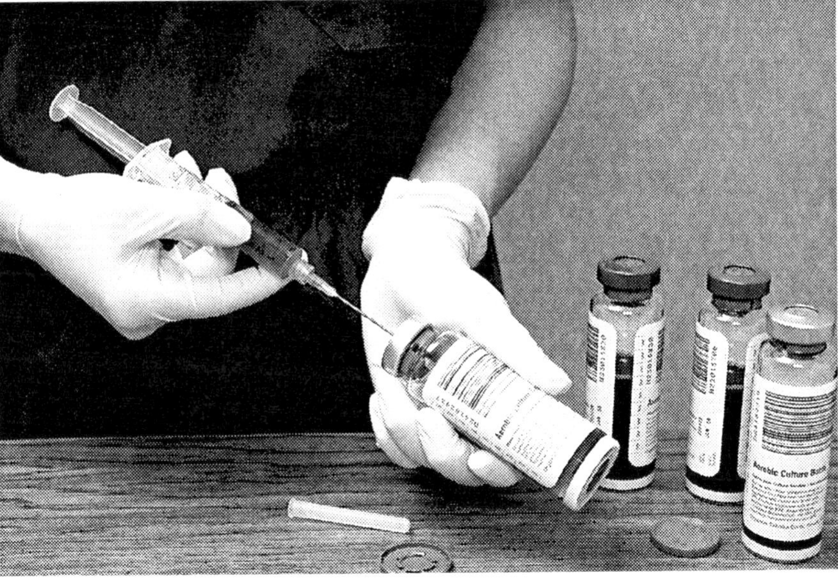

b

**Figure 5.6** (a) caregiver withdraws the patient's blood for blood cultures using a blood culture adaptor or syringe. (b) Injecting 10 cc of blood in the aerobic bottle.

19. Discard the needles in a sharps container.
20. Apply a sterile adhesive bandage to the site.
21. Clean the area and dispose of the waste in accordance with the facility's policy.
22. Label the bottles with the patient's name, the date and time, and your initials.
23. Remove and discard gloves; wash hands.
24. Finish filling out the requisitions.
25. Ensure that the blood cultures and the requisitions are delivered to the proper laboratory for testing.
26. Document and report the results to the RN or preceptor.

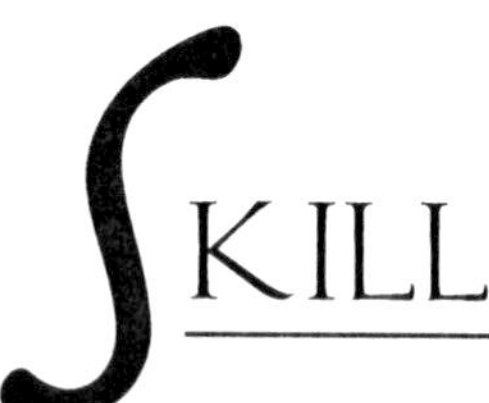

# SKILL

## Using a Lancet or a Microlance for a Microdraw or an Infant Heel Stick

***Purpose*** Microdraw, or skin puncture, is used to collect blood specimens from patients of all ages. Although small in size, these specimens are adequate for many laboratory tests. Blood collected from a skin puncture is a mixture of arterial, venous, and capillary blood. Lancets are used to collect blood from toddlers through adults. Microlances or safety flow lancets are used when performing an infant heel stick.

### Objectives

**The caregiver demonstrates the ability to do the following:**

1. Gather the correct supplies.
2. Communicate using a style that reduces the patient's anxiety, or explain procedure to the parent or guardian.
3. Maintain sterile technique.
4. Follow standard precautions.
5. Correctly prep the site.
6. Identify acceptable sites for skin puncture.
7. Collect the blood sample using the microdraw technique.
8. Apply pressure and place a sterile bandage over the site.
9. Dispose of the lancet in a sharps container.
10. Correctly label the blood sample.
11. Arrange for the blood to be taken to the laboratory.
12. Report the results of the procedure to the RN or preceptor.

### Key Terms

**Lancet** A small, extremely sharp, individually wrapped, single-use sterile, metal, or plastic object used to puncture the skin, cut the capillaries, and cause bleeding at the puncture site. Lancets come in two sizes: 2.4 mm (short-point or microlance) for use with infants or small children and 5.0 mm (long-point) for adult use.

**Microvette Collector** A preassembled system containing a capillary unit and a graduated collection tube with an attached stopper. Microvette collectors are available with or without anticoagulants and with a serum separator gel.

### Supplies/Equipment

Alcohol swab • Blood-collecting equipment • Clean gloves • Dry gauze pads • Spot adhesive bandage • Sterile disposable lancets

### Pertinent Points

- Unless there is a specific physician's order, the caregiver chooses the site for the collection of skin puncture specimens. These specimens may be obtained from the most medial or lateral portions of the plantar heel surface or the big toe in an infant or child under age 1 (Figure 5.7a).
- The sides of the middle and fourth fingers are the common sites for obtaining a microdraw on older children and adults (Figure 5.7b).
- A warm cloth can be applied to the selected site for a few minutes before sticking the site. This helps promote blood flow to the site.

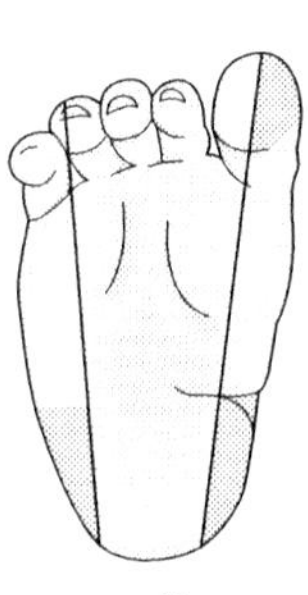


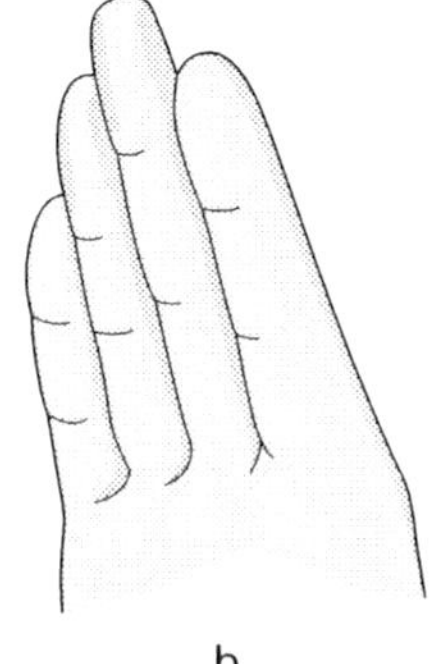


**Figure 5.7** Acceptable sites for skin puncture (shaded areas).

- There are two types of microvette collectors. Microvettes with a purple cap contain powdered ethylenediaminetetraacetic acid (EDTA), are used for CBCs, and collect up to 1 ml of blood. To ensure proper mixing, microvettes with anticoagulants should not be filled beyond 500 μl. Blood platelets have a tendency to clump; therefore, hematology specimens should be collected first. Microvettes with a red cap are available in two types: either with a plain interior or with a serum separator with gel.

## Age-Specific Considerations

Patients of all ages might benefit from microdraw, or skin puncture, as only a very small amount of blood is needed. In ambulatory or outpatient settings, it can be helpful to have a parent in the room during the procedure to comfort the infant. If the parent is upset about the procedure or is uncomfortable with the sight of blood, another caregiver should hold the child. Explain the procedure to the infant's parents before beginning the procedure to alleviate some of their concerns.

## Key Concept

Avoid using sites that are swollen or edematous or have previously been used.

## Steps

1. Wash hands.
2. Assemble the equipment.
   a. Clean gloves
   b. Alcohol swab
   c. Safety flow lancet
   d. Capillary tubes
   e. Blood label
   f. Adhesive bandage
3. Identify the correct patient.
4. Explain the procedure to the patient, parent, or guardian, emphasizing the need to hold the selected finger (adult) or foot (infant) as still as possible.
5. Put on gloves.
6. Identify acceptable sites for skin puncture. Avoid sites that are swollen or edematous or have previously been used. Clean the selected site with an alcohol swab.
7. Hold the lancet at a 45-degree angle to the surface to be punctured. Do not direct the lancet toward a bone (Figure 5.8).
8. Wipe away the first drops of blood. Collect the blood sample by gently squeezing the heel and allowing the blood to flow into the tube.

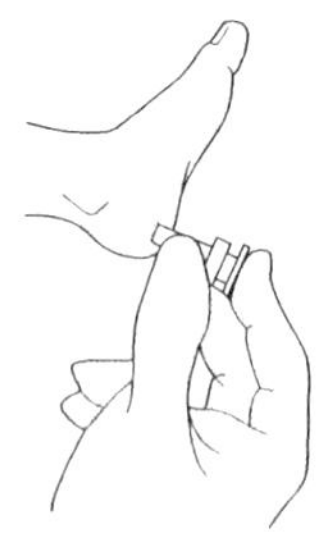
Hold lancet on site with moderate pressure.

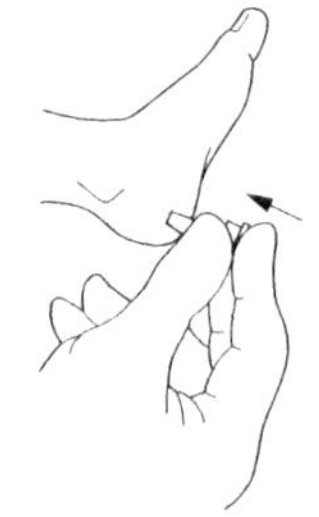
Depress plunger with index finger to make puncture.

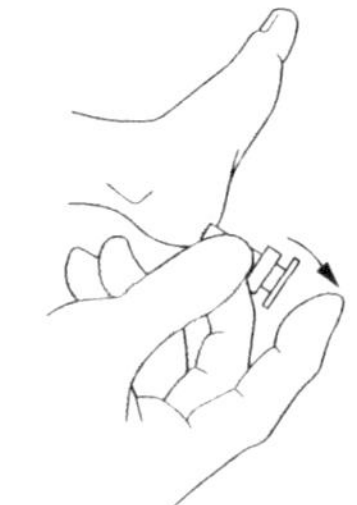
Immediately release plunger while holding lancet on site.

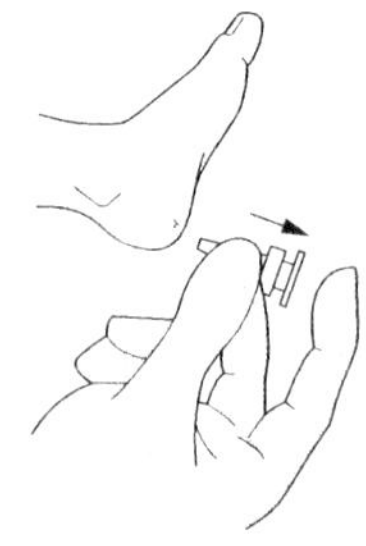
Remove lancet.

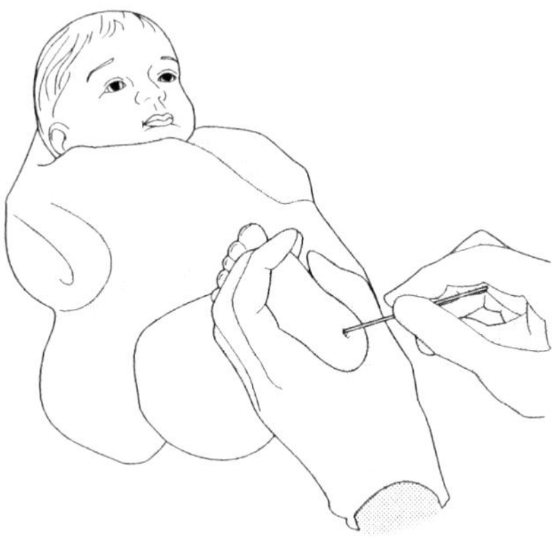
Collect blood sample by allowing the blood to flow into the tube.

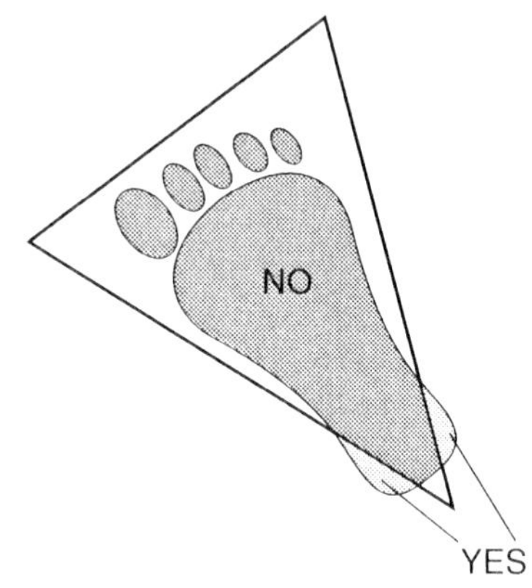


**Figure 5.8** Using a safety flow lancet for an infant microdraw.

9. Apply adhesive bandage to puncture site.
10. Discard the lancet in a sharps container.
11. Correctly label the blood sample with patient's name, date, and your initials.
12. Remove and discard gloves; wash hands.
13. Ensure that the blood sample is delivered to the proper laboratory for testing.
14. Document or notify the RN or preceptor that the blood sample has been obtained.

# Section Two
# IV Therapy

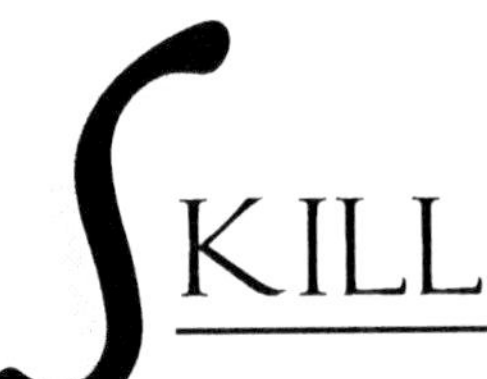

## Inserting a Heplock

**Purpose** The insertion of a tube into a patient's vein to provide direct access to the patient's bloodstream is known as intravenous (IV) therapy. A heparin lock, or heplock, is used when the continuous infusion of IV fluids is not necessary. The heplock (or saline lock) is often used for intermittent administration of IV antibiotics or other medications that the physician has ordered to be given at specific times, such as every 6 hours or PRN (whenever needed), such as for pain medications as needed. Another common use for a heplock is with unstable patients who might need emergency medications for a rapid change in condition but who do not require extra fluids.

### Objectives

**The caregiver demonstrates the ability to do the following:**

1. Receive specific instructions from the RN and check the physician's order on the patient's chart.
2. Gather the correct supplies.
3. Communicate using a style that reduces the patient's anxiety.
4. Maintain sterile technique.
5. Use standard precautions.
6. Evaluate and select the most appropriate vein.
7. Select an IV catheter that is appropriate for the size of the patient's veins and the purpose of the IV therapy.
8. Insert the IV catheter, attach the heplock adapter, flush with saline or heparin per institution policy, and correctly apply dressing.
9. Dispose of the needle in a sharps container.
10. Document the procedure correctly in the patient's chart.
11. Report the results of the procedure to the RN or preceptor.

### Key Terms

**Antecubital** Related to the space in the bend of the elbow.

**Bevel** The slanted edge at the opening of a needle or catheter.

**Distal** Farthest from the heart.

**Gauge** The size or measurement of the diameter of a needle or catheter opening (i.e., 14, 16, 18, 20, 22, 24). The larger the number, the smaller the diameter of the needle or catheter. Needles are usually sized in odd numbers; catheters, in even numbers.

**Palpation** Examination by touch, such as the examination of a vein by touch to determine its size, elasticity, and location.

**Proximal** Closest to the heart.

**Stylet** The needle inside a catheter.

## Supplies/Equipment

Intermittent injection adapter • 3-cc syringe filled with normal saline or heplock solution, per institution policy • Towel or protective pad • Tourniquet • Clean disposable gloves • Alcohol swabs or povidone–iodine swabs • IV catheter • Sterile 2×2s • Transparent dressing • Tape

## Pertinent Points

- A physician's order is required to start or discontinue a heplock.
- Because this procedure involves inserting a catheter and often medications and fluids directly into the patient's bloodstream, a strict sterile technique is required to prevent exposing the patient to a potentially life-threatening infection.
- As with an IV, when selecting a vein for a heplock, choose the distal veins first. For later heplock starts, use the more proximal portions of the vein, thereby working your way up the patient's arms through the course of therapy. This method of site selection prevents irritating fluids from being infused into previously used veins.

## Age-Specific Considerations

Patients of any age might fear being stuck with a needle. Explain the procedure and the therapy in terms that the patient can understand. Be sure to have assistance, as needed, to hold a child or a confused patient to prevent movement during the insertion. Children and geriatric patients sometimes have small or fragile veins, requiring the use of smaller catheters to start the heplock.

## Key Concept

The fluid instilled in the lock has long been a controversy in many hospitals. In recent years, many institutions have switched from the anticoagulant heparin to normal saline flushes to maintain patency. Check and follow your institution's policy.

## Steps

1. Wash hands.
2. Assemble the equipment. Prime the intermittent infusion adapter with normal saline or heplock solution.
3. Identify the correct patient.
4. Explain the procedure to the patient. Determine the patient's preference for site selection if possible. Ask patient if he or she is allergic to iodine or latex.
5. Set up the equipment on the bedside table, within easy reach.
6. Place the towel or protective pad under the patient's arm.
7. Apply the tourniquet to the patient's arm.
8. Palpate the arm and select a venipuncture site.
9. Remove the tourniquet.
10. Put on gloves.
11. Clean the chosen site with an alcohol or povidone–iodine swab, per institution policy. Use a circular motion, starting at the insertion site and moving slowly outward. Clean for 1 minute. Allow to dry. (Hair at the site may be clipped, if necessary, before cleaning.)
12. Reapply the tourniquet approximately 3 to 4 inches above the selected insertion site.
13. Stabilize the vein with the nondominant hand. Using sterile technique, hold the catheter by the hub. Insert the catheter at a 25- to 45-degree angle, with the bevel pointing up. Firmly pierce the skin.
14. Carefully advance the catheter and stylet into the vein. Observe for blood return (flashback).

15. Stabilize the stylet, and advance the catheter into the vein. Do not push the stylet, or needle portion, through the vein.
16. Place a sterile 2×2 beneath the hub of the catheter. Withdraw the stylet most of the way out of the catheter. Put slight pressure over the vein about 1 inch above the insertion site.
17. Remove the tourniquet.
18. Remove the stylet and place it in a sharps container. Attach the intermittent infusion adapter and release pressure on the vein. Many needles now have a safety button that, when pushed, removes the stylet in one motion.
19. Slowly inject normal saline or heplock solution (Figure 5.9).
20. Observe the site for signs of infiltration: swelling, skin coolness, or blanching.
21. Dress the IV site using a transparent dressing over the insertion site and tape to secure the hub. Tape tubing so it does not cross the vein being used.
22. Label the dressing with the date, the catheter size, and your initials.
23. Remove and discard gloves; wash hands.
24. Document and report the results of the procedure, as well as patient tolerance, to the RN or preceptor.

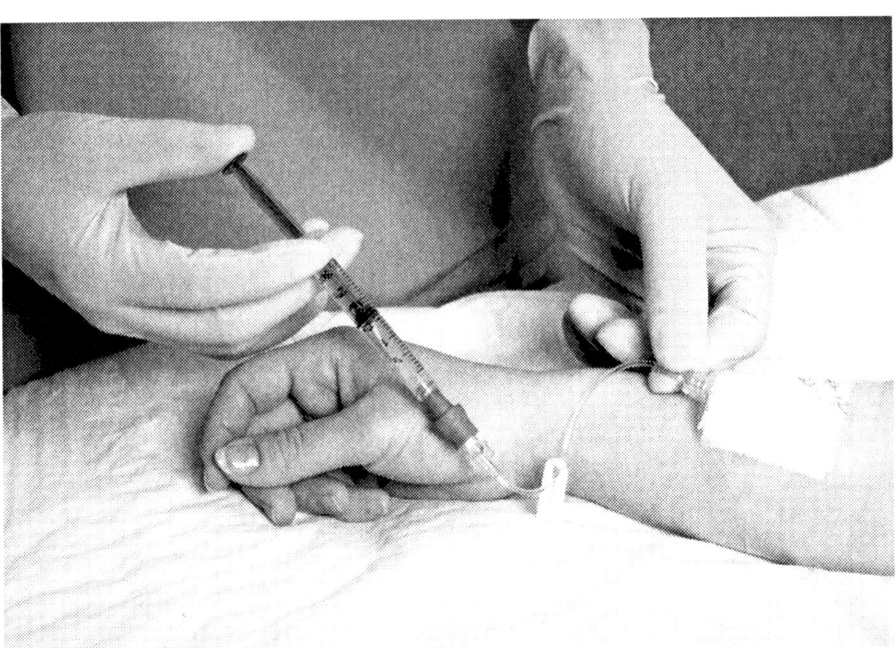

**Figure 5.9** Injecting normal saline in a heplock.

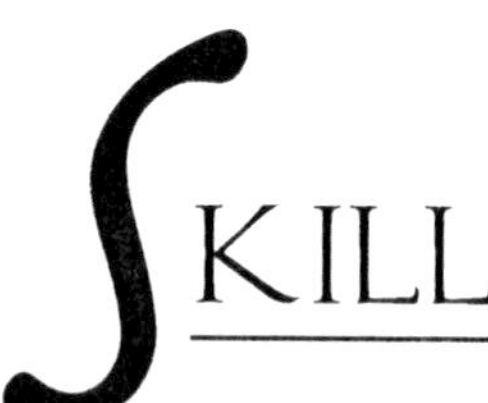

# SKILL

## Inserting a Butterfly (Winged Infusion Device)

*Purpose* The insertion of a tube into a patient's vein to supply fluid, salts, glucose, vitamins, or medications is called *IV therapy*. A butterfly device is usually used for short-term IV therapy, such as infusing chemotherapy IV push, or for difficult blood drawing.

### Objectives

**The caregiver demonstrates the ability to do the following:**

1. Receive specific instructions from the RN and/or check the physician's order on the patient's chart.
2. Identify the type of IV fluid, the size of the bag, and the flow rate ordered.
3. Gather the correct supplies.
4. Communicate using a style that reduces the patient's anxiety.
5. Maintain sterile technique and use standard precautions.
6. Correctly set up the IV bag and tubing.
7. Evaluate and select the most appropriate vein.
8. Select an IV catheter that is appropriate for the size of the patient's veins and the purpose of the IV therapy.
9. Insert the butterfly, attach the tubing, and apply the dressing correctly.
10. Set the IV rate per the physician's order.
11. Document the procedure correctly in the patient's chart.
12. Report the results of the procedure to the RN or preceptor.

### Key Terms

**Antecubital** Related to the space in the bend of the elbow.

**Bevel** The slanted edge at the opening of a needle or catheter.

**Distal** Farthest from the heart.

**Gauge** The size or measurement of the diameter of a needle or catheter opening (i.e., 19, 21, 23, 25). The larger the number, the smaller the diameter of the needle or catheter. Needles are usually sized in odd numbers, catheters in even numbers.

**Palpation** Examination by touch, such as the examination of a vein by touch to determine its size, elasticity, and location.

**Proximal** Closest to the heart.

**Spike** To insert an administration set into an IV bag or bottle.

**Venipuncture** Insertion of a needle through the skin into a peripheral vein to draw blood or insert an IV device.

### Supplies/Equipment

Butterflies of various sizes • Saline-filled syringe • Towel or protective pad • Tourniquet • Clean disposable gloves • Alcohol swabs or povidone–iodine swabs • Appropriate IV bag or bottle and IV tubing • Sterile 2×2s • Transparent dressing • Tape

## Pertinent Points

- A physician's order is required to start, change, maintain, or discontinue IV therapy.
- Because this procedure involves inserting a needle and often medications and fluids directly into the patient's bloodstream, strict sterile technique is required to prevent exposing the patient to a potentially life-threatening infection.
- Due to the inflexibility of the butterfly needle, it is used only when very frequent observation of the site is possible throughout therapy.

## Age-Specific Considerations

Patients of any age might fear being stuck with a needle, and the sight of a person coming into the room with an IV pole and other assorted equipment might produce anxiety. Explain the procedure and the therapy in terms that the patient can understand. Be sure to have assistance, as needed, to hold an infant, a small child, or a confused patient to prevent movement during the insertion.

Children and geriatric patients sometimes have small or fragile veins, requiring the use of smaller-gauge butterflies to start the IV. A child's IV must be taped very securely so that it will not become dislodged with activity or during play. A butterfly may be used to start a scalp vein IV in infants.

## Key Concept

The butterfly should not be used in veins that run over joints unless total immobilization of the joint is possible. Arm boards are frequently used for this purpose.

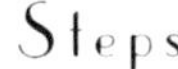

## Steps

1. Wash hands.
2. Assemble the equipment. Prime the butterfly tubing using a saline-filled syringe.
3. Identify the correct patient and ask about allergies.
4. Explain the procedure to the patient. Determine the patient's preference for site selection if possible.
5. Set up the equipment on the bedside table, within easy reach.
6. Place the towel or protective pad under the patient's arm.
7. Apply the tourniquet to the patient's arm (Figure 5.10).
8. Palpate the arm and select an insertion site. The site chosen must allow insertion into a straight length of vein; because the

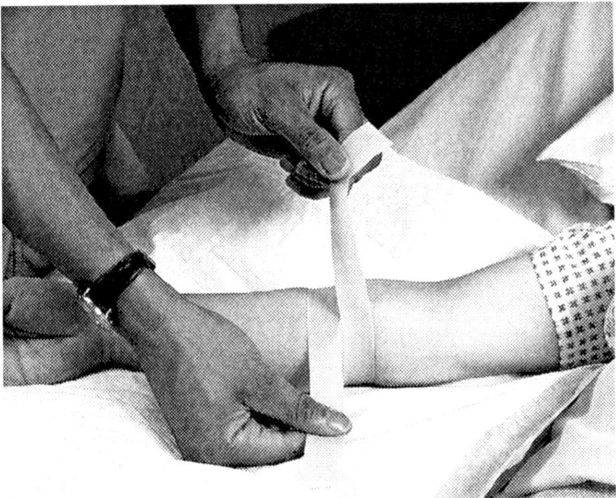

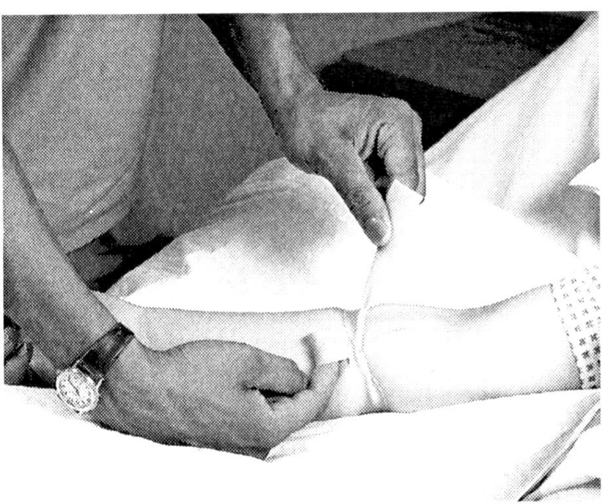

**Figure 5.10** Applying a tourniquet to the patient's arm.

butterfly is inflexible, it could easily go through a vein (Figure 5.11).

9. Remove the tourniquet.
10. Put on gloves.
11. Clean the chosen IV site with an alcohol or povidone–iodine swab, per institution policy. Use a circular motion, starting at the insertion site and moving slowly outward. Clean for 1 minute. Allow to dry. (Hair at the site may be clipped, if necessary, before cleaning.)
12. Reapply the tourniquet approximately 3 to 4 inches above the selected insertion site.
13. Stabilize the vein with the nondominant hand. Grasp the butterfly by folding the wings together with the bevel of the needle up. Firmly pierce the skin, and slide the needle into the vein up to the wings in one smooth movement.
14. Observe for blood return in the butterfly tubing.
15. Remove the tourniquet.
16. Attach the IV tubing.
17. Set the IV fluid to run at a slow rate (20 drops per minute).
18. Observe the site for signs of infiltration: swelling, skin coolness, or blanching.
19. Dress the IV site using a transparent dressing over the insertion site and tape to secure the hub and IV tubing.
20. Label the dressing with the date, the catheter size, and your initials.
21. Set the IV rate as ordered by the physician.
22. Remove and discard gloves; wash hands.
23. Document and report the results of the procedure, as well as patient tolerance, to the RN or preceptor.

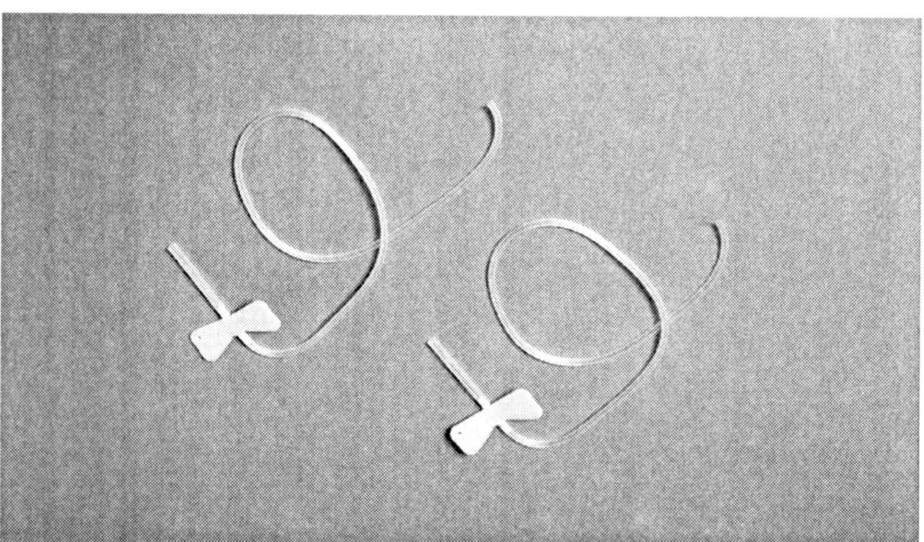

**Figure 5.11** Winged or butterfly needle.

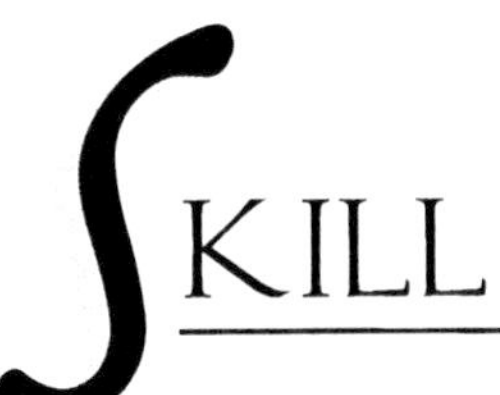

# KILL

## Inserting a Peripheral IV in an Adult

**Purpose** The insertion of a tube into a patient's vein to provide direct access to the patient's bloodstream is called *IV therapy*. The IV route may be used to supply fluid when patients are unable to take adequate amounts by mouth, to provide salts needed to maintain electrolyte balance, to provide glucose as fuel for metabolism, to provide water-soluble vitamins and medications, and to establish a lifeline for rapidly needed medications.

### Objectives

**The caregiver demonstrates the ability to do the following:**

1. Receive specific instructions from the RN and check the physician's order on the patient's chart.
2. Identify the type of IV fluid, the size of the bag, and the flow rate ordered.
3. Gather the correct supplies.
4. Communicate using a style that reduces the patient's anxiety.
5. Maintain sterile technique and follow standard precautions.
6. Correctly set up the IV bag and tubing.
7. Evaluate and select the most appropriate vein.
8. Select an IV catheter that is appropriate for the size of the patient's veins and the purpose of the IV therapy.
9. Insert the IV catheter, attach the tubing, and apply the dressing correctly.
10. Dispose of the needle in a sharps container.
11. Set the IV rate per the physician's order.
12. Document the procedure correctly in the patient's chart.
13. Report the results of the procedure to the RN or preceptor.

### Key Terms

**Antecubital** Related to the space in the bend of the elbow.

**Bevel** The slanted edge at the opening of a needle or catheter.

**Distal** Farthest from the heart.

**Gauge** The size or measurement of the diameter of a needle or catheter opening (i.e., 14, 16, 18, 20, 22, 24). The larger the number, the smaller the diameter of the needle or catheter. Needles are usually sized in odd numbers; catheters, in even numbers.

**Palpation** Examination by touch, such as the examination of a vein by touch to determine its size, elasticity, and location.

**Proximal** Closest to the heart.

**Spike** To insert an administration set into an IV bag or bottle.

**Stylet** The needle inside a catheter.

**Venipuncture** Insertion of a needle through the skin into a peripheral vein to draw blood or insert an IV device.

## Supplies/Equipment

Appropriate IV bag or bottle and IV tubing, primed • Towel or protective pad • Tourniquet • Clean disposable gloves • Alcohol swabs or povidone–iodine swabs • IV catheters of various sizes • Sterile 2×2s • Transparent dressing • Tape

## Pertinent Points

- A physician's order is required to start, change, maintain, or discontinue IV therapy.
- Because this procedure involves inserting a catheter and often medications and fluids directly into the patient's bloodstream, strict sterile technique is required to prevent exposing the patient to a potentially life-threatening infection.
- If the duration of the IV therapy is expected to be long (i.e., more than a few hours), several factors must be taken into account when choosing the site. If patients are to be able to feed, bathe, and dress themselves, the caregiver should take into account their ability to move their hand or arm after the IV is placed. Thus, the antecubital space and any site over a joint are used only as a last resort for long-term IV therapy.

## Age-Specific Considerations

Patients of any age might fear being stuck with a needle, and the sight of a person coming into the room with an IV pole and other assorted equipment might produce anxiety. Explain the procedure and the therapy in terms that the patient can understand. Be sure to have assistance, as needed, to hold a confused patient to prevent movement during the insertion. Geriatric patients sometimes have small or fragile veins, requiring the use of smaller catheters to start the IV.

## Key Concepts

- There is variation throughout the United States in who may start IVs or infuse fluids. Check with your employer or instructor.
- When selecting an initial IV site, use the distal veins first. For subsequent IV starts, choose the more proximal portions of the vein, thereby working your way up the patient's arms through the course of therapy. This method of site selection prevents irritating fluids from being infused into previously used veins.
- Use caution as you advance the catheter into the vein. Do not push the stylet, or needle portion, into the vein.

## Steps

1. Wash hands.
2. Assemble the equipment. Prime the IV tubing. (RN may be needed to do this.)
3. Identify the correct patient and ask about allergies.
4. Explain the procedure to the patient. Determine the patient's preference for site selection if possible.
5. Set up the equipment on the bedside table, within easy reach.
6. Place the towel or protective pad under the patient's arm.
7. Apply the tourniquet to the patient's arm (Figure 5.10).
8. Palpate the arm and select an IV site.
9. Remove the tourniquet.
10. Put on clean exam gloves.
11. Clean the chosen IV site with an alcohol or povidone–iodine swab, per institution policy. Use a circular motion, starting at the insertion site and moving slowly outward (Figure 5.12a). Clean for 1 minute. Allow to dry. (Hair at the site may be clipped, if necessary, before cleaning.)

12. Reapply the tourniquet approximately 3 to 4 inches above the selected insertion site.
13. Stabilize the vein with the non-dominant hand (Figure 5.12b). Using sterile technique, hold the catheter by the hub. Insert the catheter at a 25- to 45-degree angle, with the bevel pointing up. Firmly pierce the skin (Figure 5.12c).
14. Carefully advance the catheter and stylet into the vein (Figure 5.12d). Observe for blood return (flash-back).
15. Stabilize the stylet, and advance the catheter into the vein. Do not push the stylet, or needle portion, into the vein.
16. Place a sterile 2×2s beneath the hub of the catheter. Withdraw the stylet most of the way out of the catheter. Put slight pressure over the vein about 1 inch above the insertion site.
17. Remove the tourniquet.
18. Remove the stylet, and place it in a sharps container. Attach the IV tubing and release pressure on the vein (Figure 5.12e). Many needles now have a safety button that, when pushed, will retract the stylet into the handle.
19. Open the IV fluid to run at a slow rate.
20. Observe the site for signs of infiltration: swelling, skin coolness, or blanching.
21. Dress the IV site using a transparent dressing over the insertion site and tape to secure the hub and IV tubing (Figure 5.12f). Tape the tubing so that it does not cross the vein being used.
22. Label the dressing with the date, the catheter size, and your initials.
23. Set the IV rate to run at a slow rate (20 drops per minute).
24. Remove and discard gloves; wash hands.
25. Document and report the results of the procedure, as well as patient tolerance, to the RN or preceptor.

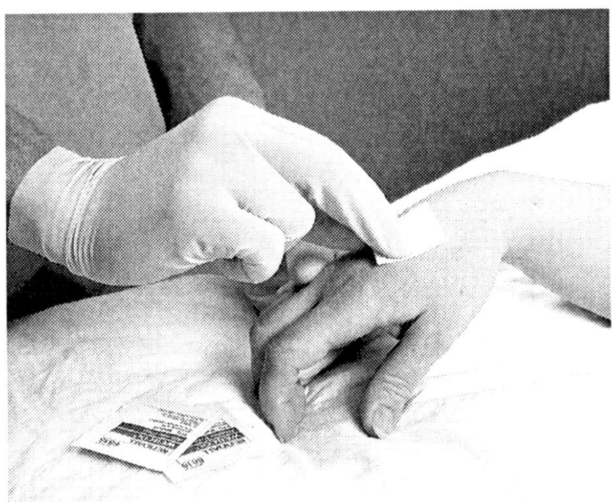

a

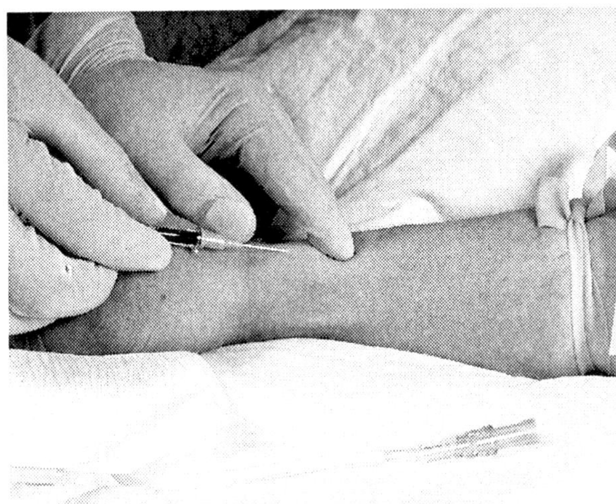

b

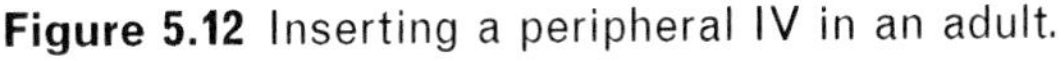

**Figure 5.12** Inserting a peripheral IV in an adult.

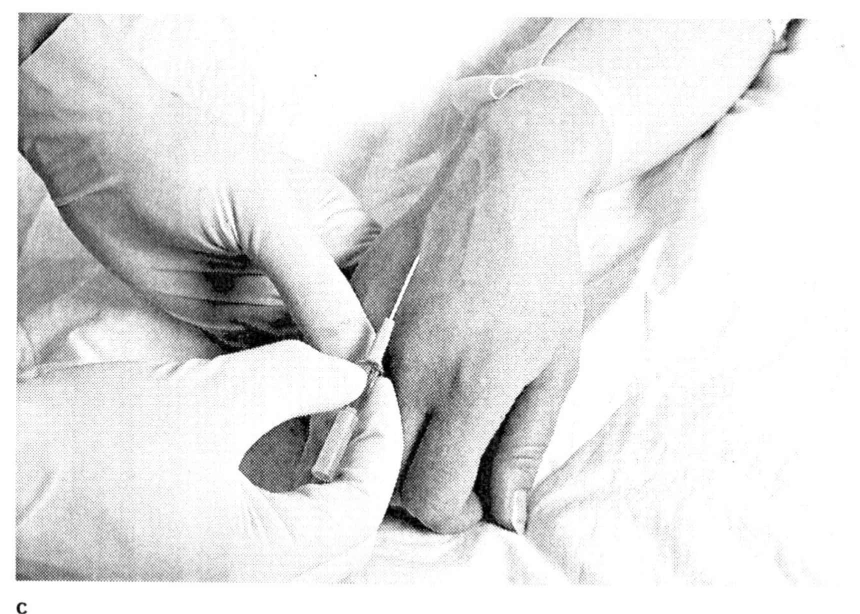

c

d

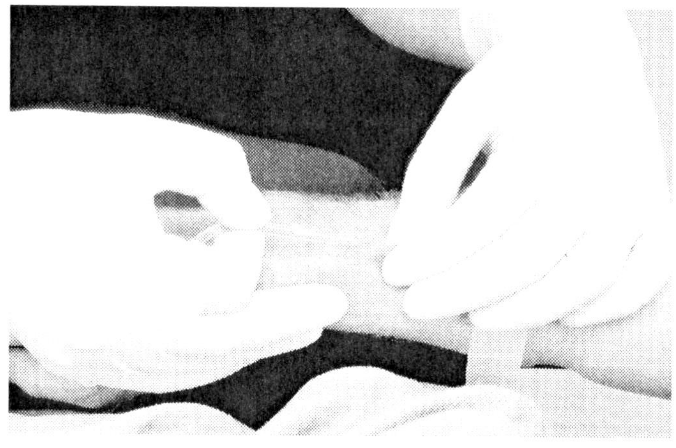

e

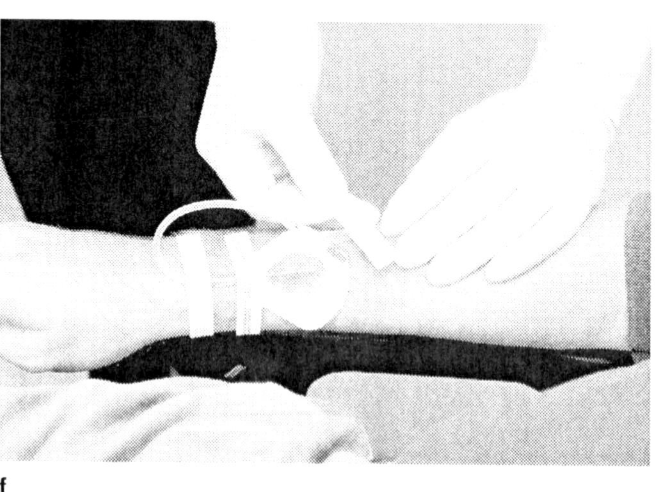

f

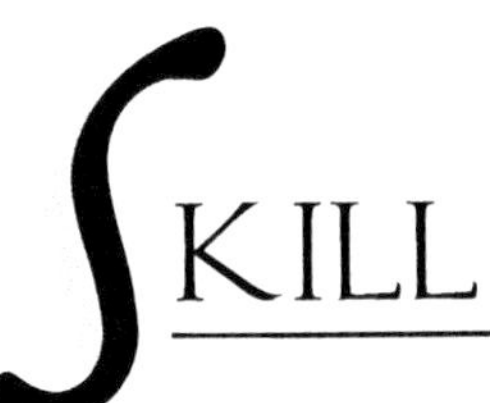

# SKILL

## Inserting a Peripheral IV in a Child

***Purpose*** The insertion of a tube into a patient's vein to provide direct access to the patient's bloodstream is called IV therapy. Pediatric patients become dehydrated more easily than adults. IV fluids are often used to replace fluids and electrolytes lost through fever, vomiting, or diarrhea.

### Objectives

**The caregiver demonstrates the ability to do the following:**

1. Receive specific instructions from the RN and check the physician's order on the patient's chart.
2. Identify the type of IV fluid, the size of the bag, and the flow rate ordered.
3. Gather the correct supplies.
4. Communicate using a style that reduces the patient's anxiety.
5. Maintain sterile technique and follow standard precautions.
6. Correctly set up the IV bag and tubing.
7. Evaluate and select the most appropriate vein.
8. Select an IV catheter that is appropriate for the size of the patient's veins and the purpose of the IV therapy.
9. Ensure adequate assistance to hold the child securely.
10. Insert the IV catheter, attach the tubing, and apply the dressing correctly.
11. Dispose of the needle in a sharps container.
12. Set the IV rate per the physician's order.
13. Document the procedure correctly in the patient's chart.
14. Report the results of the procedure to the RN or preceptor.

### Key Terms

**Antecubital** Related to the space in the bend of the elbow.

**Bevel** The slanted edge at the opening of a needle or catheter.

**Distal** Farthest from the heart.

**Gauge** The size or measurement of the diameter of a needle or catheter opening (i.e., 14, 16, 18, 20, 22, 24). The larger the number, the smaller the diameter of the needle or catheter. Needles are usually sized in odd numbers, catheters in even numbers.

**Palpation** Examination by touch, such as the examination of a vein by touch to determine its size, elasticity, and location.

**Proximal** Closest to the heart.

**Spike** To insert an administration set into an IV bag or bottle.

**Stylet** The needle inside a catheter.

**Venipuncture** Insertion of a needle through the skin into a peripheral vein to draw blood or insert an IV device.

## Supplies/ Equipment

Appropriate IV bag or bottle and IV tubing with volume-limiting reservoir (such as Buretrol), primed • Towel or protective pad • Pediatric tourniquet • Arm board • Tape • Sterile disposable gloves • Alcohol swabs • Small IV catheters of various sizes • Sterile 2×2s • Transparent dressing

## Pertinent Points

- A physician's order is required to start, change, maintain, or discontinue IV therapy.
- Because this procedure involves inserting a catheter and often medications and fluids directly into the patient's bloodstream, strict sterile technique is required to prevent exposing the patient to a potentially life-threatening infection.
- The most frequently used sites for pediatric patients are the dorsum of the hand, the dorsum of the foot, and the scalp veins (Figure 5.13).

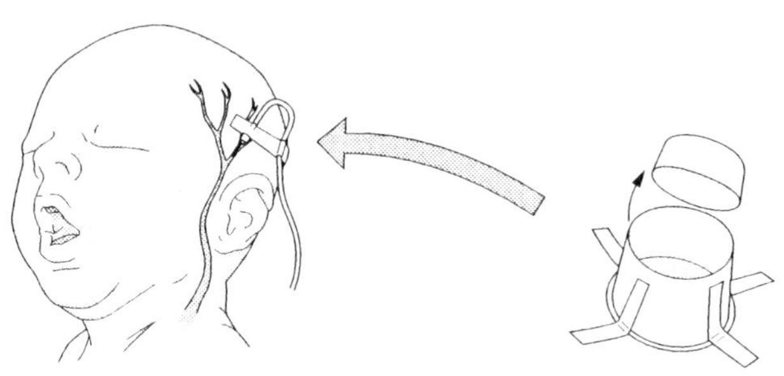

Venipuncture of scalp vein

Paper cup taped over venipuncture site for protection. A clear plastic cup may also be used.

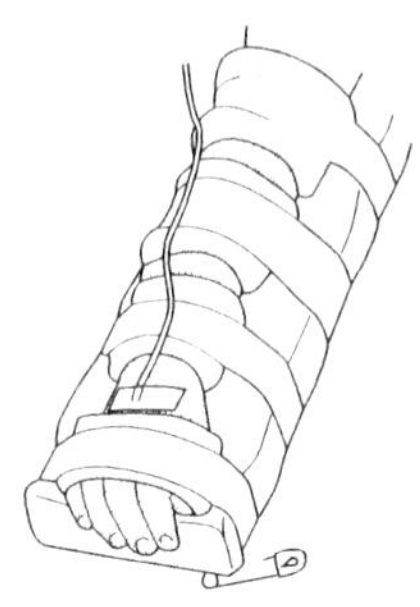

Restraint of arm when hand is site of infusion

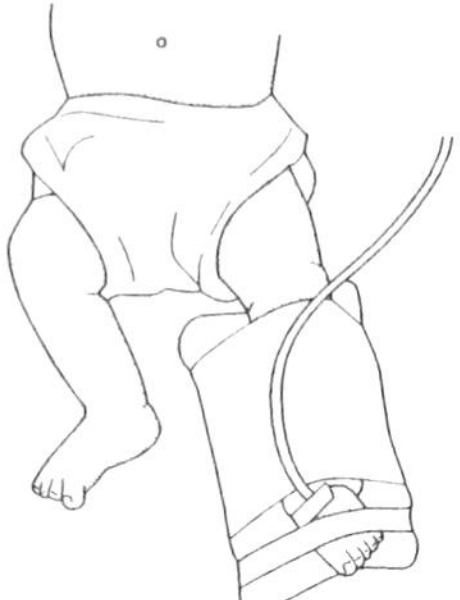

Infant's leg taped to sand-bag for immobilization

**Figure 5.13** IV sites on infant scalp, arm, and leg.

## Age-Specific Considerations

Children often fear needles. Explain the procedure and the therapy in terms that the patient can understand. Be sure to have assistance, as needed, to hold the infant or child to prevent movement during the insertion. Children often have small or fragile veins, requiring the use of small catheters (22- or 24-gauge) to start an IV. Do not tell pediatric patients that the procedure will not hurt. Be truthful, but explain that the needle will hurt only for a short time. The IV must be taped very securely so that it will not become dislodged with activity or during play.

## Key Concept

**U**se caution when advancing the catheter into the vein. Do not push the stylet, or needle portion, into the vein.

## Steps

1. Wash hands.
2. Assemble the equipment. Prime the IV tubing and fill the volume-limiting reservoir.
3. Identify the correct patient.
4. Explain the procedure to the patient. Use words that the child can understand.
5. Set up the equipment on the bedside table, within easy reach.
6. Place the towel or protective pad under the patient's arm.
7. Apply the tourniquet to the patient's arm.
8. Palpate the arm and select an IV site.
9. Remove the tourniquet.
10. Secure the arm to the arm board with tape, leaving the insertion site uncovered. Have an assistant hold the limb securely without cutting off circulation.
11. Put on gloves.
12. Clean the chosen IV site with an alcohol swab. Use a circular motion, starting at the insertion site and moving slowly outward. Clean for 1 minute. Allow to dry.
13. Reapply the tourniquet approximately 2 to 3 inches above the selected insertion site.
14. Stabilize the vein with the nondominant hand. Using sterile technique, hold the catheter by the hub. Insert the catheter at a 25- to 35-degree angle, with the bevel pointing up. Firmly pierce the skin.
15. Carefully advance the catheter and stylet into the vein. Observe for blood return.
16. Stabilize the stylet, and advance the catheter into the vein. Do not push the stylet, or needle portion, into the vein.
17. Place a sterile 2×2s beneath the hub of the catheter. Withdraw the stylet most of the way out of the catheter. Put slight pressure over the vein about 1 inch above the insertion site.
18. Remove the tourniquet.
19. Many needles now have a safety button that, when pushed, will retract the stylet into the handle. Remove the stylet and place it in the sharps container. Attach the IV tubing and release the pressure on the vein.
20. Open the IV fluid to run at a slow rate.
21. Observe the site for signs of infiltration: swelling, skin coolness, or blanching.
22. Dress the IV site using a transparent dressing over the insertion site and tape to secure the hub and IV tubing. The arm board may be removed or readjusted as necessary to secure the IV and prevent its accidental removal.
23. Label the dressing with the date, the catheter size, and your initials.
24. Remove and discard gloves; wash hands.
25. Set the IV rate as ordered by the physician.
26. Document and report the results of the procedure, as well as patient tolerance, to the RN or preceptor.

Note: IVs may also be inserted into scalp veins in infants with a physician's order. This procedure requires specialized training and preceptoring by a practitioner experienced in scalp vein IV placement.

# Recognizing Problems in IV Therapy

Complications of IV therapy can be either local or systemic. Local complications tend to be less serious or life-threatening in nature than do systemic ones. The key to managing local complications is frequent observation and assessment of the IV site, prevention by strict asepsis in starting and maintaining the IV, and teaching the patient to observe for early signs of problems.

## Infiltration

When the IV device, needle or catheter, comes out of the vein, IV fluids and medications can flow into the surrounding tissues. This is referred to as *infiltration*. When a particularly irritating drug—a vesicant—infiltrates, it is called *extravasation*.

The signs and symptoms of infiltration are coolness, blanching or paleness of the adjacent skin, swelling or tautness around the insertion site, discomfort, dependent edema, absence of a blood return, and slowing of the IV rate when infusing by gravity.

Techniques for prevention begin with appropriate site selection, selection of veins that avoid joints or can be readily stabilized, proper dressing techniques, and avoidance of high-pressure infusion pumps. Early recognition of infiltration requires frequent monitoring of the IV site and teaching the patient to report signs of infiltration immediately.

Treatment consists of stopping the infusion, discontinuing the IV, elevating the extremity, and using warm compresses to aid in the reabsorption of the fluid.

## Streaking or Phlebitis

Phlebitis or streaking is an inflammation of the interior surface of a vein. It is a common complication of IV therapy. There are two types of phlebitis: mechanical and chemical. Mechanical phlebitis is caused when the needle or catheter traumatizes the vein wall. This usually happens when the IV device is not adequately secured to the patient's skin. Chemical phlebitis results when irritating fluids or medications damage the endothelial cells of the vein wall.

The signs and symptoms of phlebitis are redness, warmness to the touch, local swelling, and palpable venous cord. The formation of phlebitis is affected by insertion techniques, vein condition, the type and pH of medications infused, the rate and dilution of infusates, and the fluids being infused.

Prevention techniques include using large veins for irritating medications, choosing the smallest IV needle or catheter appropriate for the therapy, rotating the site every 72 hours, stabilizing the IV device, infusing medications slowly and diluting irritating medications, using an in-line filter, and practicing a strict aseptic technique when starting and maintaining the IV.

Treatment of phlebitis consists of stopping the IV, removing the IV needle or catheter, and applying warm compresses for comfort. Subsequent IV starts should always be proximal to the previous site of phlebitis.

## Ecchymosis or Hematoma

The formation of an ecchymosis, a hematoma, or bruise, at the venipuncture site is usually related to caregiver technique. Bruising can be caused by nicking the vein during an unsuccessful venipuncture attempt, by failing to apply pressure over the venipuncture site after the blood draw, or after discontinuing an IV device.

Prevention includes proper device insertion and the application of pressure over the site after removal of the device.

The signs and symptoms of a hematoma are a darkening or discoloration under the skin at the venipuncture site, swelling at the site, tenderness, and discomfort.

Hematomas can be prevented with the appropriate use of pressure over an IV site after discontinuing the IV device, pressure after blood draws, and care to prevent pushing the needle through the vein during venipuncture.

If the patient develops a hematoma, stop the venipuncture attempt at once and put pressure over the developing hematoma. Have the patient elevate the extremity to maximize venous return. Careful observation of the venipuncture site when the vein is being pierced will allow the caregiver to discover a hematoma formation early and prevent the further extension of the hematoma. The discoloration will gradually fade, and the blood will be reabsorbed over a period of days to weeks.

## IV-Related Infection

Needle or catheter contamination is the most frequent cause of IV-related infection. This is a localized infection at the site of the IV insertion.

The signs and symptoms of IV-related infection include redness, swelling, exudate at the IV insertion site, increased temperature, and elevated white blood cell counts.

Local infections are preventable by maintaining strict aseptic technique during insertion, changing the IV site and tubing at Centers for Disease Control and Prevention (CDC)-recommended intervals, and careful maintenance of the IV site and dressing during therapy.

If localized infection is suspected, remove the dressing from the IV site. If the symptoms of infection exist, remove the IV device and culture the catheter tip and any purulent drainage from around the site. Notify the patient's physician at once and send the specimens to the lab for culture as ordered by the physician.

## Systemic Complications

The most common systemic complication of peripheral IV therapy is septicemia, which is an invasion of the blood by microorganisms.

The signs and symptoms of septicemia are chills, fever, and malaise. This is a life-threatening problem, and if suspected must be reported to the physician immediately. Prompt treatment greatly increases the patient's chance for recovery.

Prevention includes good hand washing and strict aseptic technique during line insertion and maintenance. Filtration of infusate (with a 0.2-micron bacterial-retentive filter) also helps prevent septicemia.

Treatment depends on the results of the culture and must be ordered by the physician on a case-specific basis.

## Tissue Sloughing

Tissue sloughing is a serious complication of IV therapy. When sloughing occurs, necrotic tissue forms or separates from viable or healthy tissue.

The signs and symptoms include tissue necrosis.

Prevention includes appropriate selection of the site and device, proper stabilization of the device, and frequent checks for signs of infiltration. This is particularly important when irritating solutions or drugs, such as those used to treat cancer (chemotherapy agents), are being administered.

# CHAPTER 6

# ECG MONITORING, ARRHYTHMIA RECOGNITION, AND ADVANCED CARDIAC CARE SKILLS

## INTRODUCTION

More and more, nurses and nursing support staff are being asked to perform skills for a growing population of patients with cardiovascular disease. Advanced cardiac skills are becoming necessary tools for caregivers in a variety of settings, from the acute care hospital to the home care environment.

This chapter includes information on the basic anatomy and physiology of the heart as well as preparing caregivers to perform necessary skills:

*ECG Monitoring and Arrhythmia Recognition*

- Basic Anatomy and Physiology of the Heart
- The Electrocardiogram
- Components of the ECG
- Setting Up Continuous Three- or Five-Lead Cardiac Monitoring and Telemetry
- Recognizing ECG Rhythms That Require RN Notification or Intervention

*Additional Advanced Cardiac Care Skills*

- Caring for the Patient with an Arterial Line
- Changing an Arterial Line Dressing
- Withdrawing Blood from an Arterial Line
- Removing an Arterial Line
- Palpating Dorsalis Pedis and Posterior Tibial Pulses
- Removing a PTCA Femoral Sheath
- Performing a Postcardiac Catheterization Check

Section One

# ECG Monitoring and Arrhythmia Recognition

## Basic Anatomy and Physiology of the Heart

The heart is a pump that propels oxygen-rich blood to all parts of the body. The human heart has been masterfully designed to respond quickly and efficiently to our physical needs.

This section prepares caregivers to do the following:

1. Describe the basic anatomy and physiology of the heart.
2. Acquire a basic understanding of the conduction system.
3. Relate waveforms on an electrocardiogram to heart action.

### Key Terms

**Arrhythmia** A variation from the normal sinus rhythm.

**Atrial** Pertaining to an atrium.

**Atrium** One of two upper chambers of the heart. (Plural is *atria.*)

**Atrioventricular (AV) Node** An area of cardiac muscle fibers lying on the posterior floor of the right atrium that conducts impulses from the atria to the bundle of His. It can also act as a pacemaker of the heart.

**Conduction System** The cardiac muscle fibers that normally conduct impulses rapidly through the heart to cause depolarization and then contraction to occur. They include the Sinoatrial (SA) node, the AV node, the bundle of His, the right and left bundle branches, and the Purkinje fibers.

**Depolarization** The spread of an impulse through a chamber of the heart (atrium or ventricle). causes contraction of the heart

**Intercostal Space** Space between two ribs.

**Lead** A wire attached to an electrode on the patient's skin that connects in the electrocardiogram (ECG) machine, the bedside monitor, or the telemetry device and transmits electrical information to the monitor or recorder.

**Myocardial Infarction** A condition in which an area of the heart is deprived of oxygen and the cells die.

**Myocardium** The middle layer of heart muscle.

**Pacemaker (pacer)** The site in the heart that initiates the impulses that are spread throughout the cardiac tissue and cause contraction to occur. Normally, the pacemaker of the heart is the SA node, which is located in the right atrium.

**Pacemaker Cells** A specialized group of cells able to initiate impulses that set the rate of the heartbeat and spread to other areas of the heart.

**Precordial** Pertaining to an area of the chest over the heart and over the lower portion of the sternum.

**Repolarization** The recovery period of a chamber of the heart after it has contracted.

**Ventricles** One of two lower chambers of the heart.

**Ventricular** Pertaining to a ventricle.

The heart functions to pump blood to the lungs and to the rest of the body. It supplies oxygen- and nutrient-rich blood throughout the body through the circulatory system. The heart consists of four chambers. The two upper chambers are the right and left atria. The two lower chambers are the right and left ventricles. The right atrium receives blood from the superior vena cava and the inferior vena cava. It contracts to supply the right ventricle with blood, which passes through the tricuspid valve. The right ventricle contracts to move unoxygenated blood along through the pulmonic valve and the pulmonary arteries to the lungs, where the blood receives oxygen. The oxygenated blood then travels back through the pulmonic veins to the left atrium and through the mitral valve to the left ventricle. The left ventricle is responsible for pumping the blood through the aortic valve and aorta to the rest of the body. During ventricular relaxation, blood is supplied to the coronary arteries, which supply oxygenated blood and nutrients to the heart muscle itself (Figure 6.1).

· Pericardium outside layer double layer sac of the heart
· Myocardium thickest, actual muscular portion of the heart
· Endocardium innermost section, protective covering of myocardium

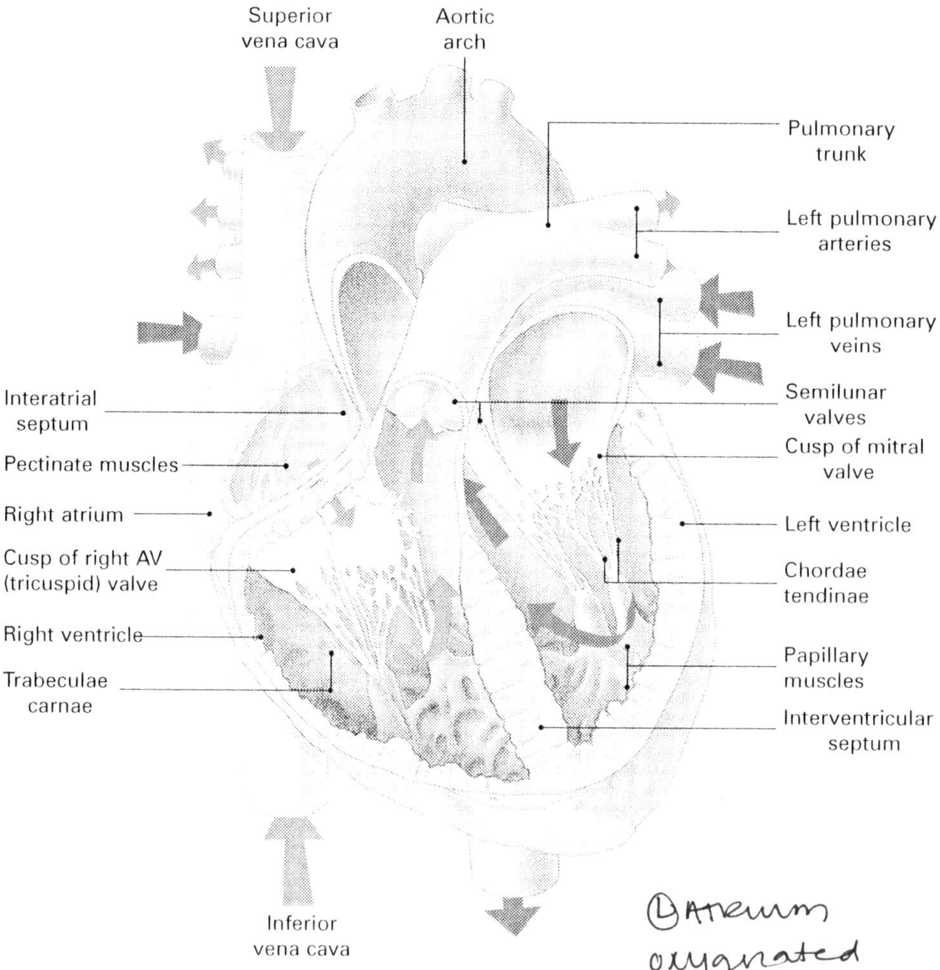


**Figure 6.1** Blood flow through the heart.

(R) Atrium receiving chambers of the heart (R) - deoxygenated blood from superior vena cava from the body

(L) Atrium oxygenated blood from lungs from pulmonary vein

Pulmonary artery is the only artery to carry deoxygenated blood

The coronary circulation consists of two main branches: the left and right coronary arteries. The left main coronary artery divides into the left anterior descending artery (LAD) and the left circumflex artery (LCA) with many additional smaller branches. The LAD supplies blood to the anterior wall of the left ventricle, to most of the intraventricular septum, and to the bundle branches of the electrical system. The circumflex artery supplies blood to the left atrium, to a portion of the lateral wall of the left ventricle, to the posterior wall of the left ventricle in some people, and, in a small percentage of people, to the SA and the AV nodes. The right coronary artery (RCA) supplies blood to the right atrium, the right ventricle, and, in the majority of hearts, to the SA and AV nodes (Figure 6.2).

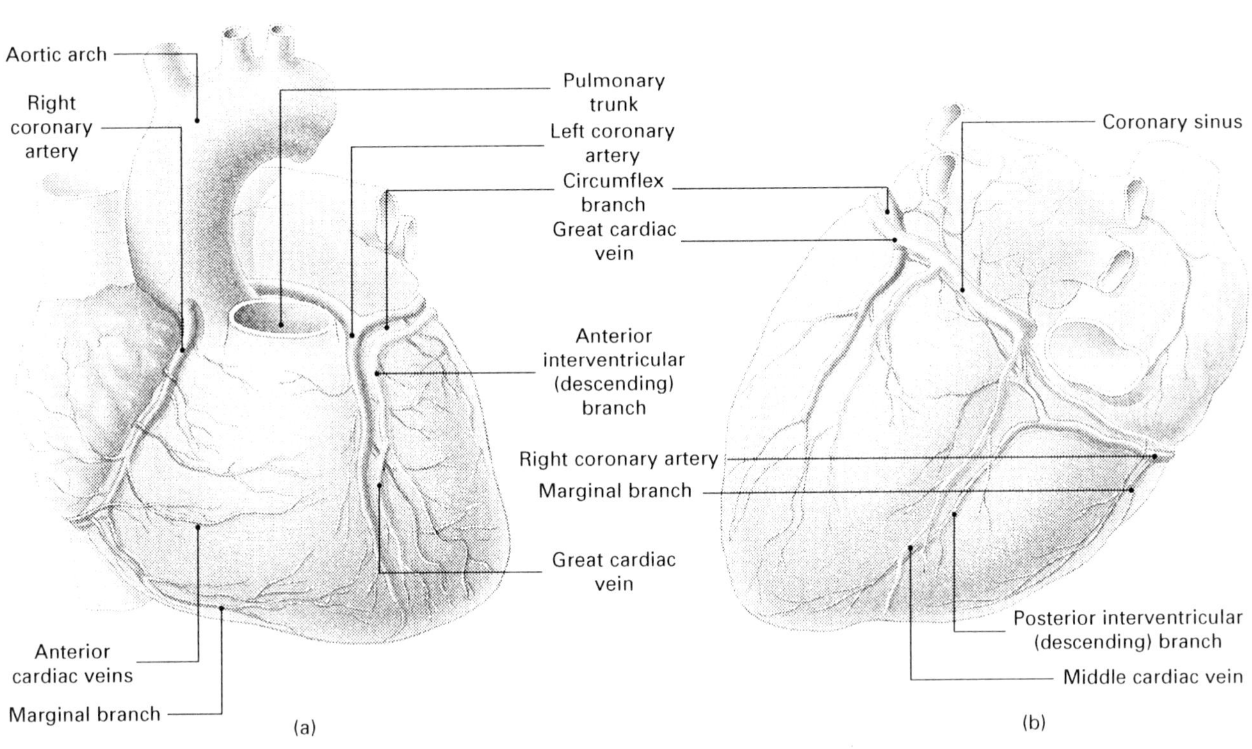


**Figure 6.2** The coronary circulation; (a) anterior; (b) posterior.

SA node has a range of 60-100
AV node will delay impulses to allow (R) atrium to empty.

Pulmonic ejects blood into pulmona art.

Aorta pumps blood into aorta

Vena cava → (R) atrium → tricuspid valve → (R) ventricle → pulmonary artery → lungs → pulmonary veins → (L) atrium → bicuspid valve → (L) ventricle → aorta (systemic)

LV → systemic

## The Conductive System

In a normally functioning heart, the SA node acts as the pacemaker of the heart, initiating electrical impulses and spreading the impulse down through the rest of the conduction system, causing depolarization of the muscle cells and, ultimately, contraction of the atria and ventricles. The electrical impulse travels from the SA node through the internodal pathways to the AV node. The AV node delays the impulses from the atria for a short time, allowing for atrial emptying. The impulse then travels through the bundle of His to the right and left bundle branches and, finally, to the Purkinje fibers, which spread throughout the ventricles (Figure 6.3).

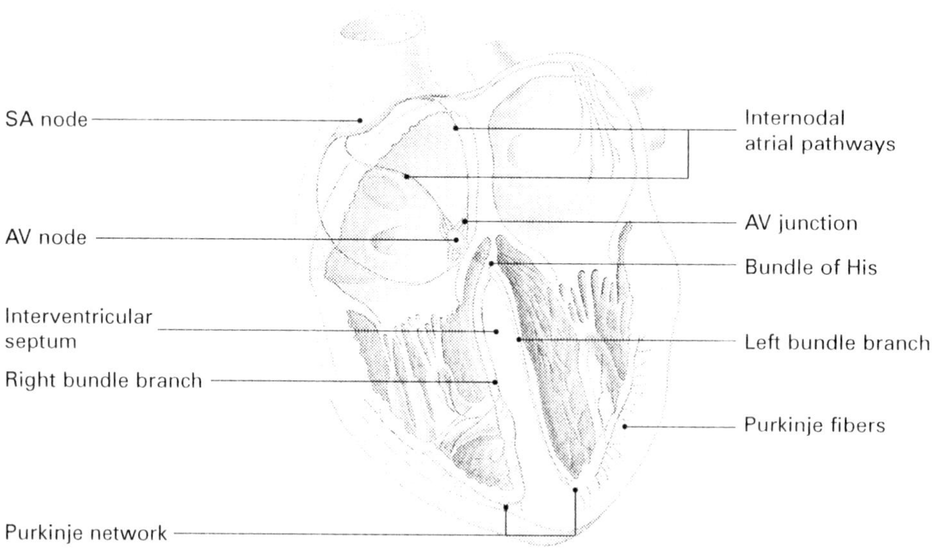


**Figure 6.3** The cardiac conductive system.

## The Electrocardiogram

The terms *ECG* and *EKG* both refer to an electrocardiogram. EKG comes from the German spelling (*elektrokardiogram*); and ECG reflects the English spelling (*electrocardiogram*). Throughout this text, we use the term ECG.

The first ECG was reported by Willem Einthoven in the early 1900s. He placed leads on the arms and legs of his subject and measured the electrical activity of the heart with a galvanometer.

ECG monitoring may be done in twelve different leads. Leads I, II, and III are known as bipolar limb leads. Bipolar means that two electrodes, a negative and a positive attached to two extremities, are used to permit a view of the electrical activity from a frontal plane (Figure 6.4). To eliminate electrical interference, a third lead, or ground lead, is commonly used. The three leads, aVR, aVL, and aVF, are unipolar leads. They look at the heart in a horizontal plane. A unipolar lead is made by attaching a positive electrode on the skin and connecting it with a zero reference point that is made by the machine as it internally connects the extremity electrodes. The

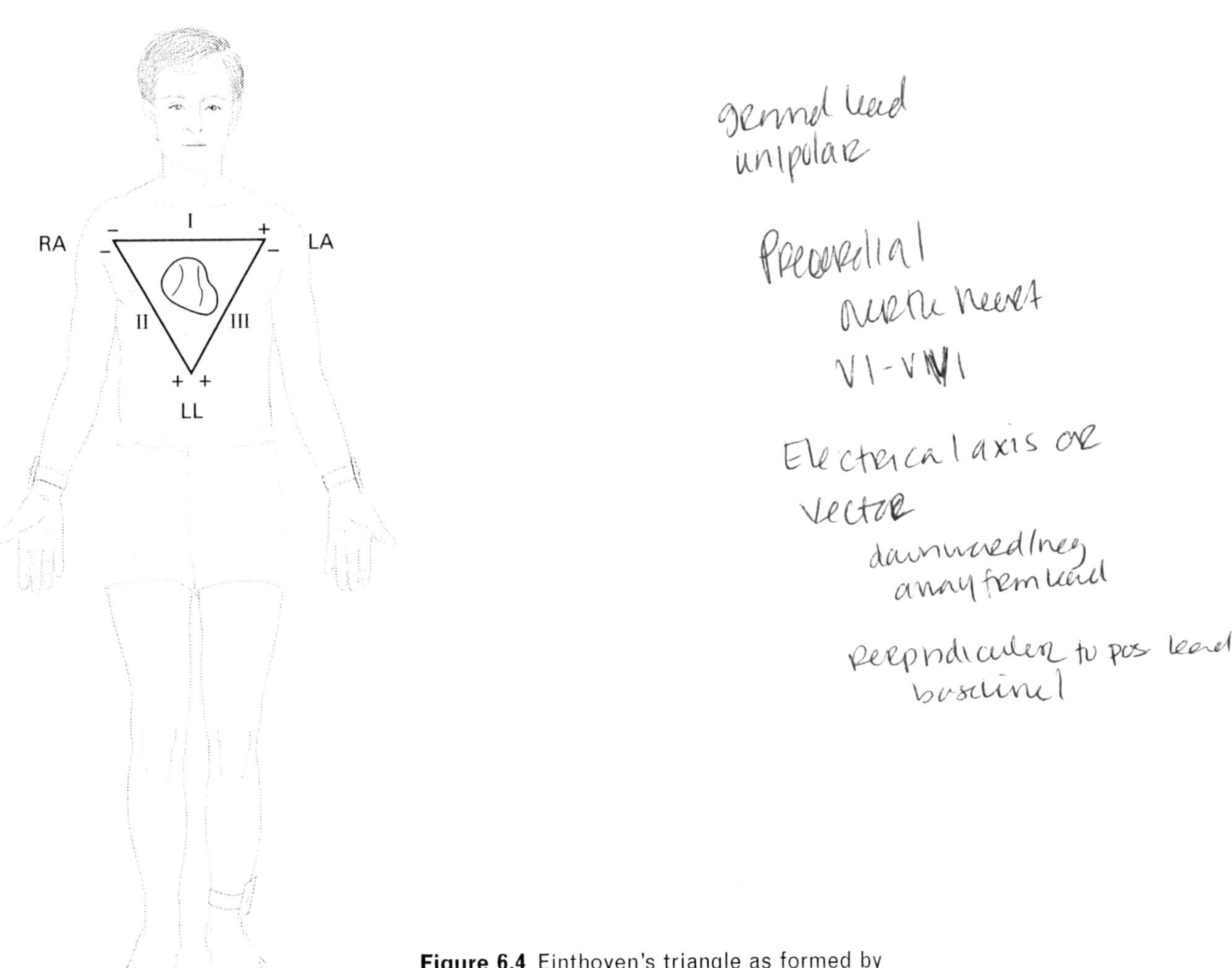


**Figure 6.4** Einthoven's triangle as formed by Leads I, II, and III.

augmented leads are made by attaching a positive electrode to one of the three extremity leads (the left arm, the right arm, or the left leg). The chest leads ($V_1$–$V_6$) are also unipolar leads. They are known as the precordial leads. Electrodes are placed across the chest in each of the six specified precordial locations.

## Electrical Axis or Vector

All of the electrical forces in the heart can be combined into a single vector, or force, that has both magnitude and direction. This vector is usually represented by an arrow. The main vector in a normal heart is downward to the left foot because this is the direction of the normal electrical pathway. If the wave of electrical activity flows toward a positive lead, the pattern will be upright, or positive. If the wave of electrical activity flows away from the positive lead, the pattern will be negative, or inverted. If the wave of electricity flows perpendicular to the positive electrode, the pattern will be isoelectric (Figure 6.5).

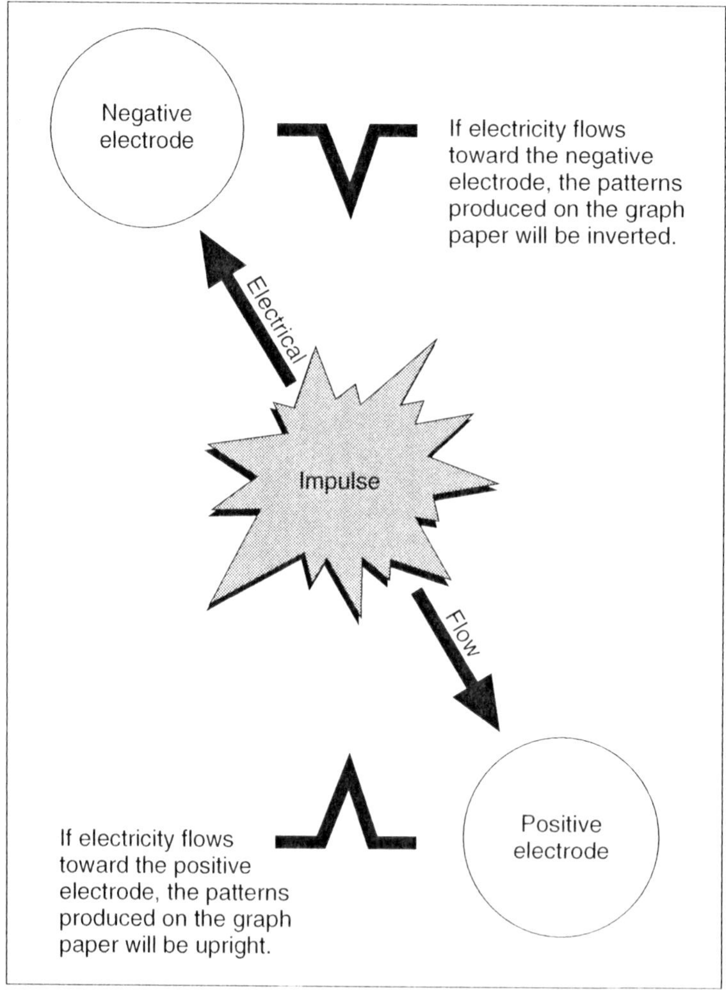


**Figure 6.5** Wave of depolarization.

## Components of the ECG

An ECG consists of several components. The P wave is small, rounded, and upright. It represents atrial contraction. It is normally the first movement away from the isoelectric line, or baseline, of the ECG. The Q wave is the first negative deflection following a P wave. The R wave is the first positive deflection in the QRS complex following a P wave. The S wave is the first negative complex following the R wave. The S wave normally returns to the isoelectric line before the next wave is seen. The T wave is the next rounded upright wave, and it represents ventricular repolarization (relaxation). The QRS complex is a combination of the Q, R, and S waves. All three waves do not always need to be present for it to be called a QRS complex. The QRS complex represents ventricular depolarization (contraction). The QRS interval is normally 0.06 to 0.11 seconds. The ST segment begins at the end of the QRS and ends at the beginning of the T wave. The PR interval shown in Figure 6.6 represents the time from atrial contraction to the onset of ventricular contraction. The PR interval is measured from the beginning of the P wave to the beginning of the QRS complex. The normal duration of this interval is 0.12 to 0.20 seconds.

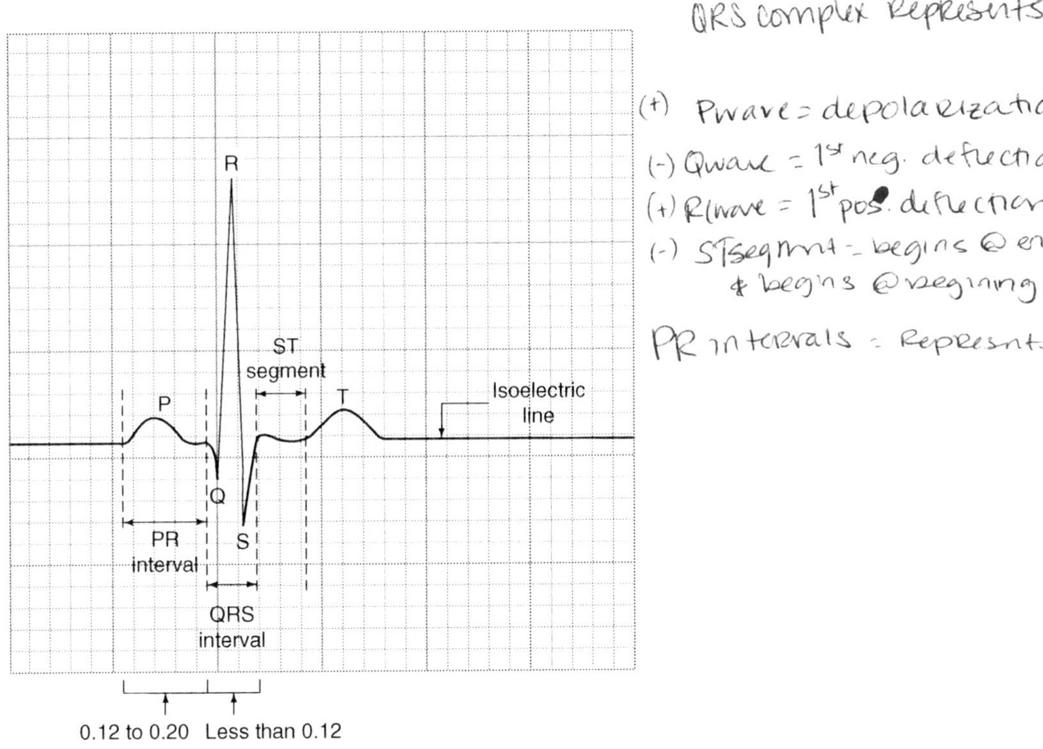


**Figure 6.6** The ECG.

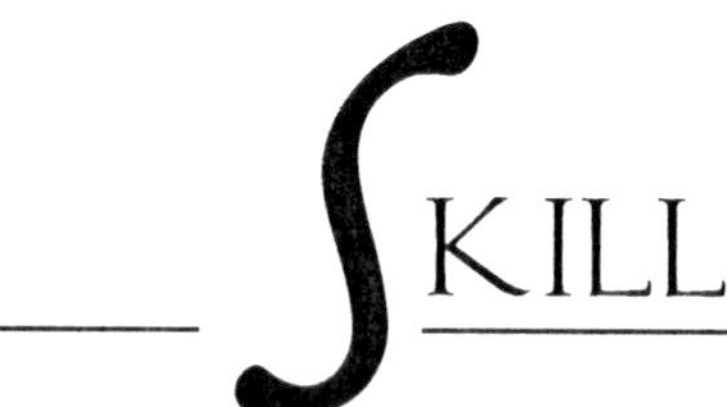

# SKILL

## Setting Up Continuous Three- or Five-Lead Cardiac Monitoring and Telemetry

***Purpose*** Continuous cardiac monitoring and telemetry are useful diagnostic tools for patients who have had cardiac abnormalities or might be at risk for them. Continuous cardiac monitoring can be performed with a three- or a five-lead setup. The patient is connected to a hardwire monitor with a display at a central monitoring station. Telemetry units, on the other hand, are portable. Their lead wires are connected to a unit that the patient wears in a pocket or a pouch. They offer the advantage of allowing the patient to ambulate without wires connected to a hardwire unit.

### Objectives

**The caregiver demonstrates the ability to do the following:**

1. Gather the correct supplies.
2. Communicate using a style that reduces the patient's anxiety.
3. Set up five-lead hardwire monitoring.
4. Set up three- or five-lead telemetry monitoring.
5. Determine heart rate and regularity.
6. Describe the process of obtaining an ECG.
7. Report the results of the procedure to the RN or preceptor.

### Key Terms

**Augmented** Made larger; increased.

**Bigeminy** The state of having an ectopic beat that occurs every other beat.

**Caliper** A tool used to assist in measuring heart rate and rhythm on an ECG strip.

**Couplets** Two abnormal beats that occur in a row.

**Ectopic** Situated somewhere other than in the normal place.

**Ectopy** Abnormal beats.

**Electrode Gel** A gelatinous substance that is used with the ECG electrodes to transmit a good-quality signal to the ECG monitor.

**Hardwire Monitoring** A monitoring system by which the patient is physically connected to a monitoring device that displays the ECG rhythm at the bedside.

**Isoelectric Line** The flat area of an ECG where no electrical impulse is detected. Also called baseline.

**Multifocal** Pertaining to two or more ectopic beats that look different from one another.

**Premature Beat** A cardiac contraction that occurs before the next normal beat is expected.

**Rhythm Strip** A long (6- to 12-second) ECG recording of one or more leads during cardiac monitoring.

**Stylus** The needle-like instrument that writes the heart rhythm onto ECG paper.

**Telemetry** A system in which the patient is attached to ECG leads and a portable transmitter that sends radio signals to a central monitor where the patient's ECG can be viewed.

**Unifocal** Pertaining to two or more ectopic beats that look alike.

**Supplies/Equipment**

Soap and water • Clippers or scissors to remove hair (if needed) • Pregelled electrodes • Five-lead hardwire monitoring system or three- or five-lead telemetry monitoring system • Carrying pouch or holder for telemetry monitoring unit

**Pertinent Points**

## Monitoring Methods

Hardwire monitoring usually uses a five-lead system. One end of the leads attaches to a monitor in the patient's room. Lead wires then connect to adhesive electrodes placed on the skin. Five-lead systems offer selection options so that the observer is able to monitor in more than one lead without changing the electrode setup on the chest. Typically, the white lead is on the right arm, the black lead is on the left arm, the green lead (which represents the right foot) is on the right lower abdomen just above the iliac crest, the red lead (representing the left foot) is on the left lower abdomen just above the iliac crest, and the brown lead is in the fourth intercostal space to the right of the sternum (the $V_1$ position).

A telemetry system uses a portable receiver that transmits ECG data to a central monitoring station. With this system, the patient is able to move about without being confined by wires attached to a monitor in the room. The chest leads connect to a small box that is usually carried in a pouch that the patient wears around the neck or waist.

Five-lead telemetry systems (Figure 6.7) can monitor patients simultaneously in two leads, depending on the monitoring system used (Figure 6.8). Most computers are designed to decide which leads to use for whichever lead you choose. Lead $MCL_1$, the modified chest lead, is a bipolar lead that simulates lead $V_1$ of the twelve-lead ECG. This lead can be helpful in differentiating supraventricular tachycardia

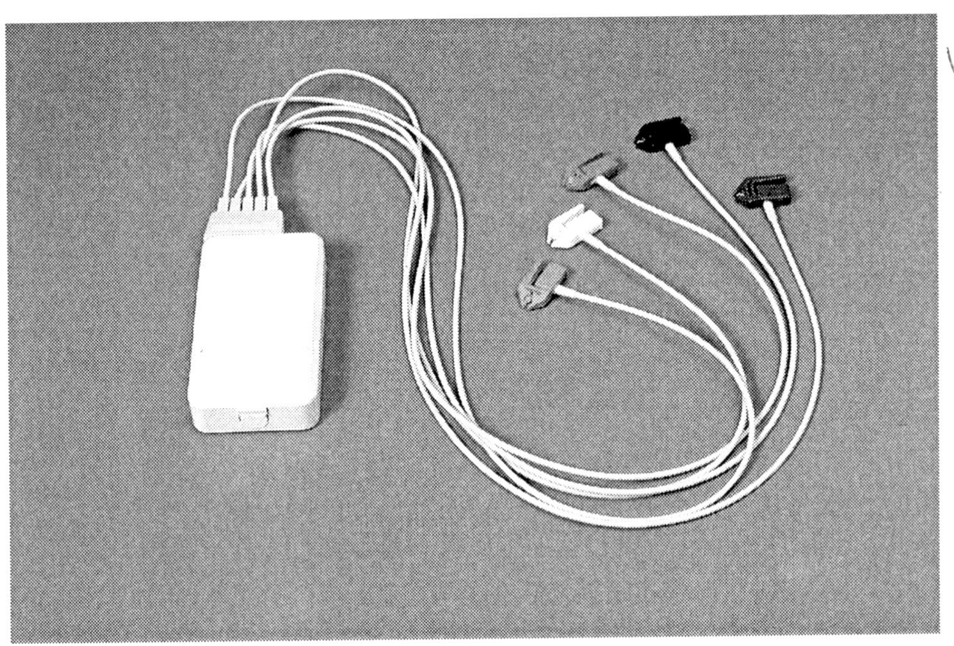

vII is most looked at.

**Figure 6.7** Telemetry and leads.

green = (R) leg "clouds over grass"
white = (R) arm "smoke over fire"
(Red) = left leg vI - v VI
Brown - 4th int. cost space (R) of sternum vIV
Black = (L) arm

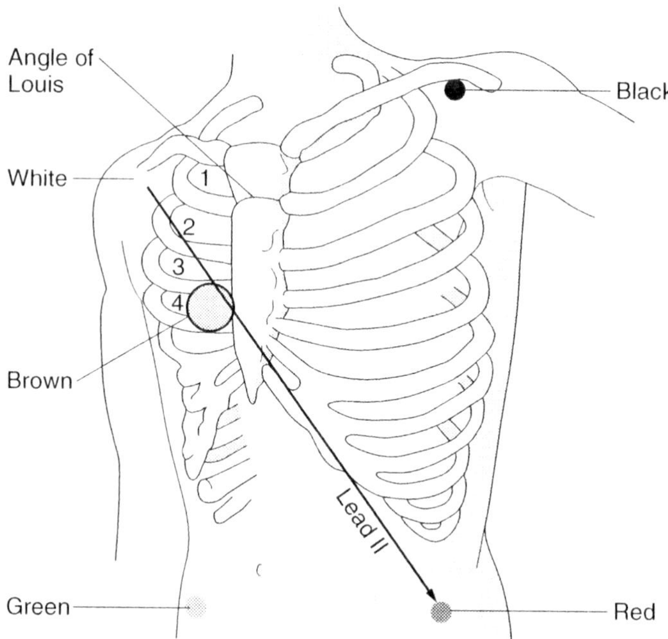


**Figure 6.8** Telemetry setup using a five-lead cable (Lead II).

(SVT) from ventricular tachycardia (VT). To monitor using $MCL_1$, the brown lead should be in the $V_1$ position (the fourth intercostal space, to the right of the sternum). $MCL_6$ simulates $V_6$ of the twelve-lead ECG. To monitor in $MCL_6$, the brown lead should be in the $V_6$ position (the fifth intercostal space, at the midaxillary line).

Three-lead telemetry systems consist of a positive lead and a negative lead, with an additional neutral, or ground, lead. Lead I has a negative lead on the right arm and a positive lead on the left arm (Figure 6.9). Lead II has a negative lead on the right arm and a positive pole at the left lower abdomen (Figure 6.10). $MCL_1$ has a negative lead on the left arm, with the positive lead at the fourth intercostal space to the right of the sternum (Figure 6.11).

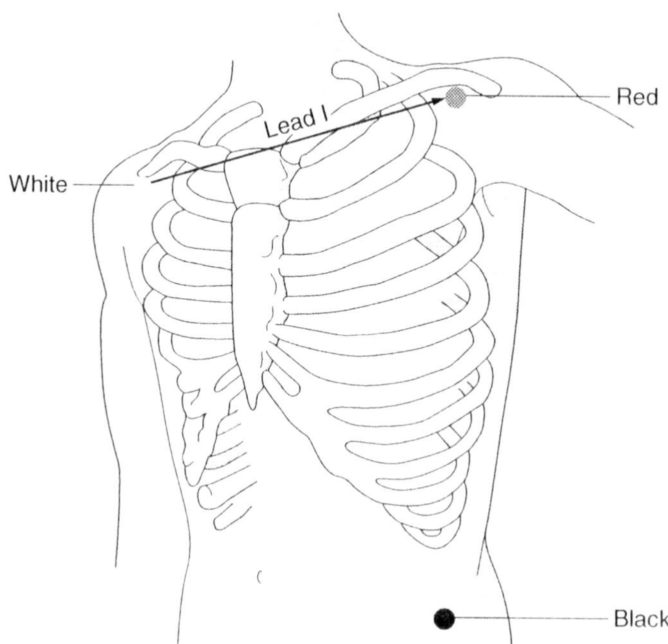


**Figure 6.9** Three-lead telemetry (Lead I).

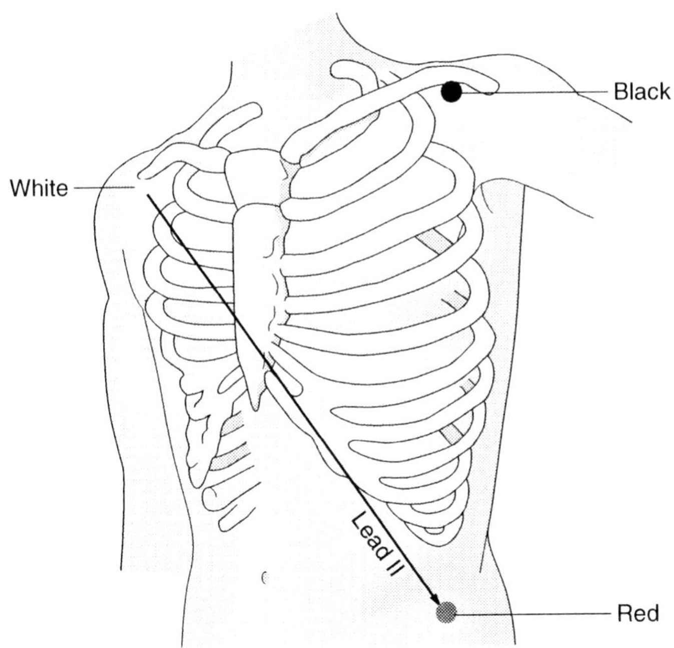


**Figure 6.10** Three-lead telemetry (Lead II).

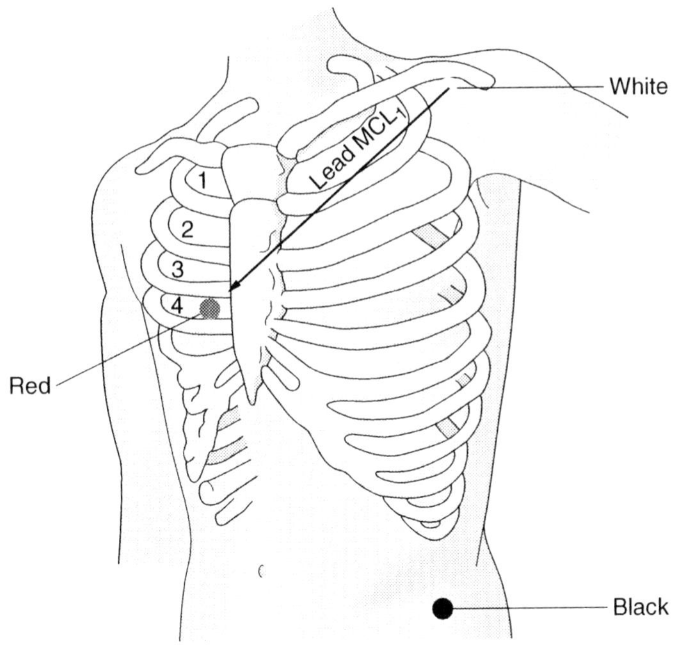


**Figure 6.11** Three-lead telemetry ($MCL_1$).

## The ECG Graph Paper

The paper that records ECG electrical activity is a grid. It records the time in seconds along the horizontal lines, and the voltage (the size of the activity) in millimeters (mm) along the vertical lines. The smallest size box represents 0.04 seconds. There are 1,500 small boxes in a minute (Figure 6.12).

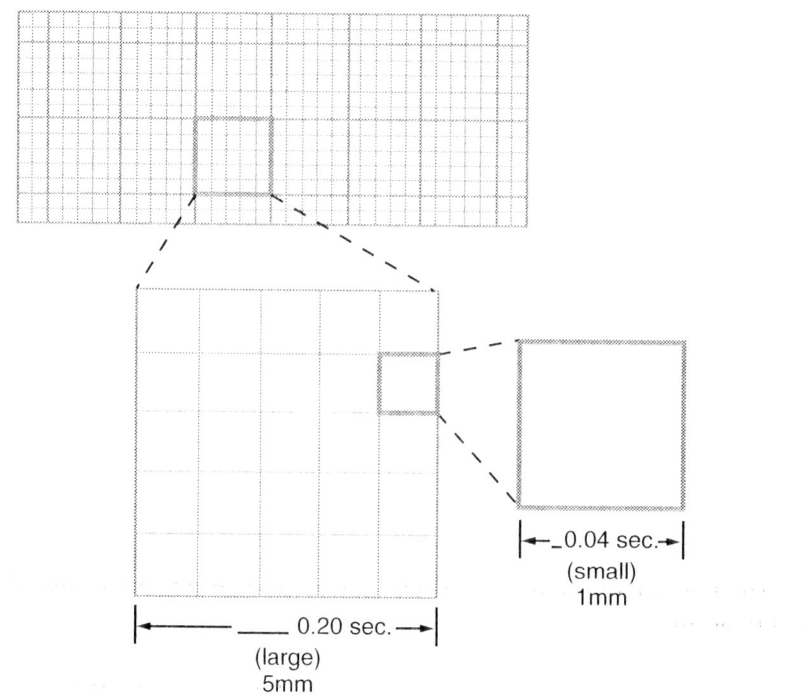


**Figure 6.12** ECG graph paper measures electrical activity of the heart and the time it takes to complete each part of that activity.

## Determining Heart Rate and Regularity

Heart rate can be calculated by different methods. The 6-second interval method is the easiest way to calculate heart rate. It can be used if the heart rate is regular or irregular. There are usually short marks in 3-second intervals at the top of the ECG graph paper (Figure 6.13). The heart rate is calculated by counting the number of R waves in a 6-second interval and multiplying this number by 10. For example, in Figure 6.13, there are six QRS complexes in the 6-second interval.

$$6 \times 10 = 60 \quad \text{beats per minute}$$

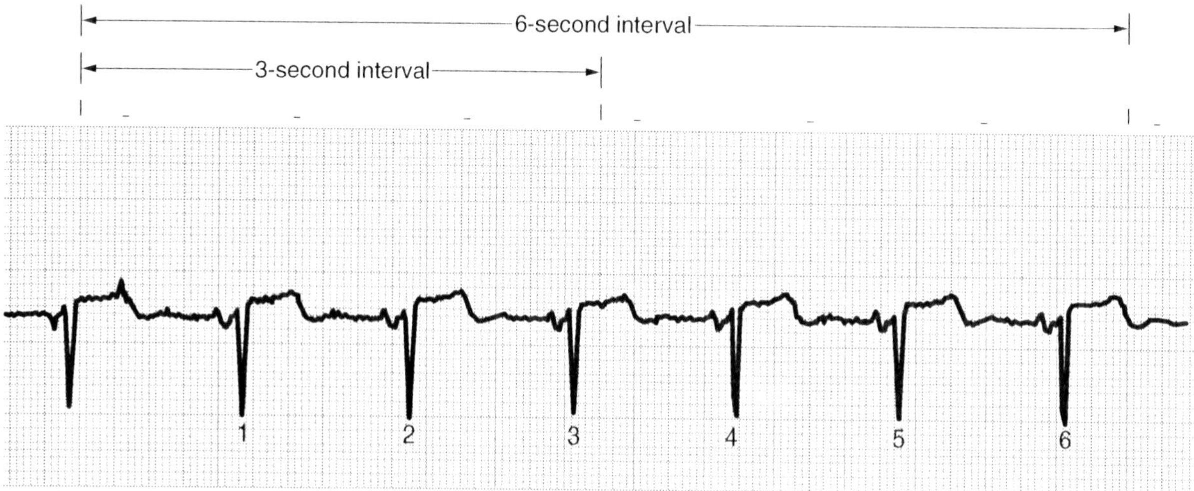


**Figure 6.13** Three- and 6-second intervals.

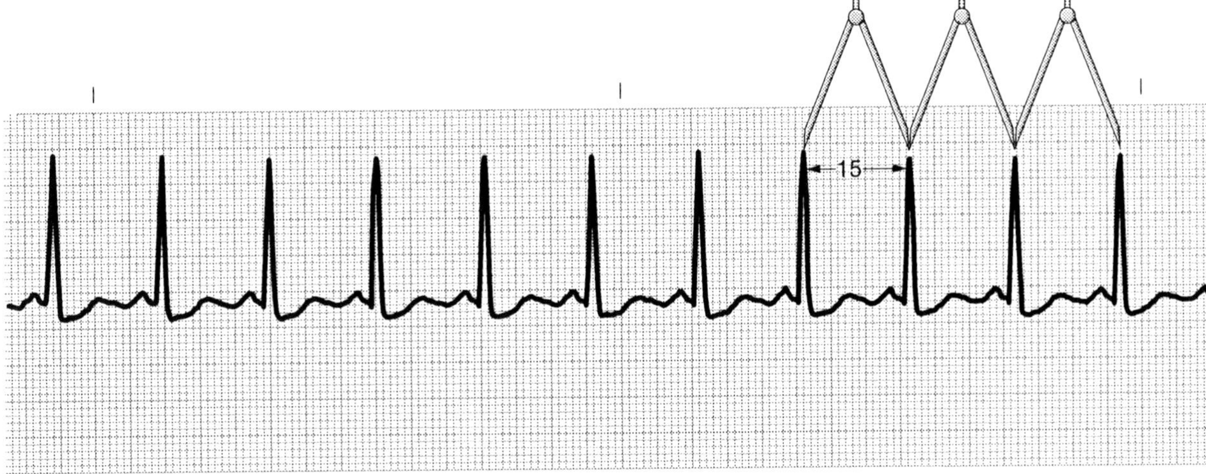


**Figure 6.14** Heart rate = 1,500 ÷ (no. of small squares from R to R).

ONLY

The R-to-R interval method (Figure 6.14) can be used with regular rhythms and is very accurate. With this method, use calipers to measure the number of boxes between two consecutive R waves. For example, in Figure 6.14, there are fifteen small boxes between the R waves. Remember, there are 1,500 boxes in a minute.

$$\text{Heart rate} = \frac{1{,}500}{\text{No. of small boxes from R to R}}$$

$$\frac{1{,}500}{15} = 100 \text{ beats per minute}$$

| #R–R | HR |
|---|---|
| 20 | 75 |
| 40 | 38 |
| 15 | 100 |

Atrial rate can be determined by measuring the distance between consecutive waves using the same method.

Calipers can also be used to determine the regularity of the rhythm. The tips of the calipers are placed on the peaks of the R waves. Without moving the distance between the peaks of the calipers, the R-to-R intervals are compared across the ECG paper.

### Age-Specific Considerations

Pediatric and infant electrodes are available for children. Older adults, infants, and those patients with very sensitive skin might benefit from hyperallergenic electrodes. Check the skin of these patients for a rash or signs of irritation. Adult female patients who have very large breasts may need to have their left breast lifted to place the $V_4$ or $V_5$ electrode in the correct position.

### Key Concept

The following might help you remember where the color leads are placed:

White = white is right (right chest below clavicle)
Black = opposite of right (left chest below clavicle)
Green = go! (accelerator pedal for driving a car—right upper iliac crest)
Red = stop! (brake on a car—left upper iliac crest)
Brown = fourth intercostal space to the right of the sternum

## Steps for Setting Up Five-Lead Hardwire Monitoring

1. Wash hands.
2. Identify the correct patient.
3. Explain the procedure to the patient.
4. Assemble the equipment.
5. Prepare the patient's skin:
   a. Wash with soap and water; rinse and allow to dry. (Repeat with electrode change every 24 hours.)
   b. Clip excess hair if necessary.
6. Apply electrodes (use electrodes of the same brand and age):
   a. Check that the electrodes have fresh, moist gel.
   b. Attach the lead clip to the electrode.
   c. Apply the five electrodes, placing the lower electrodes just above the iliac crest bilaterally. Use the lead selector for the preferred lead.
7. Check for the characteristics of a good ECG signal:
   a. Stable baseline.
   b. QRS tall, narrow, and monophasic.
   c. T wave less than one-third the height of the R wave.
   d. P wave smaller than the T wave.
8. Obtain a rhythm strip:
   a. Observe for a good ECG signal.
   b. Locate and activate the record button on the monitor.
9. Document and report the results to the RN or preceptor.

## Steps for Setting Up Three- or Five-Lead Telemetry Monitoring

1. Wash hands.
2. Identify the correct patient.
3. Explain the procedure to the patient.
4. Assemble the equipment.
5. Prepare the patient's skin:
   a. Wash with soap and water; rinse and allow to dry. (Repeat with electrode change every 24 hours.)
   b. Clip excess hair if necessary.
6. Apply electrodes (use electrodes of the same brand and age):
   a. Check that the electrodes have fresh, moist gel.
   b. Attach the lead clip to the electrode.
   c. Apply the five electrodes for Lead II and $MCL_1$, placing the lower electrodes just above the iliac crest bilaterally.
7. Operate the transmitter safely:
   a. Check the battery (zinc lasts 6 days versus 3 days for alkaline).
   b. Use a regular 9-volt alkaline battery when the patient showers.
   c. Demonstrate the disconnect/connect function.
   d. Instruct patient about how to use the nurse call button. (The button can run a strip from the room. The caregiver may teach the patient to use it in specific cases only; please use discretion!)
   e. Secure the transmitter safely in the patient's carrying pouch or holder.
8. Check for the characteristics of a good ECG signal:
   a. Stable baseline.
   b. QRS tall, narrow, and monophasic.
   c. T wave less than one-third the height of the R wave.
   d. P wave smaller than the T wave.
9. Obtain a rhythm strip:
   a. Observe for a good ECG signal.
   b. Locate and activate the record button on the monitor.
10. Document and report the results to the RN or preceptor.

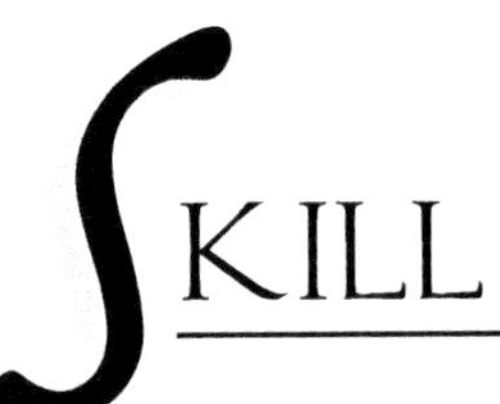

# SKILL

## Recognizing ECG Rhythms That Require RN Notification or Intervention

***Purpose*** Early recognition and reporting of life-threatening arrhythmias are necessary for timely treatment by the health care team. It is important to identify a characteristic normal heart rhythm in order to differentiate it from abnormal rhythms (Table 6.1).

### Objectives

**The caregiver demonstrates the ability to do the following:**

1. Recognize the components of normal sinus rhythm.
2. Recognize various arrhythmias.
3. Identify life-threatening arrhythmias.

### Pertinent Points

- In *normal sinus rhythm,* the impulse is generated from the sinus node, which acts as the pacemaker of the heart. The heart rate is between 60 and 100 beats per minute, and the rhythm is regular. All intervals and waveforms are normal (Figure 6.15).

| | |
|---|---|
| Rate: | 60–100 beats per minute |
| Rhythm: | Regular |
| P wave: | Round, upright |
| PR interval: | 0.12–0.20 seconds |
| QRS interval: | 0.06–0.11 seconds |

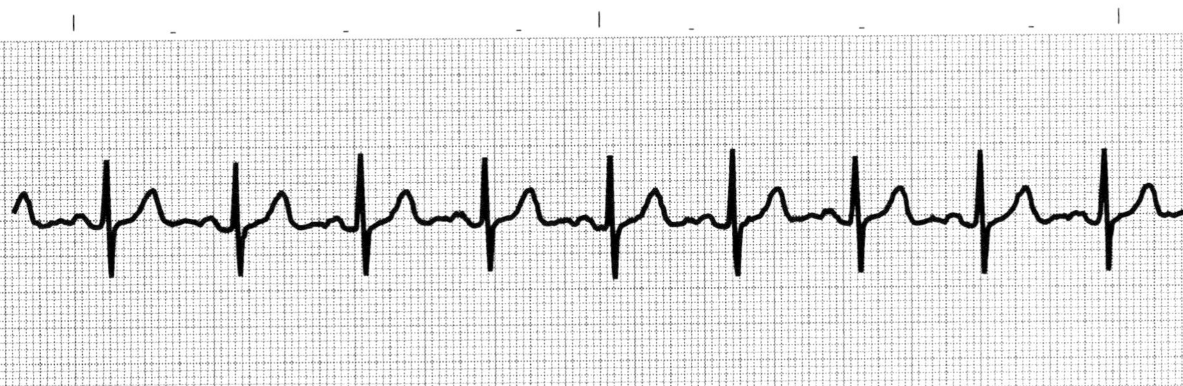

**Figure 6.15** Normal sinus rhythm.

## Table 6.1 ECG Rhythm Comparison Chart

| Rhythm | Atrial Rate (Beats Per Min) | Atrial Rhythm | Ventricular Rate (Beats Per Min) | Ventricular Rhythm | P Waves | PR Interval (Sec) | QRS Interval (Sec) |
|---|---|---|---|---|---|---|---|
| Normal sinus rhythm (SR) | 60–100 | Regular | 60–100 | Regular | Present; round, upright | 0.12–0.20 | 0.06–0.11 |
| Sinus bradycardia (SB) | Less than 60 | Regular | Less than 60 | Regular | Normal | Normal | Normal |
| Sinus tachycardia (ST) | Greater than 100 | Regular | Greater than 100 | Regular | Normal | Normal | Normal |
| Sinus arrhythmia | 60–100 | Irregular | 60–100 | Irregular | Normal | Normal | Normal |
| Sinus arrest | Normal to slow | Irregular with pauses | Normal to slow | Irregular with pauses | Absent during pause | Normal with conducted beat; absent with pause | Normal |
| Wandering atrial pacemaker | Normal to slow | Irregular | Normal to slow | Irregular | Vary in size and shape; might be absent | Varies | Normal |
| Premature atrial contraction (PAC) | Depends on underlying rhythm | Irregular due to PAC | Depends on underlying rhythm | Irregular due to PAC | Differs from that of sinus beat | Normal but differs from sinus interval | Normal |
| Atrial fibrillation | Varies; F waves very rapid, up to 360 per min | Irregularly irregular | Varies | Irregular | Absent; F (fibrillation) waves | None | Usually normal |
| Atrial flutter | 250–400 | Regular | 60–150 | Usually regular | Absent; F (flutter) waves | None | Normal |
| Premature junctional contraction (PJC) | Depends on underlying rhythm | Irregular due to premature beat | Depends on underlying rhythm | Irregular due to premature beat | Might be absent, inverted, before or after QRS | Less than 0.12 | Normal |
| Junctional rhythm | If seen, atrial rate is equal to ventricular rate | Regular, if seen | 40–60 | Regular | Might be absent, inverted, before or after QRS | Less than 0.12 | Normal |
| Paroxysmal supraventricular tachycardia (PSVT) | 150–250 | Regular; might not be able to determine atrial activity | 150–250 | Regular | Might be concealed in previous T wave | Might be impossible to measure | Normal |
| First-degree AV block | Depends on underlying rhythm | Depends on underlying rhythm | Depends on underlying rhythm | Depends on underlying rhythm | Normal | Greater than 0.20 | Normal |
| Second-degree block—Mobitz I (Wenckebach) | Usually normal | Regular | Slower than atrial | Irregular | Normal shape | Progressive lengthening until QRS is dropped | Normal |

| Rhythm | Atrial Rate (Beats Per Min) | Atrial Rhythm | Ventricular Rate (Beats Per Min) | Ventricular Rhythm | P Waves | PR Interval (Sec) | QRS Interval (Sec) |
|---|---|---|---|---|---|---|---|
| Second-degree block—Mobitz II | Normal | Regular | Slower than atrial | Irregular | Normal | Consistent for conducted beats | Greater than 0.12 |
| Third-degree block | Usually normal | Regular; no relationship to ventricular rhythm | Slower than atrial | Regular; no relationship to atrial rhythm | Normal | No relationship to QRS | Greater than 0.12 |
| Premature ventricular contraction (PVC) | Depends on underlying rhythm | Irregular due to premature beat | Depends on underlying rhythm | Irregular due to premature beat | Absent | Absent | Greater than 0.12; wide and bizarre |
| Ventricular tachycardia (V Tach) | None | None | 150–250 | Regular | Absent | Absent | Greater than 0.12 |
| Ventricular fibrillation (V Fib) | Cannot be determined | None | Cannot be determined | Chaotic | Absent | Absent | Cannot be determined |
| Asystole | None | None | None | None | Absent | Absent | Absent |
| Idioventricular rhythm | None | None | 20–45 | Might be irregular | Absent | Absent | Greater than 0.12; wide and bizarre |
| Ventricular paced rhythm | None | None | Set on the pacemaker | Preset backup rate—Regular | Usually absent | Not measured | Greater than 0.12 |

- In *sinus bradycardia,* the impulse originates from the SA node, as in normal sinus rhythm, but the rate is slower. The decrease in heart rate is significant when the patient relates symptoms associated with this decrease, such as a decrease in systolic blood pressure, dizziness, light-headedness, or syncope (fainting). Sinus bradycardia is normal during sleep and in trained athletes (Figure 6.16).

| | |
|---|---|
| Rate: | Less than 60 beats per minute |
| Rhythm: | Regular |
| P wave: | Normal |
| PR interval: | Normal |
| QRS interval: | Normal |

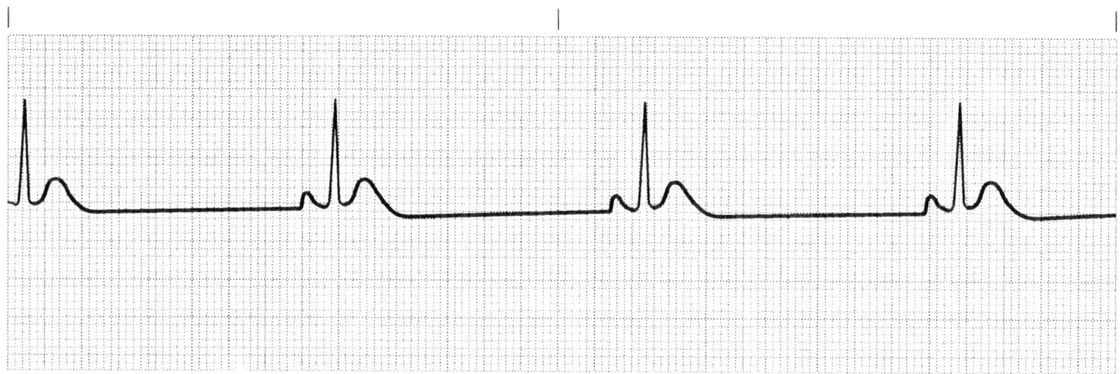

**Figure 6.16** Sinus bradycardia.

- The onset and termination of *sinus tachycardia,* or rapid heart rate, are usually gradual. The impulse originates from the SA node. Sinus tachycardia can be a normal response to exercise or emotion. In healthy individuals, it is an arrhythmia that usually does not need to be treated (Figure 6.17).

| | |
|---|---|
| Rate: | Greater than 100 beats per minute |
| Rhythm: | Regular |
| P wave: | Normal |
| PR interval: | Normal |
| QRS interval: | Normal |

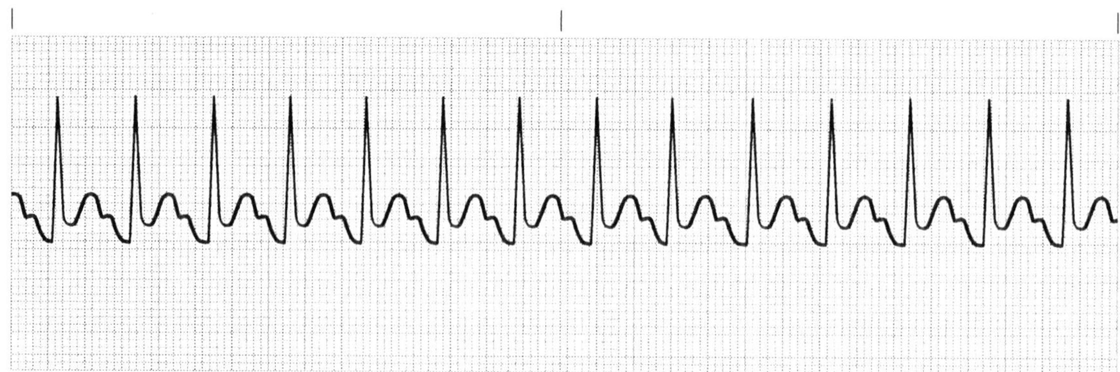

**Figure 6.17** Sinus tachycardia.

- *Sinus arrhythmia,* or irregular rhythm, is commonly related to respiration. It is normally seen in children, young adults, and the elderly. The heart rate increases with inspiration and decreases with expiration (Figure 6.18).

| | |
|---|---|
| Rate: | Usually 60–100 beats per minute |
| Rhythm: | Irregular |
| P wave: | Normal |
| PR interval: | Normal |
| QRS interval: | Normal |

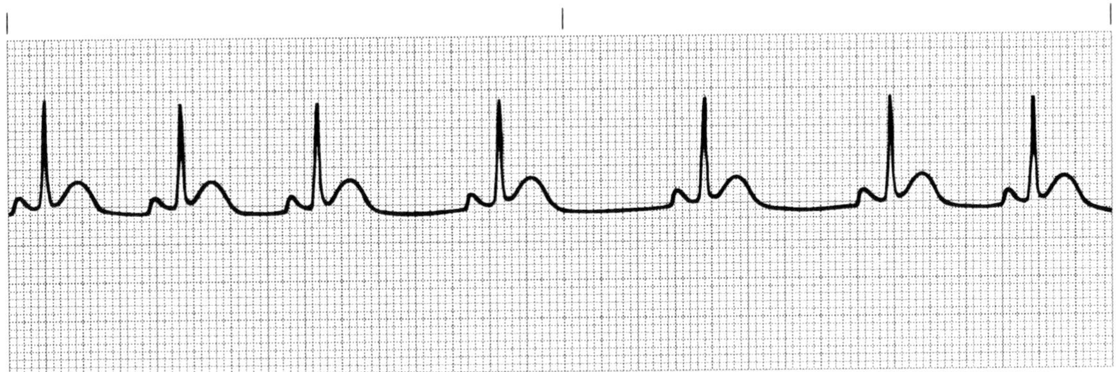

**Figure 6.18** Sinus arrhythmia.

- *Sinus arrest* occurs when the electrical impulse is not generated by the SA node, and a P wave is not seen. A pause in the rhythm will be seen until the SA node fires another beat or an escape rhythm is generated by another area of the heart in response to this pause. The length of the pause is not an interval of the normal R-to-R rhythm (Figure 6.19).

| | |
|---|---|
| Rate: | Usually 60–100 beats per minute, but might be slower if pauses are frequent |
| Rhythm: | Irregular when the pauses occur |
| P wave: | Normal with the conducted beats; absent with the pauses |
| PR interval: | Normal with the conducted beats; absent with the pauses |
| QRS interval: | Normal |

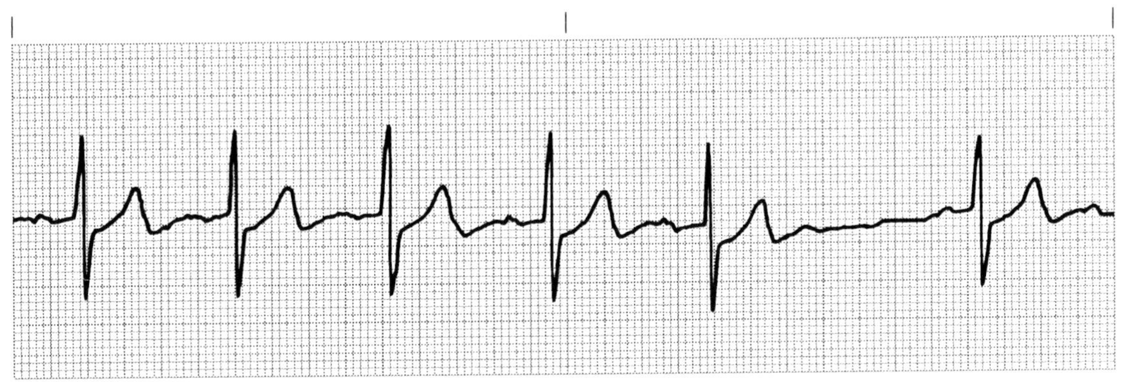

**Figure 6.19** Sinus arrest.

- *Wandering atrial pacemaker* occurs when the pacemaker of the heart moves from the SA node to the atria and to the AV node. The rate slows as the impulse shifts from a higher area of the heart, such as the SA node, to a slower area of the heart, such as the AV node. This arrhythmia does not usually require treatment (Figure 6.20).

| | |
|---|---|
| Rate: | Usually 60–100 beats per minute, but might be slower |
| Rhythm: | Irregular as impulse shifts |
| P wave: | Shape changes as pacemaker changes from one site to another; might even be absent when the beat originates within AV node |
| PR interval: | Varies |
| QRS interval: | Normal |

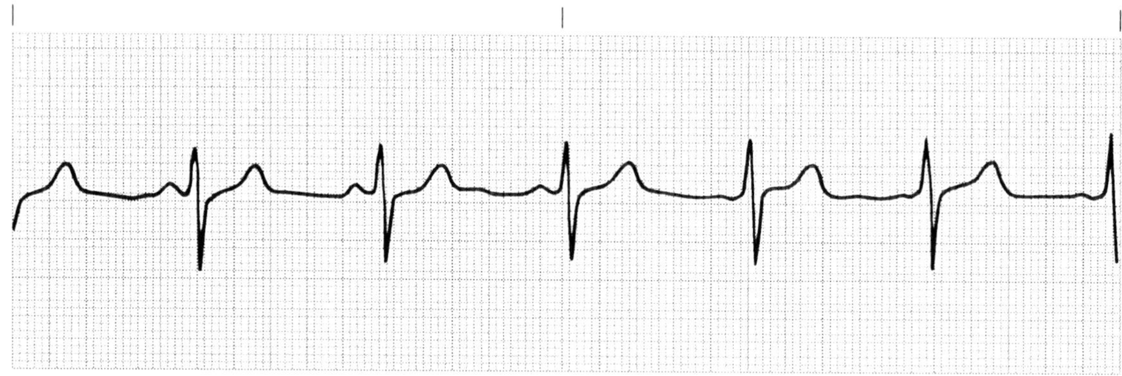

**Figure 6.20** Wandering atrial pacemaker.

- *A premature atrial contraction* (PAC) occurs when an impulse originates from outside the SA node and occurs somewhere in the atria. The impulse occurs earlier than the next expected sinus beat and is therefore considered to be premature. Single PACS can occur in healthy hearts and do not require treatment. In patients with heart disease, multiple PACS can precipitate other dysrhythmias, such as atrial fibrillation, atrial flutter, and paroxysmal (sudden onset) atrial tachycardia (PAT). Three or more PACS in a row are considered to be PAT. Heart rates with PAT can be between 150 and 250 (Figure 6.21).

| | |
|---|---|
| Rate: | Depends on underlying rhythm |
| Rhythm: | Irregular with the PACS |
| P wave: | With the PAC, can be a different shape from the sinus P wave |
| PR interval: | Within normal limits, but usually different from the sinus PR interval |
| QRS interval: | Normal |

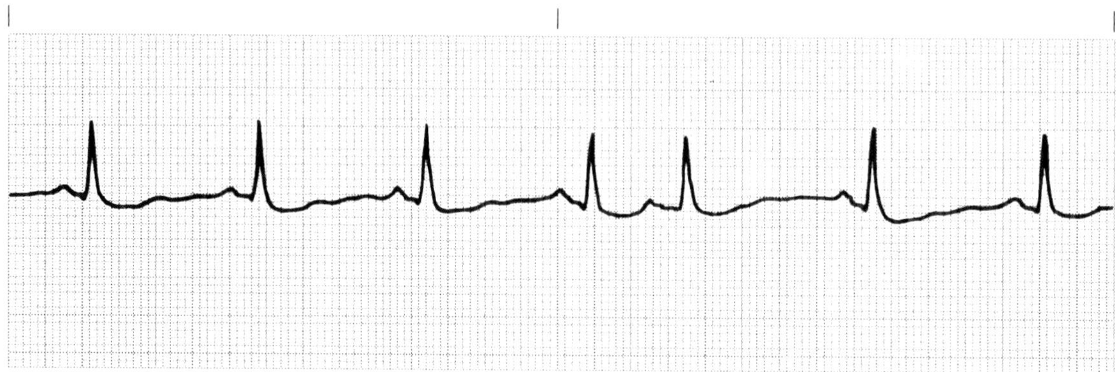

**Figure 6.21** Premature atrial contractions.

- *Atrial fibrillation* has a characteristic of being "irregularly irregular." The pacemaker of the heart comes from multiple sites in the atria. This activity is erratic, causing the baseline to appear very irregular and chaotic. The F waves, or atrial activity, usually do not resemble normal P waves. The AV node randomly conducts some of these impulses down through the rest of the conduction pathway, causing the irregular rhythm (Figure 6.22).

| | |
|---|---|
| Rate: | Ventricular rate can vary from bradycardia to tachycardia; F waves occur very rapidly, up to 360 per minute |
| Rhythm: | Irregularly irregular |
| P wave: | Absent; F waves seen (chaotic baseline) |
| PR interval: | None |
| QRS interval: | Usually normal, but can be wide if a conduction disturbance is present |

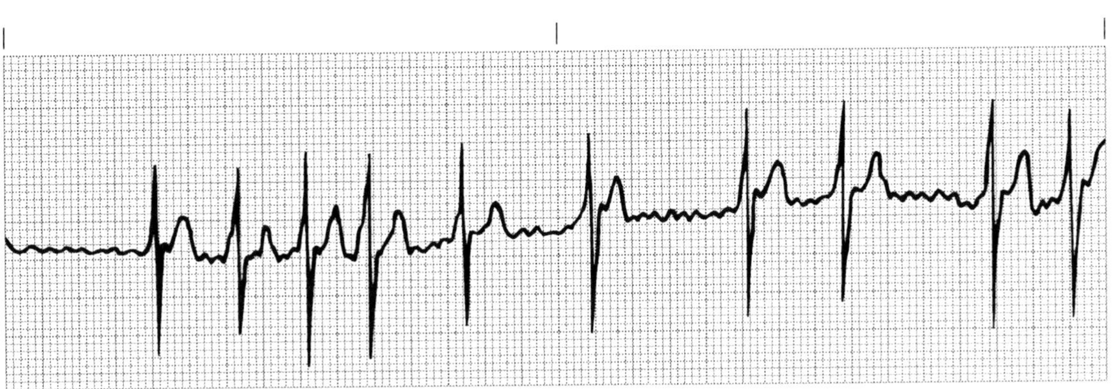

**Figure 6.22** Atrial fibrillation.

- *Atrial flutter* is a repetitive firing of a stimulus in the atria. The rhythm of the firing is regular and creates an unmistakable "sawtooth" monitor pattern. The origin of this focus is not from the sinus node, but from another area in the atria. The ventricles are unable to respond to each atrial stimulus. The AV node filters some of the atrial stimuli and sends only some of the stimuli on to the ventricles to be conducted. Typically, the conduction is expressed as a ratio of the number of atrial beats compared to ventricular conducted beats—for example, 2:1 (two P waves preceding every QRS), 3:1 (three P waves to every QRS), and so on (Figure 6.23).

| | |
|---|---|
| Rate: | Ventricular rate is usually 60–150 beats per minute; flutter waves occur very rapidly, up to 400 per minute |
| Rhythm: | Usually regular |
| P wave: | Absent; flutter waves seen ("sawtooth" baseline) |
| PR interval: | None |
| QRS interval: | Normal |

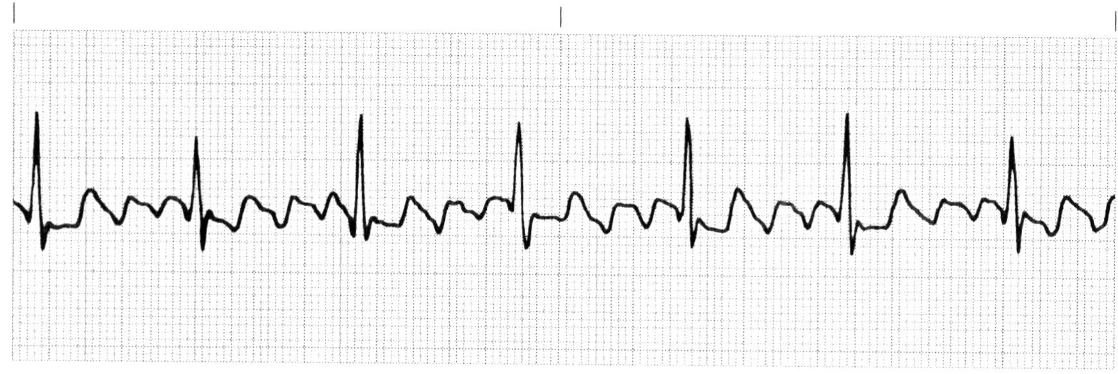

**Figure 6.23** Atrial flutter.

- *A premature junctional contraction* is a beat that originates at the AV junction (AV node). The beat comes before the next expected regular beat. Because the stimulus is not initiated at the sinus node, it does not have a characteristic P wave. Instead, there might be no P wave at all, or the P wave may look inverted or biphasic (like an S on its side). The P wave might be seen in the ST segment (Figure 6.24).

| | |
|---|---|
| Rate: | Depends on underlying rhythm |
| Rhythm: | Irregular due to premature beat |
| P wave: | Might be absent, inverted, before or after QRS |
| PR interval: | Less than 0.12 seconds |
| QRS interval: | Normal |

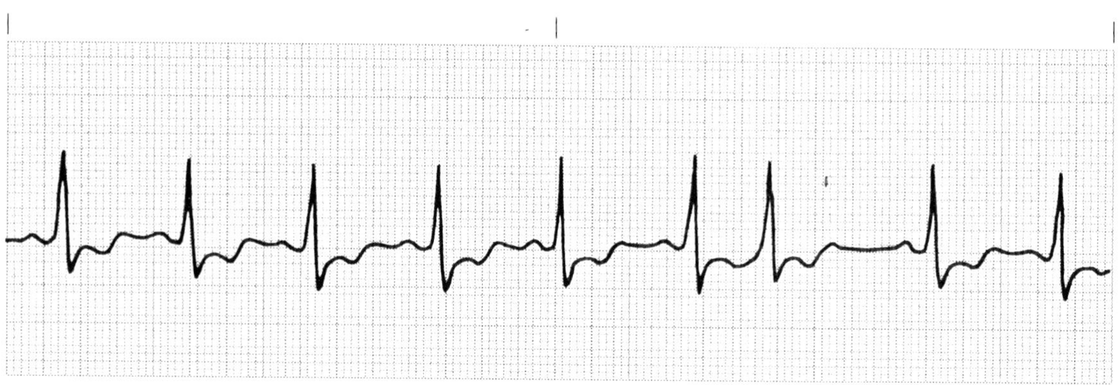

**Figure 6.24** Premature junctional contractions.

- *A junctional rhythm* is a characteristically slow rhythm that originates at the AV junction. In this rhythm, the AV junction assumes the role of pacemaker for the heart. P waves are absent, inverted, or biphasic. The QRS is usually narrow. The rate of a junctional rhythm is usually 40 to 60 beats per minute. A junctional rate is considered accelerated if the rate falls between 60 and 100 beats per minute (Figure 6.25).

| | |
|---|---|
| Rate: | Ventricular rate is usually 40–60 beats per minute |
| Rhythm: | Regular |
| P wave: | Might be absent, inverted, before or after the QRS |
| PR interval: | Less than 0.12 seconds |
| QRS interval: | Normal |

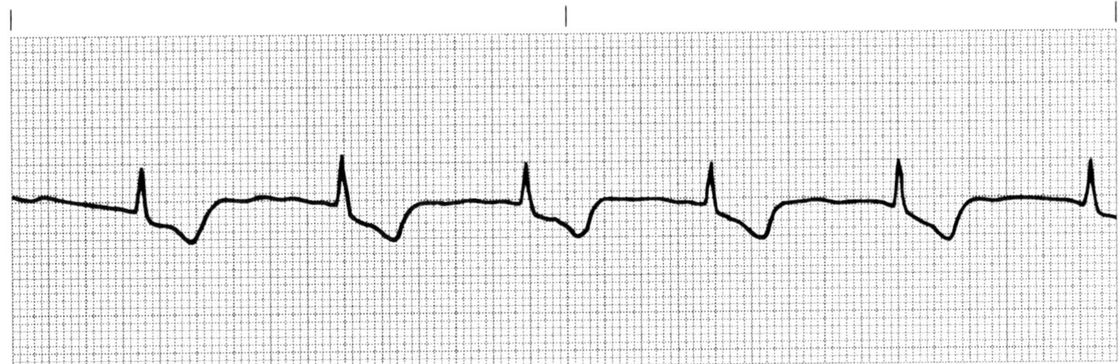

**Figure 6.25** Junctional rhythm.

- *Paroxysmal supraventricular tachycardia* describes a narrow QRS complex rhythm that originates above the ventricles but not from the SA node. The rate exceeds 100 beats per minute, and the rhythm is usually regular (Figure 6.26).

| | |
|---|---|
| Rate: | Ventricular rate is 150–250; might be unable to determine atrial rate |
| Rhythm: | Ventricular rhythm is regular |
| P wave: | Might be concealed in previous T wave |
| PR interval: | Might be impossible to measure |
| QRS interval: | Normal |

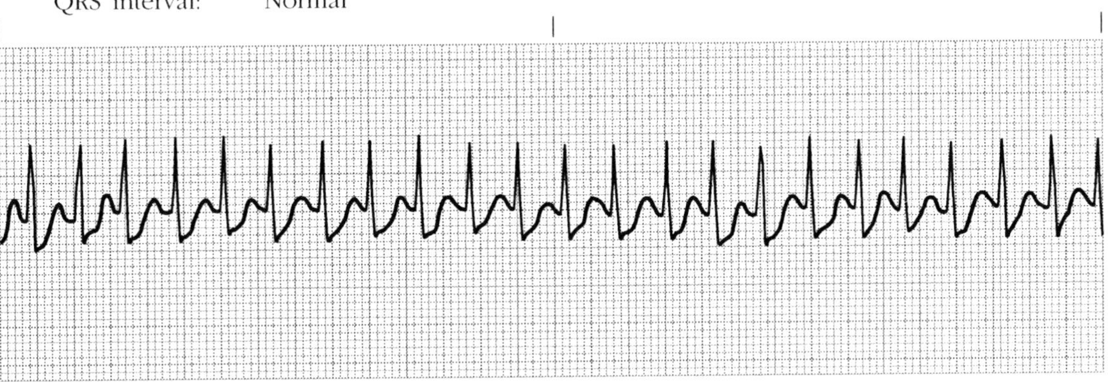

**Figure 6.26** Paroxysmal supraventricular tachycardia.

- *A first-degree AV block* exists when the length of the PR interval exceeds 0.20 seconds (five small ECG boxes; Figure 6.27.)

| | |
|---|---|
| Rate: | Depends on underlying rhythm |
| Rhythm: | Depends on rate; identify underlying rhythm as tachycardia, bradycardia, or sinus rhythm with the first degree AV block |
| P wave: | Normal |
| PR interval: | Greater than 0.20 seconds |
| QRS interval: | Normal |

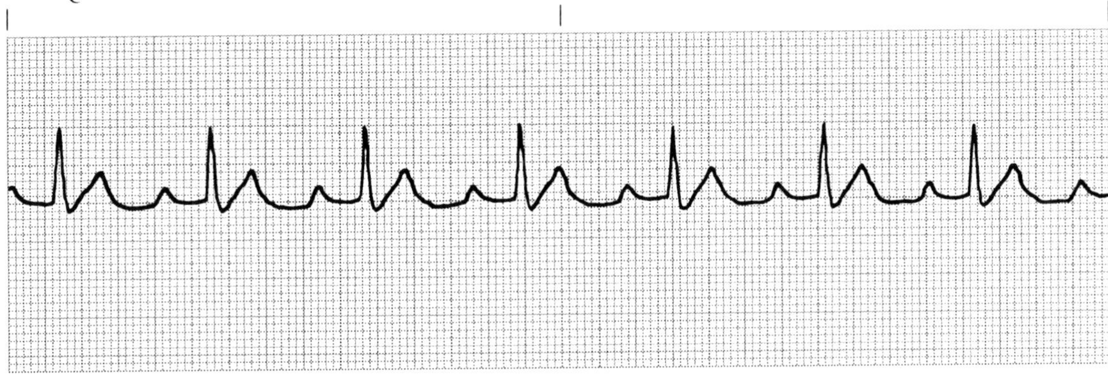

**Figure 6.27** First-degree AV block.

- *Second-degree block—Mobitz I (Wenckebach)* is described as a rhythm in which the PR interval progressively lengthens until a P wave does not generate a QRS. The cycle then resumes with progressively lengthening PR intervals until another P wave does not generate a QRS (Figure 6.28).

| | |
|---|---|
| Rate: | Ventricular is slower than atrial; atrial is usually normal |
| Rhythm: | Ventricular is irregular; atrial is regular |
| P wave: | Normal |
| PR interval: | Progressive lengthening until QRS is dropped |
| QRS interval: | Normal |

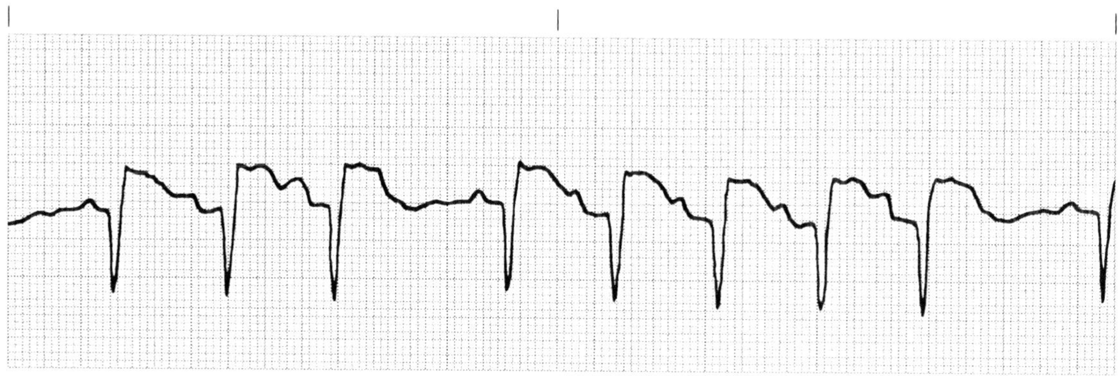

**Figure 6.28** Second-degree AV block—Mobitz I (Wenckebach).

- *Second-degree block—Mobitz II* is characterized by a prolonged PR interval with a periodically dropped QRS (P wave but no QRS). The PR interval does not progressively increase, as seen in Mobitz I (Wenckebach). The R-to-R interval with the conducted beat is consistently the same. The QRS is usually wide due to a conduction disturbance in the bundle of His (Figure 6.29).

| | |
|---|---|
| Rate: | Ventricular is slower than atrial; atrial is normal |
| Rhythm: | Ventricular is irregular; atrial is regular |
| P wave: | Normal |
| PR interval: | Consistent for conducted beats |
| QRS interval: | Greater than 0.12 seconds |

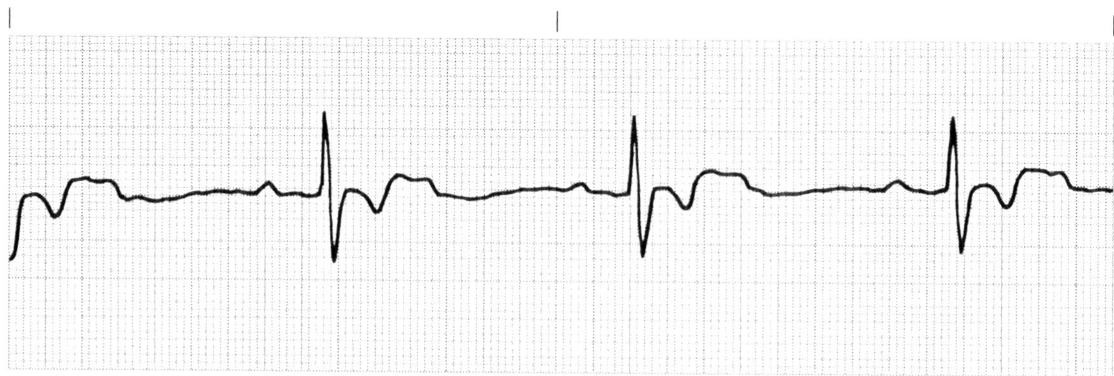

**Figure 6.29** Second-degree AV block—Mobitz II.

- In *third-degree block*, the QRS complex may appear normal; the atria and ventricles beat in a regular rhythm but are totally independent of one another. The ventricles beat at a rate slower than the atria. The rhythm can be life-threatening if the ventricular rate is not sufficient to maintain cardiac output (Figure 6.30).

| | |
|---|---|
| Rate: | Ventricular is slower than atrial; atrial is usually normal |
| Rhythm: | Both ventricular and atrial are regular but totally independent |
| P wave: | Normal |
| PR interval: | No relationship of P wave to QRS |
| QRS interval: | Greater than 0.12 seconds |

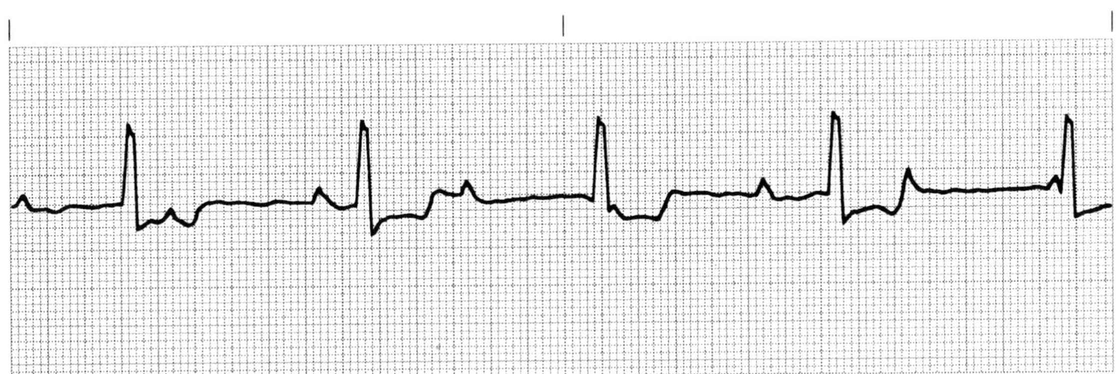

**Figure 6.30** Third-degree block.

- *Premature ventricular contractions (PVCs)* originate from stimuli in an irritable wall of the ventricle. The QRS complex is wide and not preceded by a P wave. The stimulus comes before the next expected regular beat and is usually followed by a compensatory pause. This compensatory pause is defined as the time the sinus node waits after the premature beat before initiating the next sinus beat on its previous schedule (Figure 6.31).

| | |
|---|---|
| Rate: | Depends on underlying rhythm |
| Rhythm: | Irregular due to premature beat |
| P wave: | Absent |
| PR interval: | Absent |
| QRS interval: | Greater than 0.12 seconds; wide and bizarre |

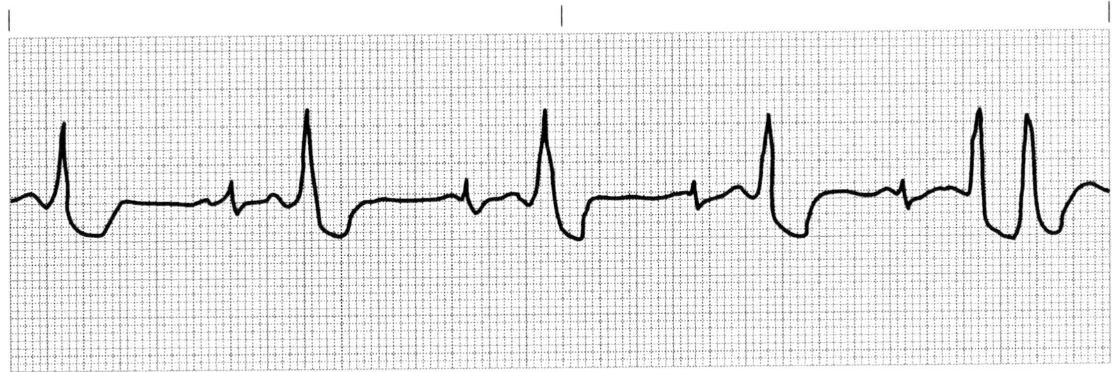

**Figure 6.31** Premature ventricular contractions.

- *Ventricular tachycardia* is a rapid series of beats (usually greater than 150 beats per minute) initiated in the ventricle. This rapid firing might not leave sufficient time for the ventricles to fill with blood after each beat, and therefore some beats might not be palpated as peripheral pulses. Left untreated, ventricular tachycardia can quickly lead to ventricular fibrillation, a life-threatening arrhythmia (Figure 6.32).

| | |
|---|---|
| Rate: | Ventricular is 150–250 beats per minute; no atrial beats seen |
| Rhythm: | Regular |
| P wave: | Absent |
| PR interval: | Absent |
| QRS interval: | Greater than 0.12 seconds |

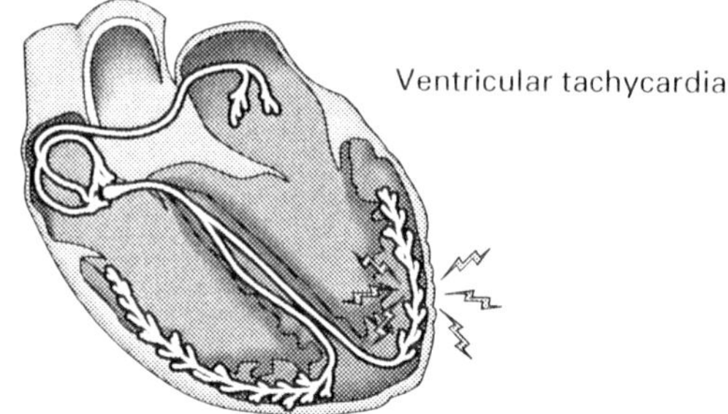


ECG tracing of ventricular tachycardia

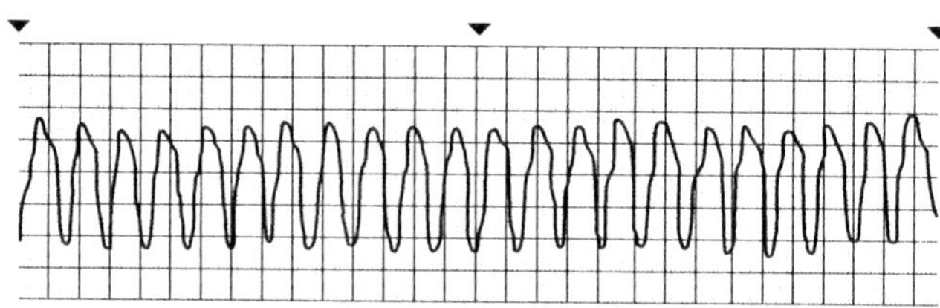

**Figure 6.32** Ventricular tachycardia.

- *Ventricular fibrillation* is a life-threatening arrhythmia characterized by a quivering of the ventricles. This is displayed as chaotic fibrillatory waves on the ECG monitor. No effective ventricular contractions take place; no peripheral pulses are felt; and if left untreated, the patient dies (Figure 6.33).

| | |
|---|---|
| Rate: | Cannot be determined |
| Rhythm: | None |
| P wave: | Absent |
| PR interval: | Absent |
| QRS interval: | Cannot be determined |

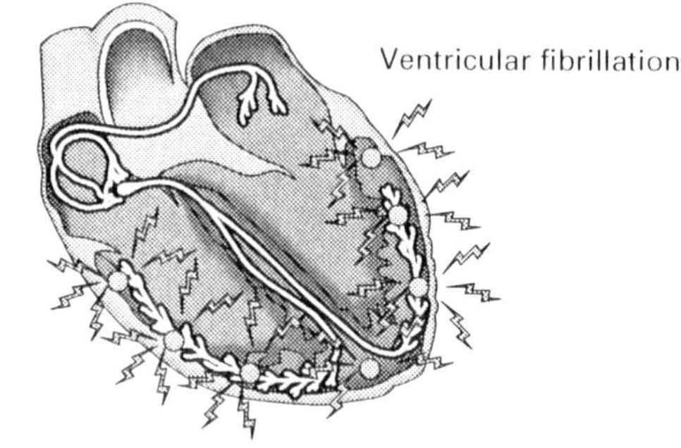


Chaotic electrical discharge as seen on an ECG tracing

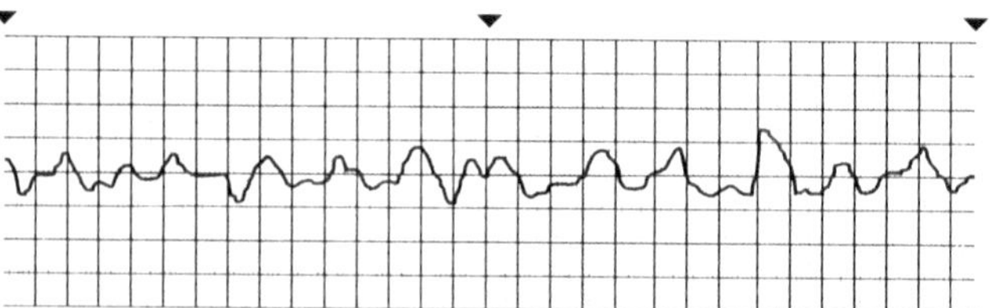

**Figure 6.33** Ventricular fibrillation.

- *Asystole* is defined as an absence of atrial or ventricular contractions. There is a characteristic flat line pattern on the monitor. Before assuming asystole, the caregiver must always assess for loose leads or other mechanical problems that might imitate asystole. True asystole is a life-threatening arrhythmia and must be treated immediately. *Ventricular asystole* is characterized by an absence of ventricular complexes, although P waves might be present (Figure 6.34).

| | |
|---|---|
| Rate: | None |
| Rhythm: | None |
| P wave: | Absent |
| PR interval: | Absent |
| QRS interval: | Absent |

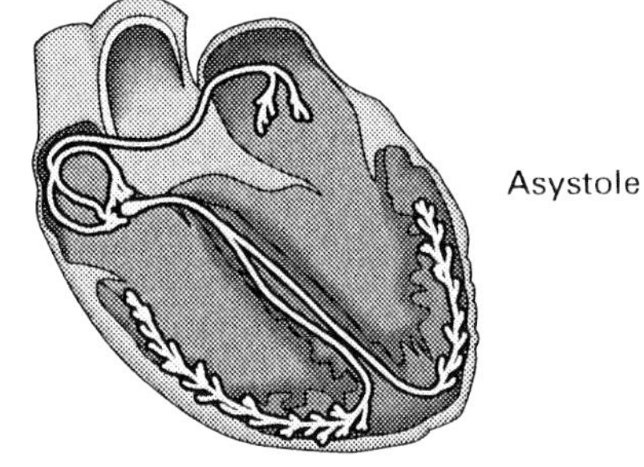


ECG tracing of asystole

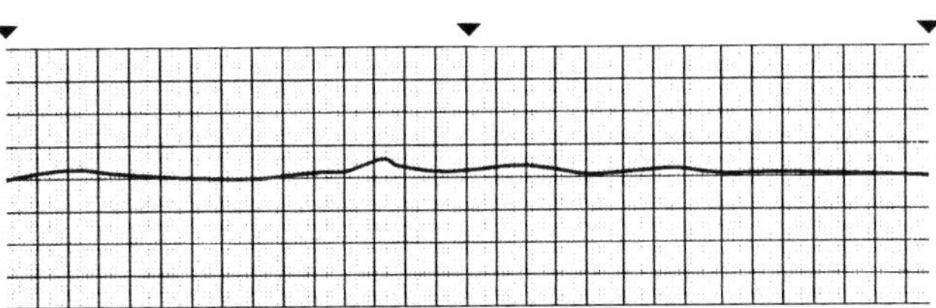

**Figure 6.34** Asystole.

- An *idioventricular rhythm* is defined as a rhythm in which the ventricles assume the role of pacemaker for the heart. The complexes are wide and slow, and no P waves are seen. The normal idioventricular rate is 20 to 45 beats per minute. This rhythm is often associated with the dying heart (Figure 6.35).

| | |
|---|---|
| Rate: | Ventricular rate is 20–45 beats per minute; no atrial rate |
| Rhythm: | Might be irregular |
| P wave: | Absent |
| PR interval: | Absent |
| QRS interval: | Greater than 0.12 seconds; wide and bizarre |

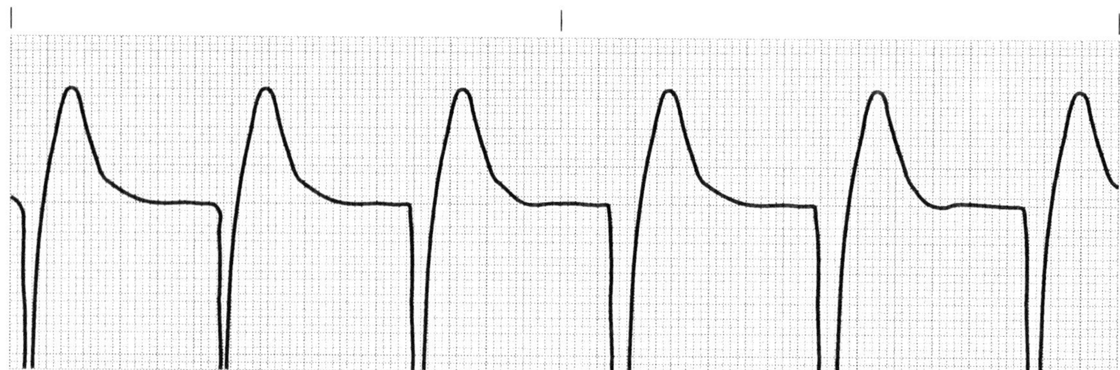

**Figure 6.35** Idioventricular rhythm.

- *Ventricular paced rhythm* is initiated by an artificial pacemaker source. A wire is implanted in the right ventricle and attached to a pacemaker generator. The pacemaker beats at a set backup rate unless it senses that the heart has its own natural beats. Characteristic spikes are noted on the ECG monitor; these are followed by QRS complexes (Figure 6.36).

| | |
|---|---|
| Rate: | When paced, the ventricular rate is the rate set on the pacemaker generator |
| Rhythm: | Paced beats are regular |
| P wave: | Usually absent in paced beats |
| PR interval: | Not measured |

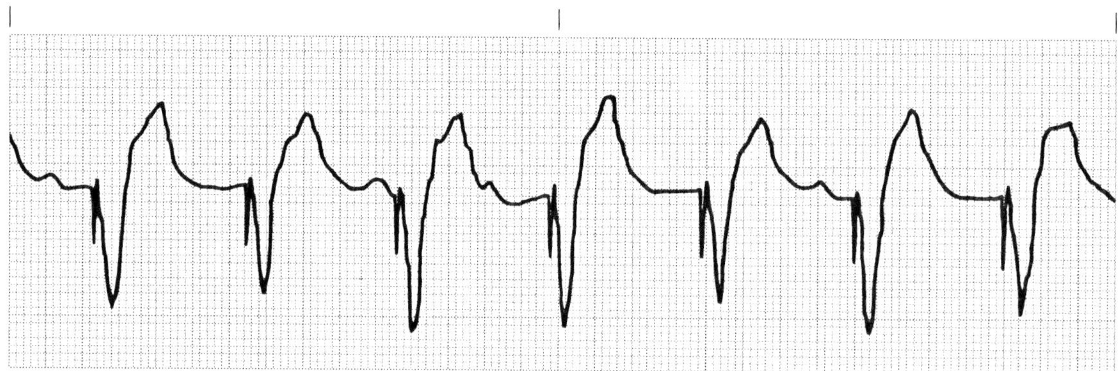

**Figure 6.36** Ventricular paced rhythm.

## Age-Specific Considerations

Heart rates might vary for children of different ages and still be considered within the normal ranges (Table 6.2). In infants, *sinus tachycardia* is usually associated with heart rates of less than 200 beats per minute. *Supraventricular tachycardia* (SVT) in infants is generally greater than 230 beats per minute. *Ventricular tachycardia* is uncommon in children unless there is structural disease, electrolyte abnormalities, or acidosis present. *Sinus bradycardia* and *AV blocks* are the most common terminal rhythms in children.

### TABLE 6.2 Normal Pediatric Heart Rates

| Age | Awake Heart Rate | Average Heart Rate | Sleeping Heart Rate |
|---|---|---|---|
| Newborn–3 months | 85–205 | 140 | 80–160 |
| 3 months–2 years | 100–190 | 130 | 75–160 |
| 2 years–10 years | 60–140 | 80 | 60–90 |
| >10 years | 60–100 | 75 | 50–90 |

Key Concept

The ECG machine records not only the electrical activity of the heart, but also the extra electrical activity or muscle movement. Loose electrodes can cause erratic electrical interference on the ECG monitor (Figure 6.37). Ensure that all leads are securely attached, and change electrode patches if necessary to ensure good contact. Sixty-cycle interference appears on the monitor as a tall band throughout all or some parts of the cardiac complex (Figure 6.38). It is caused by electrical interference in the area. Resolve this artifact by disconnecting electrical devices one at a time from the outlet until sixty-cycle interference is gone. The ground wire of that electrical device needs repair.

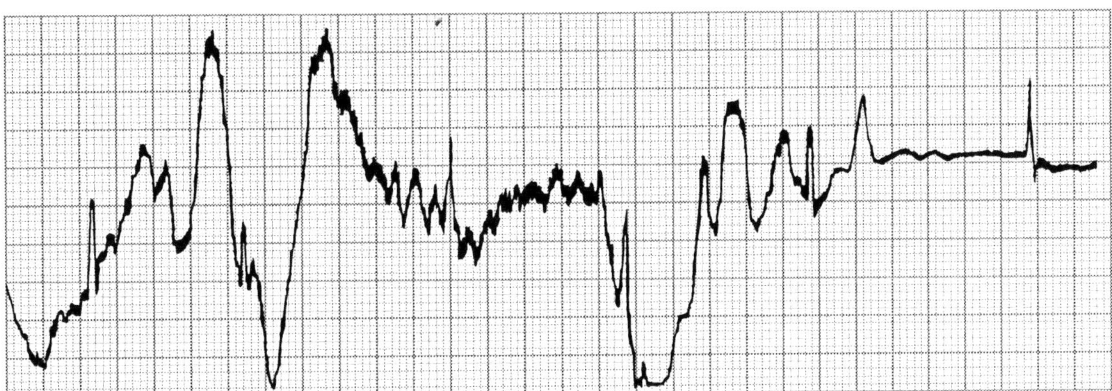

**Figure 6.37** Artifact.

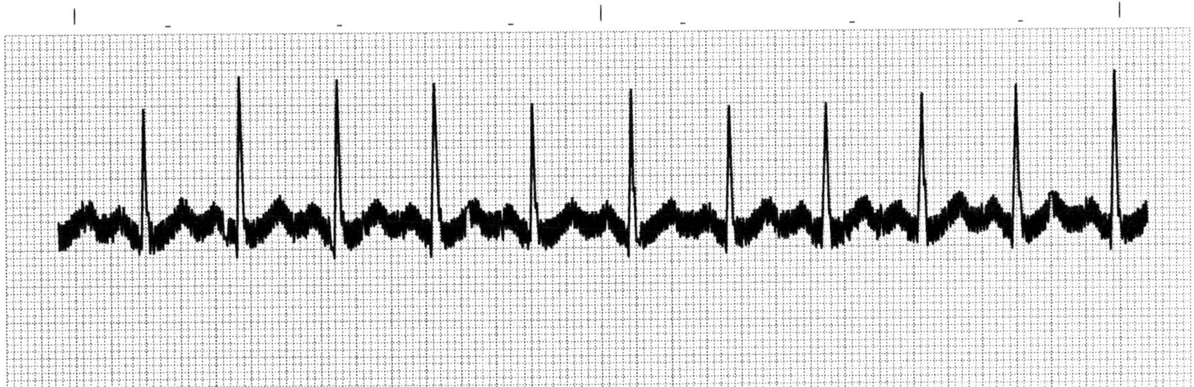

**Figure 6.38** Sixty-cycle interference.

Your instructor or preceptor will likely administer a competency test to you.

SECTION TWO

# Additional Advanced Cardiac Care Skills

## CARING FOR THE PATIENT WITH AN ARTERIAL LINE

Arterial catheters are inserted for patients who need close blood pressure monitoring or frequent blood draws. Generally, a physician places an intravenous catheter into the radial artery and sutures the catheter in place. Although most arterial catheters are placed in the radial artery, an alternate site for placement of the catheter is in the femoral artery. Once placed, the catheter is covered with a sterile occlusive dressing and is immediately connected to a monitoring system (Figure 6.39). The system includes five parts: the transducer, the fluid-filled pressure tubing, the solution, a pressure bag, and the intraflow device.

### Pertinent Points: Advantages and Risks of an Arterial Line

The use of an arterial line provides several advantages, including continuous accurate measurement of blood pressure, detection of blood pressure trends, and convenient access for blood draws. Disadvantages, however, do exist. The risk of bleeding, embolism, vessel and tissue damage, and infection must be considered.

To minimize the risk of bleeding,

- Consistently maintain the pressure at 300 mm Hg in the pressure bag.
- Ensure that all connections and stopcocks are positioned properly and securely.
- Set alarm limits to warn of decreases in blood pressure.

To avoid embolism and vessel or tissue damage,

- Notify the RN of any patient complaints of pain or numbness.
- Immobilize the extremity with an arm board.
- Fast flush for no more than 1 second at a time to avoid sending a fluid embolus through the artery.

To protect against the risk of infection,

- Ensure that dead-end caps are securely positioned on ports.
- Change dressing using sterile technique according to institution guidelines.
- Monitor the insertion site for early signs and symptoms of infection.
- Use disposable transducers.

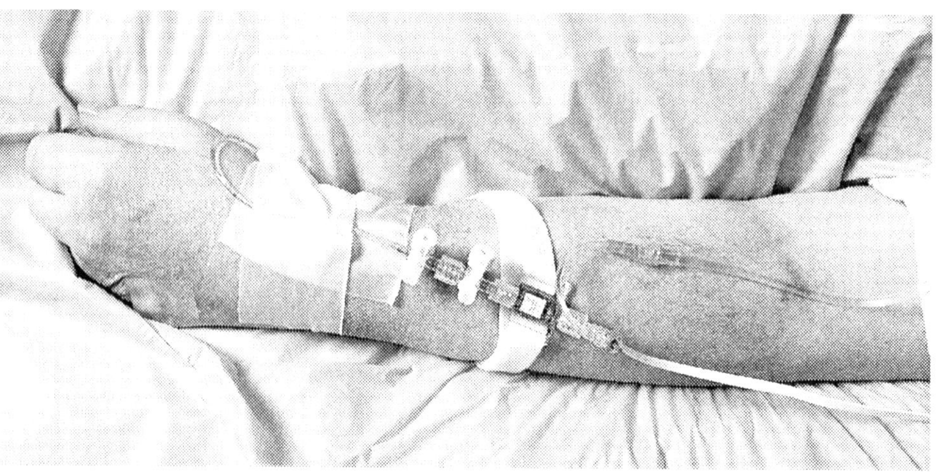

**Figure 6.39** Patient with a dressed arterial line.

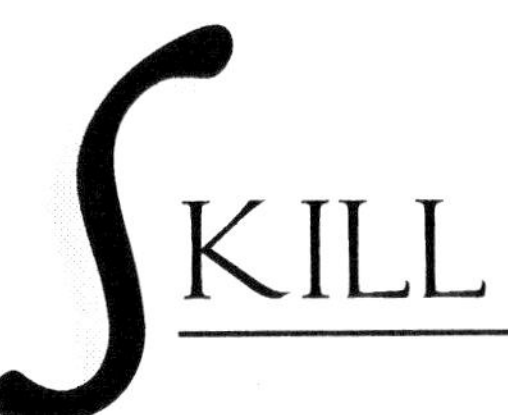

# SKILL

## Changing an Arterial Line Dressing

**Purpose** Caregivers need to be able to change an arterial line dressing whenever the dressing becomes nonocclusive, moist, or soiled. Institutional policy will also influence when a dressing is changed.

### Objectives

**The caregiver demonstrates the ability to do the following:**

1. Gather the correct supplies.
2. Communicate using a style that reduces the patient's anxiety.
3. Maintain sterile technique.
4. Change an arterial line dressing.
5. Report the results of the procedure to the RN or preceptor.

### Key Terms

**Fluid-Filled Pressure Tubing** Specialized rigid tubing that connects the vascular system (the artery) and the transducer.

**Heparinized Solution** A solution containing the drug heparin, which is used to keep the system patent.

**Intraflow Device** A device that limits the amount of continuous flow being delivered through the pressurized system yet allows the caregiver to flush the system after blood draws to keep it clear.

**Pressure Bag** A device that holds the heparinized solution under 300 mm Hg pressure to maintain flow against the patient's own arterial pressure.

**Transducer** A device that can convert pulse waves into electrical energy that is visible on a monitor as a waveform and a systolic and diastolic number.

### Supplies/Equipment

Blue pad • Mask • Clean gloves • 2×2s • Betadine pledgets • Sterile gloves • Tape (1½ inches and 1 inch)

### Pertinent Points

- When a dressing is removed, the site must be examined for signs of infection (redness, swelling, or pus). If evident, notify the physician, discontinue the arterial line, and culture the catheter tip.
- Some arterial lines are not sutured and can be accidently dislodged or removed. Should this happen, apply pressure on the artery for 5 to 15 minutes. Report immediately.

### Age-Specific Considerations

Older adults and patients with skin sensitivities should be monitored for skin rash or irritation. An arm board might provide greater support to the limb.

### Key Concept

Arterial line dressing changes are routinely performed according to facility guidelines and whenever the dressing becomes nonocclusive, moist, or soiled.

## Steps

1. Wash hands.
2. Identify the correct patient.
3. Explain the procedure to the patient.
4. Assemble the equipment (Figure 6.40a).
5. Place the blue pad under the patient's arm (or groin if the catheter is in the femoral artery).
6. Put on mask and clean gloves (Figure 6.40b).
7. Remove and discard the old dressing, being careful not to dislodge the catheter (Figure 6.40c).
8. Remove and discard gloves. Wash hands if it is agency policy.
9. Drop 2×2s and betadine pledgets on a sterile field.
10. Put on sterile gloves.
11. Check the site for signs of infection and irritation. (Report findings to the RN.)
12. Clean the insertion site in a circular motion with a betadine pledget; repeat (Figure 6.40d). Allow the betadine to dry.
13. Secure the tubing to the skin with tape; cover with 2×2s and additional tape (Figure 6.40e).
14. Write the date and time and your initials on the dressing (Figure 6.40f).
15. Remove and discard gloves; wash hands.
16. Document and report the results to the RN or preceptor.

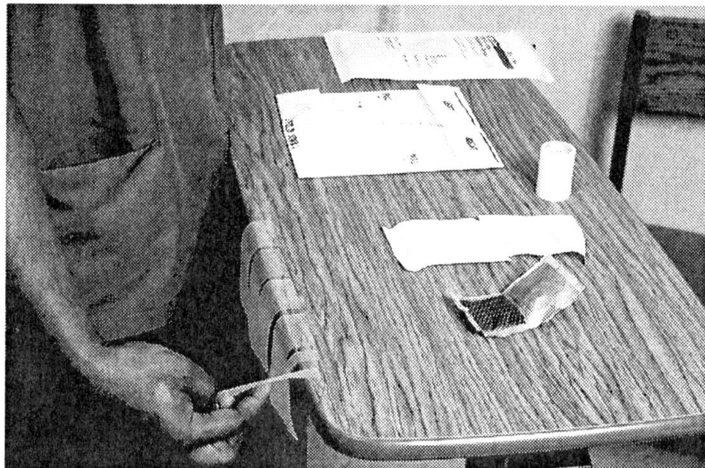

a

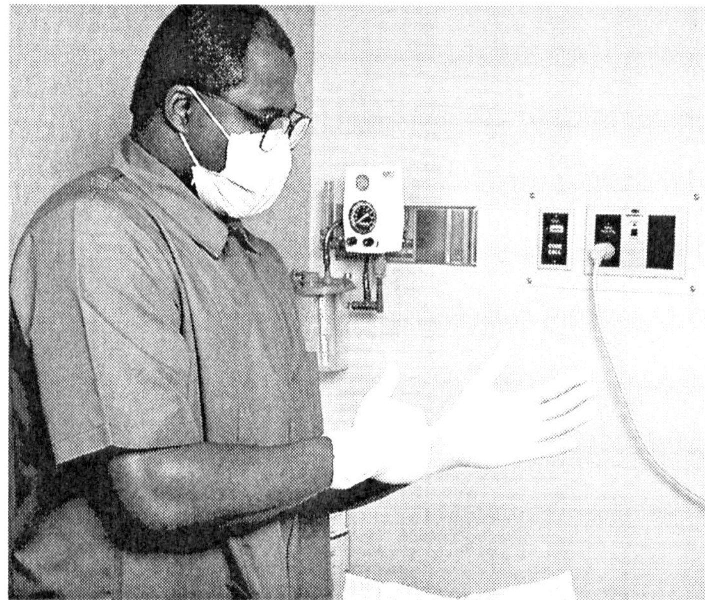

b

**Figure 6.40** Assembling the equipment.

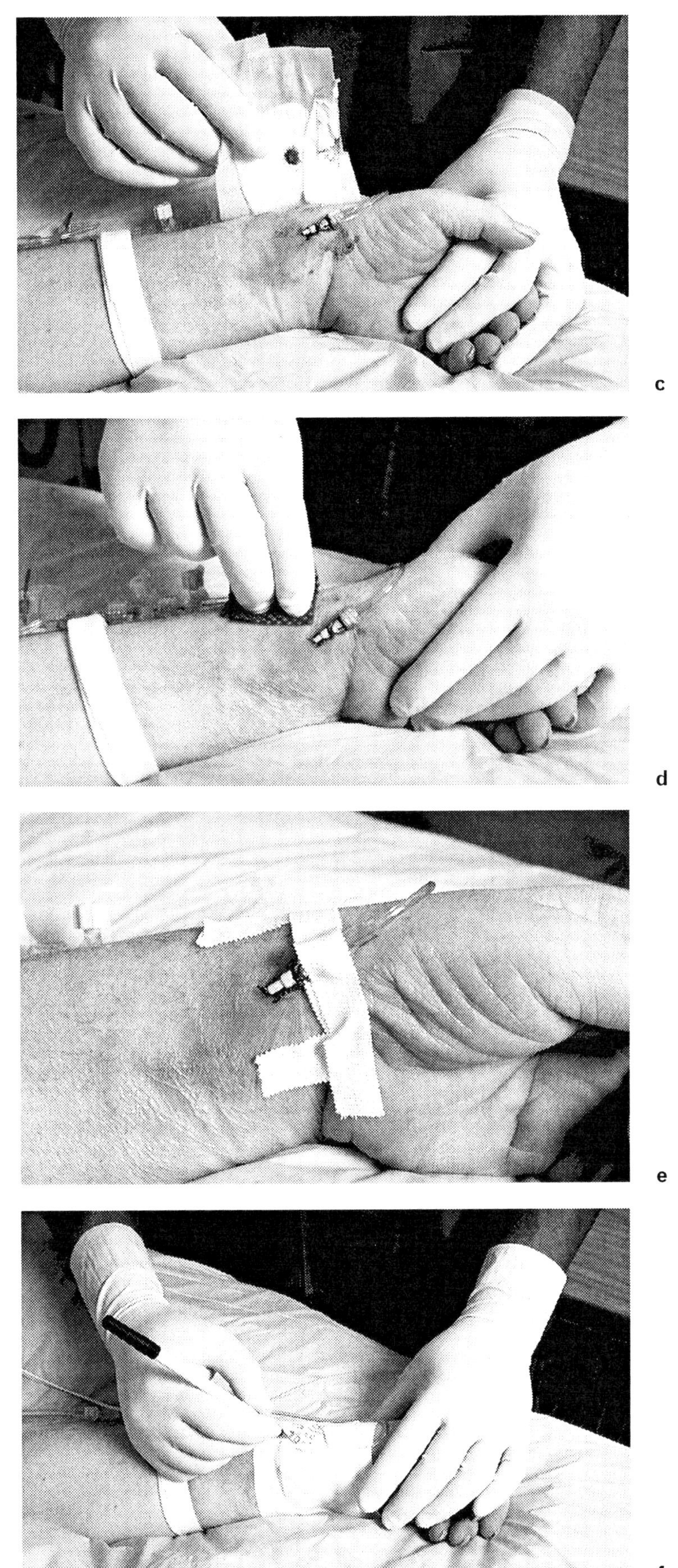
c
d
e
f

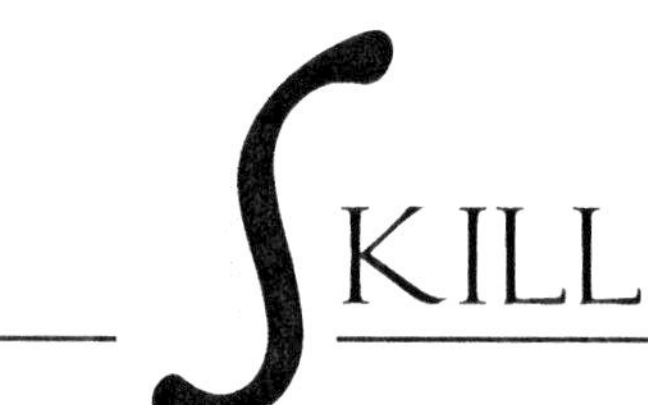

# Withdrawing Blood from an Arterial Line

**Purpose** Arterial lines allow convenient access to obtain frequently ordered blood specimens from unstable cardiac patients. The caregiver obtains blood samples from the arterial line stopcock port. The blood can be collected with a vacutainer or a syringe.

## Objectives

**The caregiver demonstrates the ability to do the following:**

1. Gather the correct supplies.
2. Communicate using a style that reduces the patient's anxiety.
3. Maintain sterile technique.
4. Obtain an arterial line blood sample.
5. Report the results of the procedure to the RN or preceptor.

## Key Terms

**Transducer** A device that can convert pulse waves into electrical energy that is visible on a monitor as a waveform and a systolic and diastolic number.

**Fluid-Filled Pressure Tubing** Specialized rigid tubing that connects the vascular system (the artery) and the transducer.

**Heparinized Solution** A solution containing the drug heparin, which is used to keep the system patent.

**Pressure Bag** A device that holds the heparinized solution under 300 mm Hg pressure to maintain flow against the patient's own arterial pressure.

**Intraflow Device** A device that limits the amount of continuous flow being delivered through the pressurized system yet allows the caregiver to flush the system after blood draws to keep it clear.

## Supplies/Equipment

Clean gloves • Lab slips stamped with patient name, date, time, and unit phone number • Blood tubes and/or heparinized syringe for specimens • Alcohol wipes • Vacutainer holder with protected needle adapter or syringe • Syringe or red-top tube for discard • 2×2s or medicine cup • Plastic bag • Ice, if drawing blood gas specimens

## Pertinent Point

Arterial blood gas specimens must be transported to the lab on ice to obtain valid results. Some arterial lines are not sutured in place. Follow agency policies and procedures to avoid contamination or problems.

Key Concept

The portion of blood that is mixed with the heparinized saline solution must not be used or sent as the test sample. Discard 3 cc of blood for all tests, unless drawing coagulation studies.

If drawing numerous tests with coagulation studies, at least 10 cc of blood must be obtained before drawing the coagulation studies. If coags are the only tests needed, use a 10-cc red-top for the discard tube, then proceed with drawing the coagulation studies.

Put the blood sample into labeled tubes. For multiple tubes, fill red (or yellow) first, then blue, and then purple.

Steps

1. Wash hands.
2. Identify the correct patient.
3. Explain the procedure to the patient.
4. Assemble the equipment and apply gloves.
5. Label the appropriate tubes with patient name, date, time, and unit phone number.
6. Suspend the monitor alarm.
7. Remove the Luer Lok cap from the distal stopcock and maintain sterility (Figure 6.41a).
8. Wipe the open end of the stopcock with an alcohol wipe and allow to dry (Figure 6.41b).
9. Perform the procedure for a vacutainer blood draw:
   a. Attach the adapter and the vacutainer to the stopcock. Then place an unlabeled discard tube over the needle, and open the stopcock to the vacutainer.
   b. Discard 3 cc of blood for all tests, unless drawing coagulation studies. If drawing numerous tests with coagulation studies, obtain at least 10 cc of blood before drawing the coagulation studies. If coags are the only tests needed, use a 10-cc red-top for the discard tube, then proceed with drawing the coagulation studies.

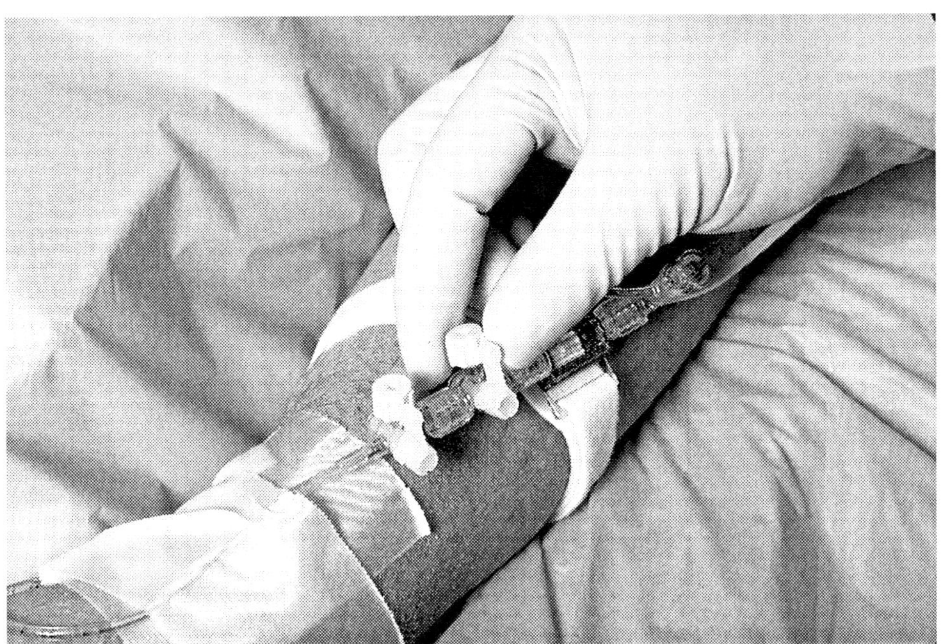

a

**Figure 6.41** Removing the cap from the distal stopcock on a four-way or Luer Lok stopcock.

c. Put the blood sample into the labeled tubes. For multiple tubes, fill red (or yellow) first, then blue, and then purple.

d. Close the stopcock to the patient. Remove the vacutainer. Flush out the stopcock into a 2 × 2s or medicine cup.

e. Close the stopcock to the atmosphere.

f. Replace the dead-end cap.

g. Flush the patient line in short, 1-second increments until it is clear of blood.

h. Turn the monitor alarm back on.

i. Place blood specimens in a plastic bag.

j. Dispose of equipment.

k. Wash hands thoroughly.

l. Document on nursing flowsheet—or patient record—time blood was drawn and what specimen(s) were sent to lab.

10. Perform the procedure for a syringe blood draw:

   a. Suspend the arterial line alarm.

   b. Attach the discard syringe to the stopcock, and open the stopcock to the syringe (Figure 6.41c).

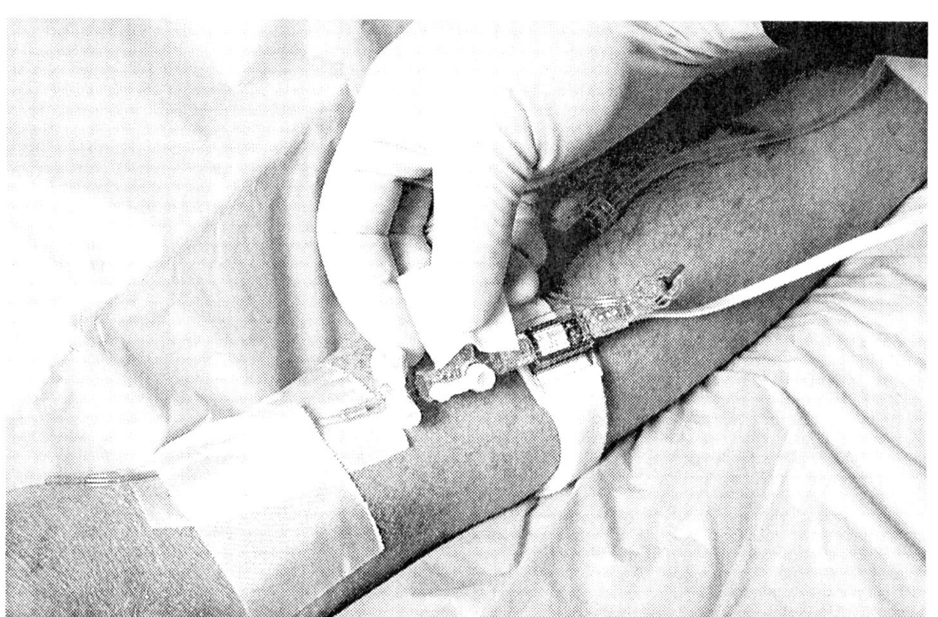

b

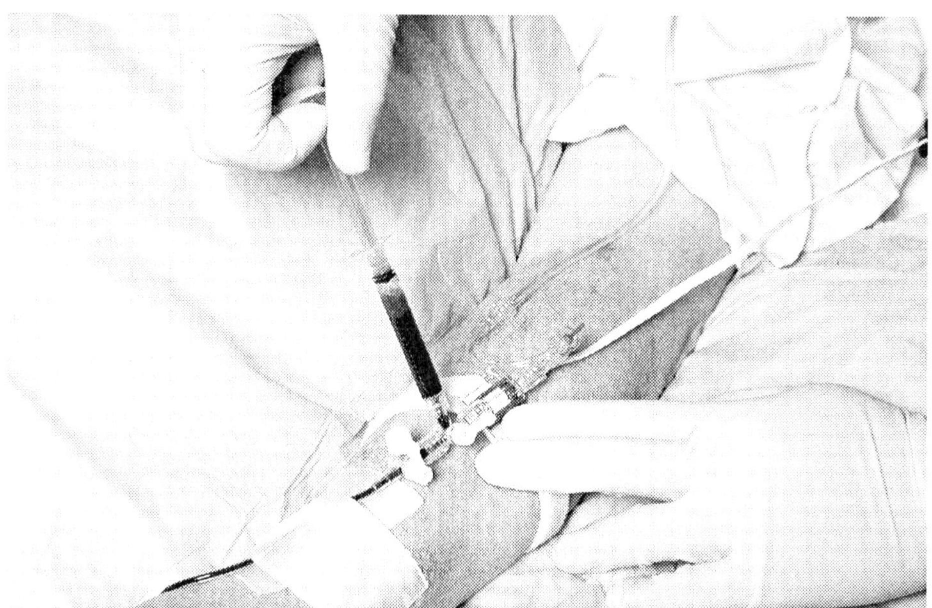

c

**c.** Discard 3 cc of blood for all tests, unless drawing coagulation studies. If drawing numerous tests with coagulation studies, obtain at least 10 cc of blood before drawing the coagulation studies. If coags are the only tests needed, use a 10-cc red-top for the discard tube, then proceed with drawing the coagulation studies.

**d.** Turn the stopcock to a 45-degree angle. Then remove the syringe (Figure 6.41d).

**e.** Attach the sample syringe and open the stopcock to withdraw the blood sample (Figure 6.41e). Be careful of accidental disconnection with non–Leur-Lok syringes. Repeat as necessary, closing the stopcock to a 45-degree angle between syringe changes.

**f.** Close the stopcock to the patient and flush out the stopcock into a 2×2s or medicine cup (Figure 6.41f).

**g.** Close the stopcock to the atmosphere. Apply the dead-end cap.

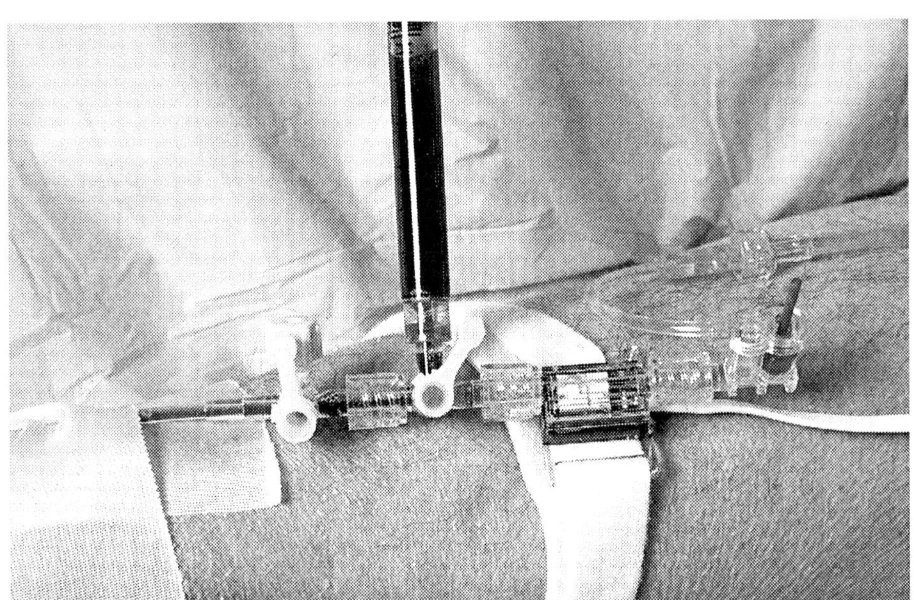

d

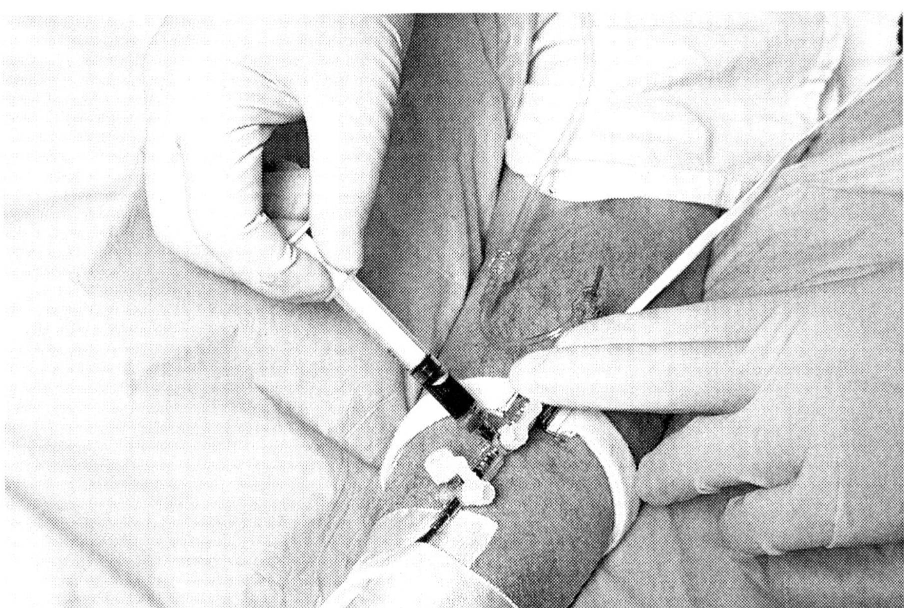

e

h. Replace the dead-end cap (Figure 6.41g).

i. Flush the patient line in short, 1-second increments, until it is clear of blood (Figure 6.41h).

j. Turn the monitor alarm back on.

k. Transfer blood from the syringes into labeled tubes.

l. Place blood specimens in a plastic bag.

m. Dispose of equipment (Figure 6.41i).

11. Remove and discard gloves; wash hands.

12. Document on the nursing flow sheet what time the blood was drawn and what specimens were sent to the lab.

13. Report the results to the RN or preceptor.

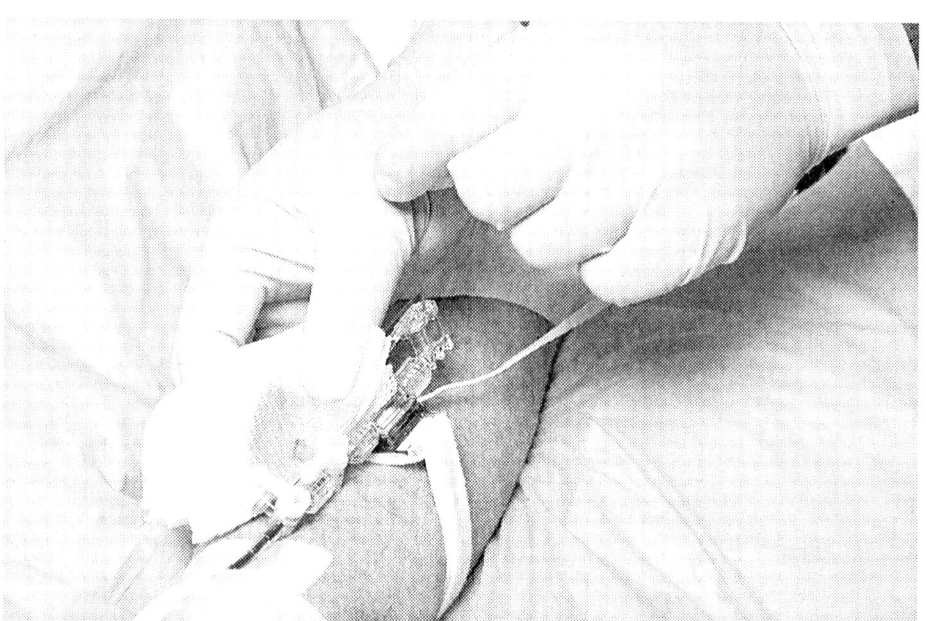

f

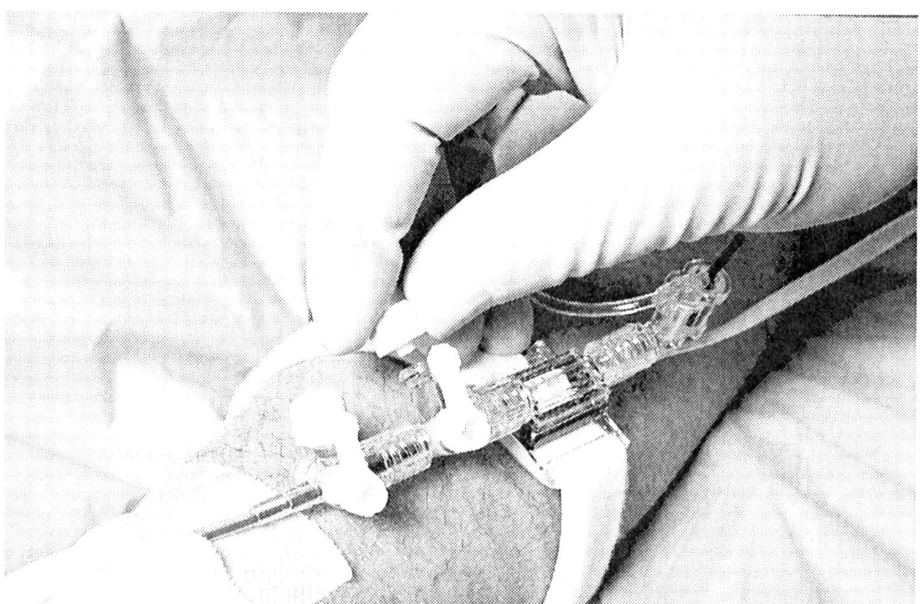

g

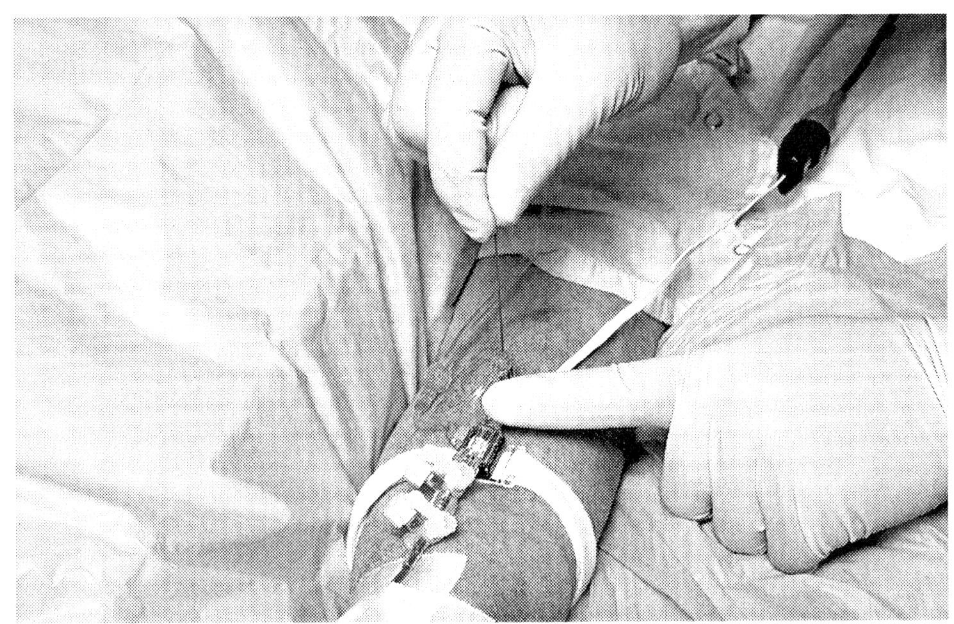

h

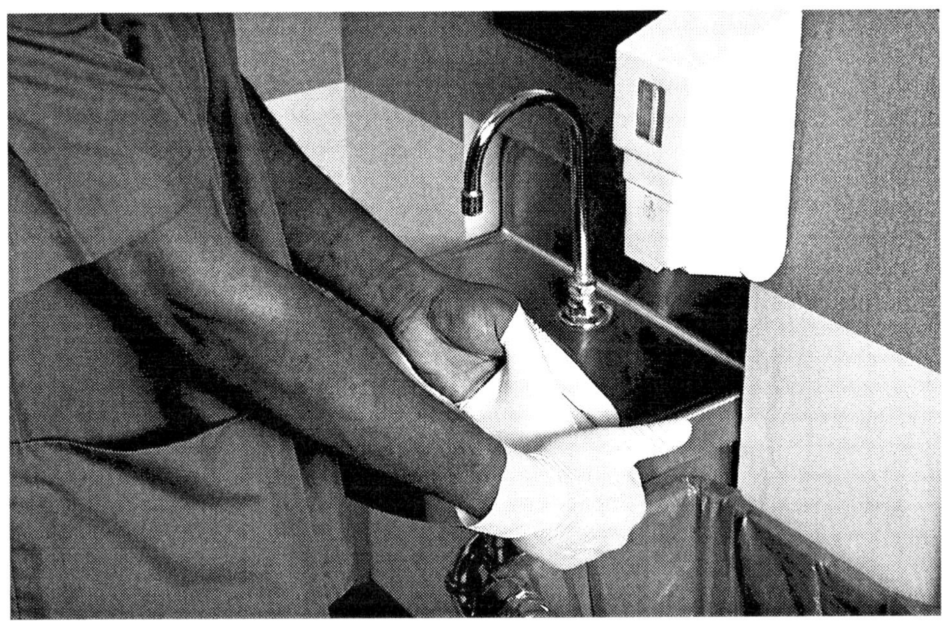

i

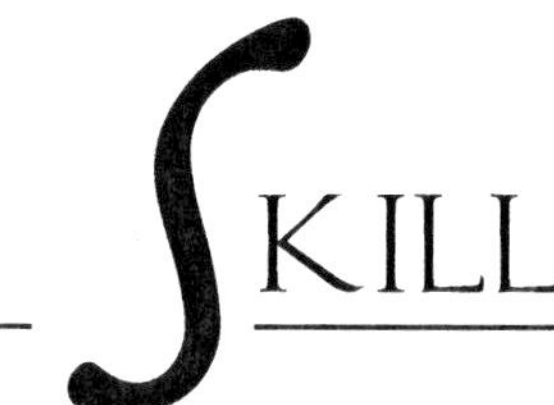

# SKILL

## Removing an Arterial Line

***Purpose*** Caregivers remove arterial lines when the patient no longer requires one or when there is evidence of an infection.

### Objectives

**The caregiver demonstrates the ability to do the following:**

1. Gather the correct supplies.
2. Communicate using a style that reduces the patient's anxiety.
3. Maintain sterile technique.
4. Correctly remove an arterial line catheter and apply a pressure dressing.
5. Respond appropriately to possible complications.
6. Report the results of the procedure to the RN or preceptor.

### Key Terms

**Transducer** A device that can convert pulse waves into electrical energy that is visible on a monitor as a waveform and a systolic and diastolic number.

**Fluid-filled Pressure Tubing** Specialized rigid tubing that connects the vascular system (the artery) and the transducer.

**Heparinized Solution** A solution containing the drug heparin, which is used to keep the system patent.

**Pressure Bag** A device that holds the heparinized solution under 300 mm Hg pressure to maintain flow against the patient's own arterial pressure.

**Intraflow Device** A device that limits the amount of continuous flow being delivered through the pressurized system yet allows the caregiver to flush the system after blood draws to keep it clear.

### Supplies/Equipment

Blue pad • Clean gloves • Sterile gloves • Suture removal kit • Sterile 4×4s • Tape

### Pertinent Point

The discontinuation of an arterial line requires sterile technique.

### Age-Specific Considerations

Older adults or those patients with very sensitive or fragile skin might benefit from hyperallergenic or paper tape to secure their dressing. The dressing is applied after the arterial line is removed.

### Key Concept

Firm pressure must be maintained over the site for at least 5 minutes for radial catheters and at least 10 minutes for femoral catheters until bleeding has completely stopped. Uncontrolled arterial bleeding can result in death.

## Steps

1. Wash hands.
2. Identify the correct patient.
3. Explain the procedure to the patient.
4. Assemble the equipment.
5. Turn the arterial line monitor alarm off.
6. Place the blue pad under the patient's arm (or groin if the catheter is in the femoral artery).
7. Close the arterial catheter stop-cock to the patient (Figure 6.42a).
8. Deflate the pressure bag (Figure 6.42b).
9. Put on clean gloves.
10. Remove and discard the arterial line dressing, being careful not to dislodge the catheter.
11. Remove and discard gloves; wash hands.
12. Put on sterile gloves.

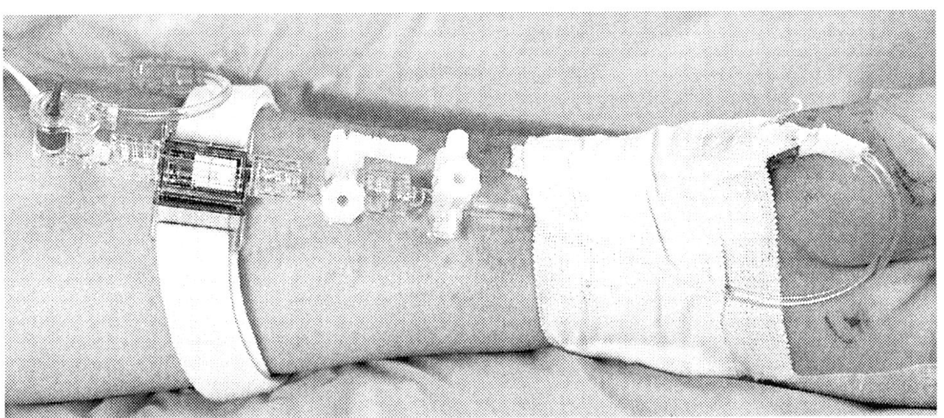

a

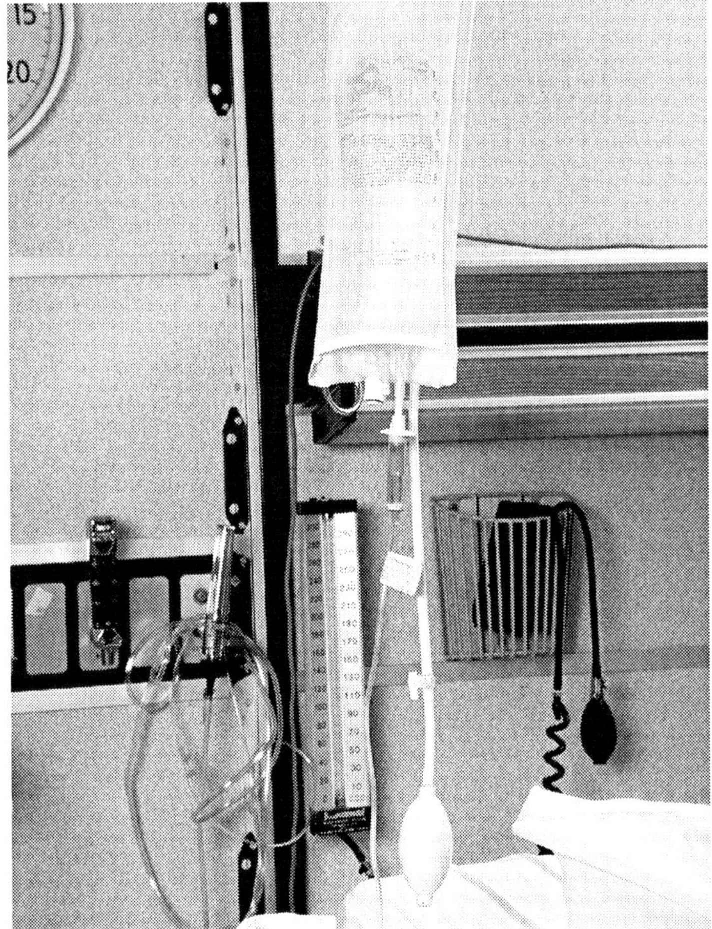

b

**Figure 6.42**
Removing an arterial line.

**13.** Cut and remove the skin sutures while stabilizing the catheter (Figure 6.42c).

**14.** Withdraw the catheter, and immediately apply firm pressure directly over the site with a 4×4s (Figure 6.42d).

**15.** Stand by as the RN assesses the integrity of the catheter and documents the condition of the site and the time of removal.

**16.** Place fingertips of one hand over the artery and apply firm pressure for a minimum of 5 minutes for radial sites and 10 minutes for femoral sites.

**17.** Check the site; if bleeding or sudden swelling occurs, reapply firm pressure for an additional 5 to 10 minutes; continue until bleeding stops.

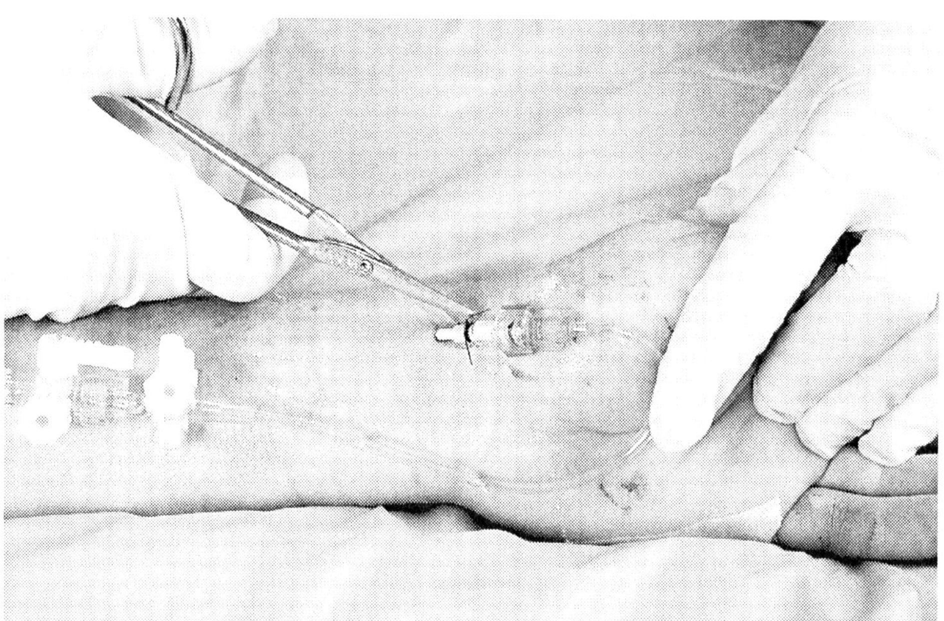

c

d

18. After the RN checks the site, place one sterile folded 4×4 (or 2×2) over the puncture site, and tape firmly to apply pressure (Figure 6.42e).
19. Write the date and time and your initials on the pressure dressing.
20. Instruct the patient to avoid putting pressure on the affected extremity for a few hours and to notify the staff whether the dressing feels warm or wet. Reapply pressure immediately for bleeding or sudden swelling. The pressure dressing may be removed after 8 hours.
21. Disconnect and discard the tubing, and empty the infusion bag into the sink.
22. Do not discard the cable or the pressure bag.
23. Dispose of the suture removal kit and any sharps in a sharps container.
24. Return the cable and the pressure bag to the appropriate place on the unit.
25. Notify the RN of any bleeding, swelling, ecchymosis, or complaints of pain or numbness.
26. Document and report the results to the RN or preceptor.

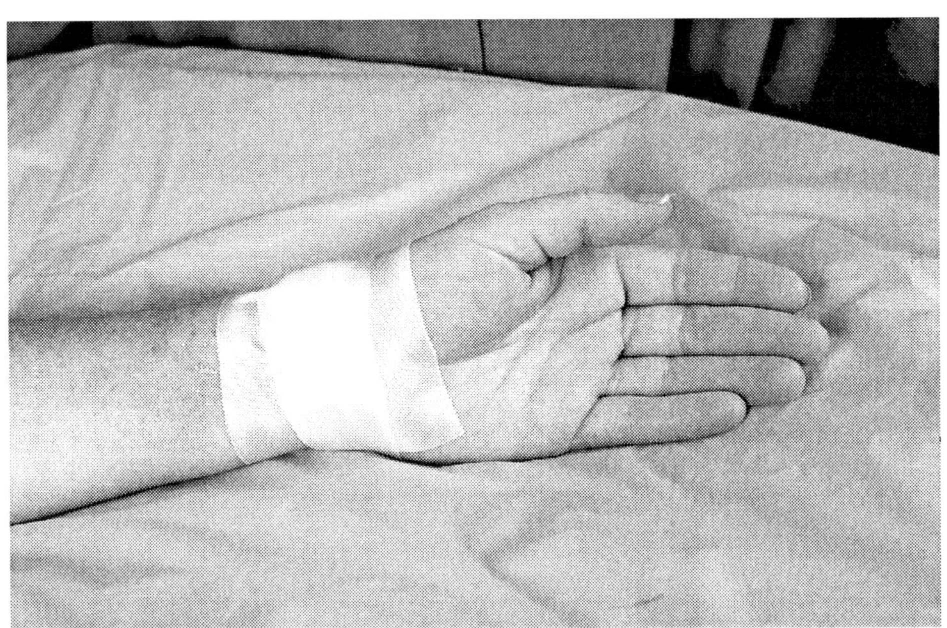

e

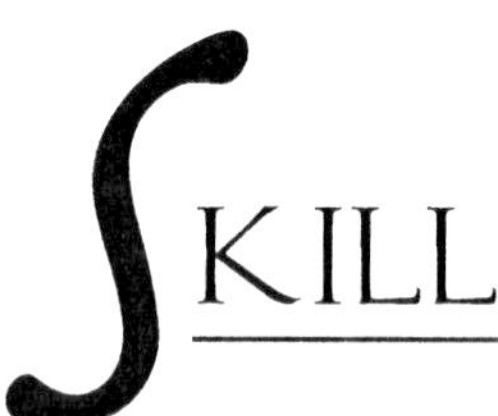

# Palpating Dorsalis Pedis and Posterior Tibial Pulses

**Purpose** The purpose of palpating the dorsalis pedis and posterior tibial pulses is to check the flow of blood or the presence of blood circulation to the feet and toes (Figure 6.43). This is very important when caring for patients with circulation disorders or patients who have had procedures that assess the status of their circulation. These pulses are located and assessed before and after the patient has the procedure.

## Objectives

**The caregiver demonstrates the ability to do the following:**

1. Gather the correct supplies.
2. Communicate using a style that reduces the patient's anxiety.
3. Correctly identify the presence of the dorsalis pedis and posterior tibial pulses.
4. Report the results of the procedure to the RN or preceptor.

## Key Terms

**Doppler** The machine that locates pulses based on the Doppler effect. There is a change in the frequency of sound waves as the probe (sensor) gets closer to the pulse of the patient. The sound decreases as the probe gets farther away from the pulse.

**Dorsalis Pedis (DP) Pulse** The pulse of the dorsalis pedis artery, which supplies blood to various muscles of the foot and toes. In about 90 percent of people, it is located between the first and second toes on the top of the foot.

**Posterior Tibial (PT) Pulse** The pulse of the posterior tibial artery, which supplies blood to a variety of muscles in the lower leg, foot, and toes. It is located in the inner aspect of the ankle, just below the anklebone.

## Supplies/Equipment

Doppler machine • Doppler jelly • Marker • Washcloth

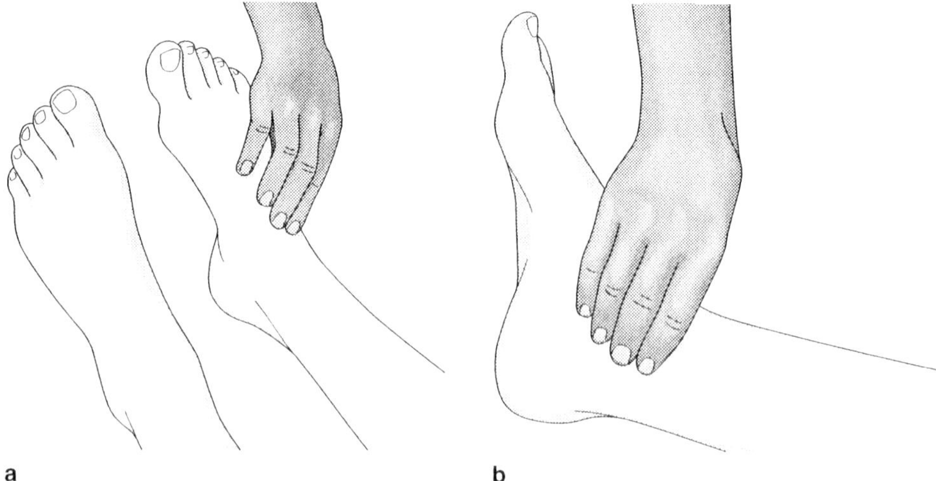


**Figure 6.43** Checking (a) dorsalis pedis pulse and (b) posterior tibial pulse.

- The DP and PT pulses can be palpated using your index and middle fingers.
- Because of chronic medical conditions—such as atherosclerosis, diabetes, and peripheral vascular disease—a patient's pulses might be very weak or impossible to palpate. In this case, a Doppler machine is used to obtain the pulses.
- Signs of reduced or poor circulation are skin that blanches slowly, skin that is very pale or dusky, and even necrotic areas on the lower legs, toes, or feet.
- The sudden absence of the DP or PT pulse after a procedure signals that an occlusion has occurred in the peripheral circulation. This is a medical emergency and requires immediate action. Notify the RN immediately. The RN will inform the physician of the patient's loss of the pulse, vital signs, and general condition.

## Pertinent Points

## Age-Specific Considerations

Due to hereditary and lifestyle factors, as people age they sometimes become more susceptible to chronic diseases that reduce the amount of blood flow throughout the body. The skin on their feet might be very fragile or thick and tough. Some people are sensitive to the coldness of the Doppler jelly. Out of respect for the seriousness of these conditions, do not rush patients. Give them time to ask questions. Be respectful at all times, and acknowledge the anxiety that is a part of all of these procedures. Inform all patients of what you are doing and why. Keep the patient's feet covered with blankets between pulse checks.

## Key Concept

The presence of the pulses indicates that an occlusion has not formed and that the circulation to the feet and toes is intact. If a pulse is lost (cannot be palpated), there has been a blockage of the circulation, often due to a blood clot.

## Steps

1. Wash hands.
2. Identify the correct patient.
3. Explain the procedure to the patient.
4. Assemble the equipment.
5. Uncover the patient's feet by untucking the sheets at the end of the bed. Leave the covers over the patient's body for warmth and privacy.
6. With a gentle but firm touch (avoid tickling), feel for the DP pulse (on the top of the patient's foot, between the first and second toes). If you are unable to palpate any pulse after trying for several minutes, use a Doppler machine:
   - **a.** Apply the Doppler jelly to the area where the DP pulse should be located.
   - **b.** Apply the Doppler pencil or sensor on the jelly. Slowly move the sensor until the pulse is audible. Listen for a whooshing sound.
   - **c.** Using the marker, note the location of the pulse with an *X* on the patient's skin (Figure 6.44a). This will help with the next pulse check (Figure 6.44b).
   - **d.** Wipe off the excess Doppler jelly with the washcloth.
7. Using the same gentle but firm touch, palpate the PT pulse (inner aspect of the ankle below the ankle bone). You might need to use the Doppler again to locate the pulse.

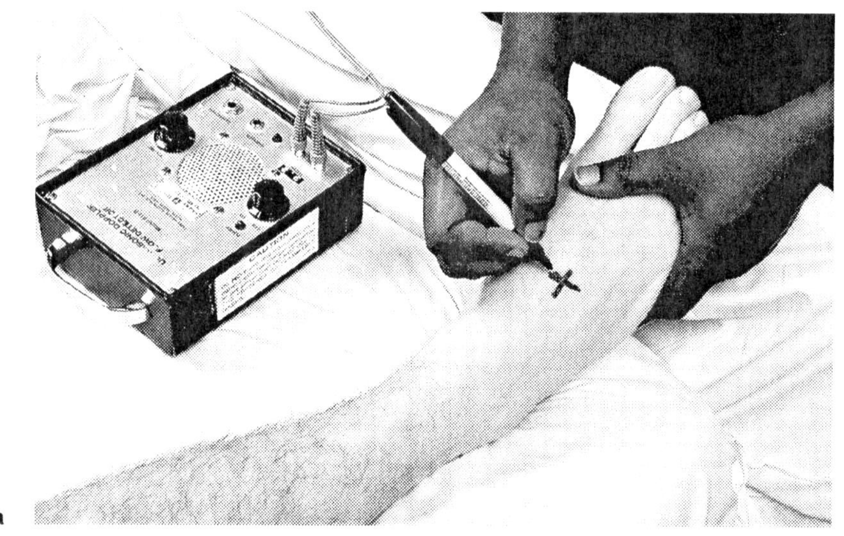

a

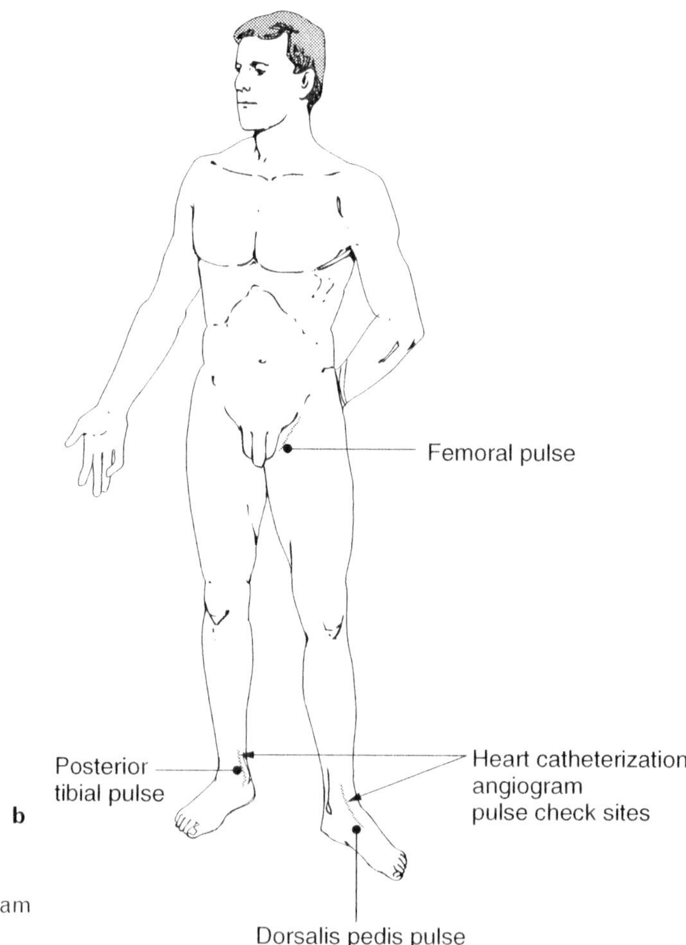


b

**Figure 6.44** (a) Marking a pulse. (b) Pulse sites to monitor during a post-heart catheterization/angiogram check.

8. Mark the location of the PT pulse with the marker on the patient's skin.
9. Turn off the Doppler. Cover the patient's feet for warmth.
10. Document the presence of the pulses by indicating whether each was positive (+) or negative (−).
11. Report the results to the RN or preceptor.

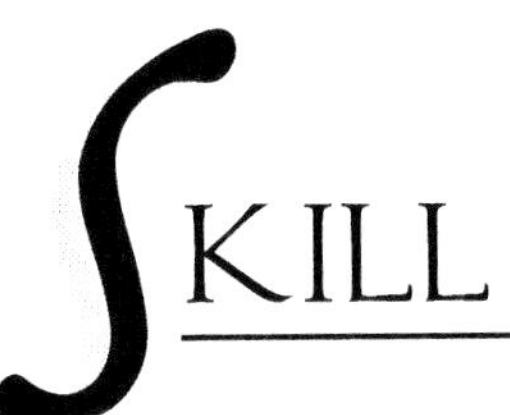

# SKILL

## Removing a PTCA Femoral Sheath

*Purpose* Percutaneous transluminal coronary angioplasty (PTCA) has been used with increasing frequency to treat patients with coronary artery disease. Many cardiac patients are sent to intermediate or progressive care units with femoral sheaths in place. Before RNs or patient care technicians (PCTs) can discontinue these lines, caregivers must demonstrate competency in manual compression and in the use of the C-clamp, which is a mechanical compression device (Figure 6.45).

### Objectives

**The caregiver demonstrates the ability to do the following:**

1. Gather the correct supplies.
2. Communicate using a style that reduces the patient's anxiety.
3. Remove a femoral sheath using manual compression.
4. Remove a femoral sheath using a C-clamp.
5. Describe possible complications associated with the procedure.
6. Report the results of the procedure to the RN or preceptor.

### Key Terms

**C-clamp** A mechanical device that holds pressure on a blood vessel.

**Femoral Sheath** A large catheter placed in the femoral artery that provides an entryway so that the balloon angioplasty catheter can be placed and threaded to the coronary arteries. The sheath is left in after removal of the angioplasty catheter until coagulation studies are near normal. The sheath is then removed.

**Hemostasis** The formation of a blood clot.

**Hematoma** A mass that forms when blood escapes the vessel and goes out into the tissues or a cavity. Bruising usually results.

**Manual Compression** A technique in which the caregiver uses the hands to compress a blood vessel to stop the bleeding.

**Vasovagal Response** A response that can occur when the vagus nerve is stimulated during compression of the femoral artery. Symptoms include a decrease in the level of consciousness; cold, clammy skin; pale skin; nausea and vomiting; decreased blood pressure; and a decrease in the heart rate.

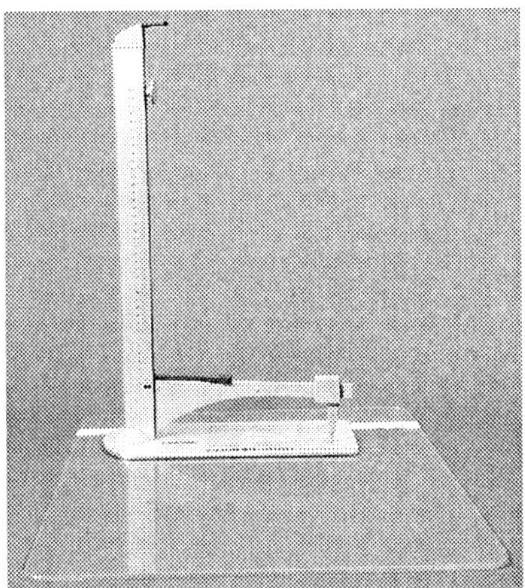

**Figure 6.45** Plexiglas board and C-clamp.

## Supplies/ Equipment

Doppler machine • Doppler jelly • Tape • Clean gloves • Sterile gloves • Suture removal kit • Sterile 4×4s • Plexiglas board, C-clamp, and sterile disc (if appropriate) • Butterfly dressing • Personal protective equipment: apron and goggles

## Pertinent Points

- Since percutaneous transluminal coronary angioplasty was first introduced in 1977, it has been used with increasing frequency to treat patients with coronary artery disease. It is estimated that more than five hundred thousand angioplasties are performed in the United States annually.
- PTCA is a nonsurgical procedure that uses a balloon to dilate the diseased coronary arteries. The balloon catheter is advanced through a larger sheath in the femoral artery. The sheath provides structural support in the artery for the catheters used in the procedure. After the PTCA, the sheath is left in place from 4 to 12 hours to allow easy access for restudy if needed. Some sheaths are removed as soon as a coagulation study—for example, an automated coagulation timer (ACT) or partial thromboplastin time (PTT)—is within a safe range to avoid bleeding complications.
- While still in place, the sheath may be used as an arterial line to draw blood for lab tests. The sheath is connected to a pressurized bag of normal saline with heparin—the same one used for radial arterial lines to maintain patency of the line. A number of different-size sheaths are made by different manufacturers. Before drawing blood to be sent to the lab, discard approximately three times the amount of dead space of the sheath (approximately 5 cc for a size 7 or 8 French). The stopcock closest to the patient can be used. For coagulation studies, six times the dead space (or approximately 10 cc) is discarded before drawing the specimen. Check the manufacturer's recommendations for the catheters used in your facility.
- Most angioplasty patients can have the sheath removed using applied pressure for approximately 15 to 30 minutes. Sandbags are sometimes used to maintain pressure to a site for lengthy time periods. In patients with an intracoronary stent (a metal device that is implanted to hold the artery open), the compression time increases from 30 to 60 minutes, depending on institution protocol. Generally, these patients receive more medications to thin the blood, causing more risk for bleeding—thus the longer compression time.
- Complications associated with this procedure include hematoma (swelling or massing of blood into the surrounding tissues), inadequate blood flow to the foot, bleeding, and vasovagal response. A vasovagal response includes any of the following symptoms: decreased level of consciousness; cold, clammy, pale skin; nausea and vomiting; decrease in blood pressure; and decrease in heart rate.
- When using the manual method, the caregiver must maintain straight wrist alignment while using either two fingers or two knuckles to apply pressure on the femoral pulse above the site.

## Age-Specific Considerations

Fewer premedication narcotics might be required before a sheath removal in an older adult due to the metabolism of these drugs in older patients. Care should be taken when lifting the C-clamp disc, as it might stick to fragile skin and cause a break in the skin. Gently break the suction of the disc against the skin, using the fingertip, before removal.

Key Concept

An RN must be present during a sheath removal to manage the patient in case he or she experiences a vasovagal response while another RN or caregiver removes the sheath. The RN must remain in the patient's room during and for at least 5 minutes after the procedure. The RN will give the patient sedation as ordered. Atropine (a medication that can increase the heart rate) can be given intravenously by the RN, along with a fluid bolus, according to established protocols.

Steps

1. Perform the procedure only after being instructed to do so by the RN. (The RN must identify whether the patient's ACT or PTT results indicate readiness to have the sheath removed.)
2. Wash hands.
3. Identify the correct patient.
4. Explain the procedure to the patient.
5. Assemble the equipment and inform the RN when ready to perform the procedure (Figures 6.46a and b).
6. Locate the dorsalis pedis pulse and secure the Doppler in place with tape (Figure 6.46c).
7. Adjust the height of the bed so that your body can be positioned directly over the patient. Place the nurse call light within easy reach.
8. Wash hands thoroughly. Put on clean gloves and personal protective equipment (apron and goggles).
9. Remove the dressing from the groin. Discard the dressing and gloves; wash hands. (Some facilities may omit the hand wash and have the caregiver immediately put on sterile gloves.)

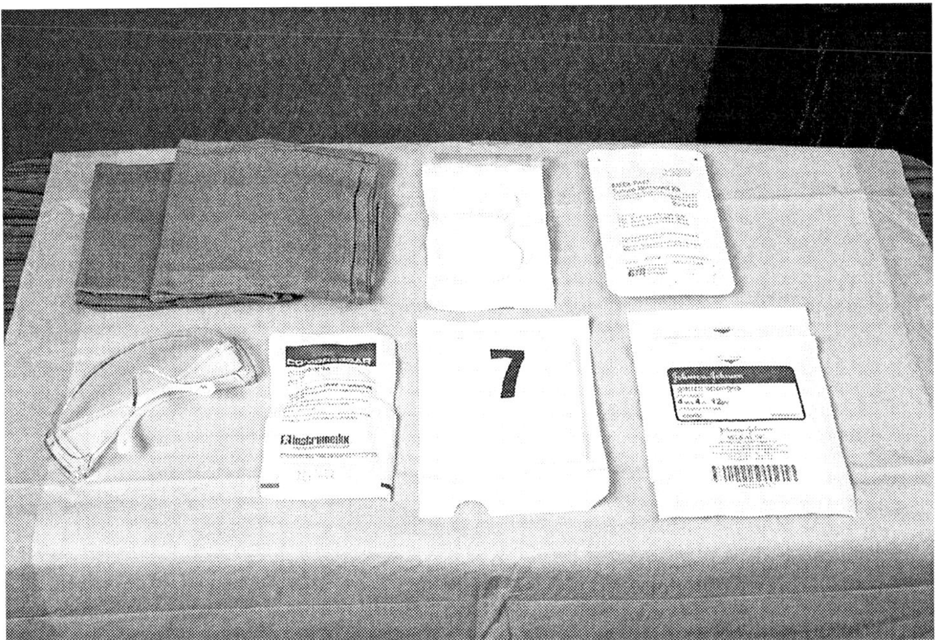


**Figure 6.46 a.** Assemble supplies and equipment including plexiglas board and C-clamp (see Figure 6.46b).

10. Put on sterile gloves and remove sutures from around the sheath site (Figure 6.46d).

11. Instruct the patient to breathe normally during sheath removal to avoid decreased heart rate due to vasovagal response.

12. Locate the femoral pulse.

13. Remove the sheath:
   a. Visualize the site.
   b. Use a single layer of gauze.
   c. Apply firm, focused pressure.
   d. Position hand correctly.
   e. Pull the sheath in one smooth, steady motion.

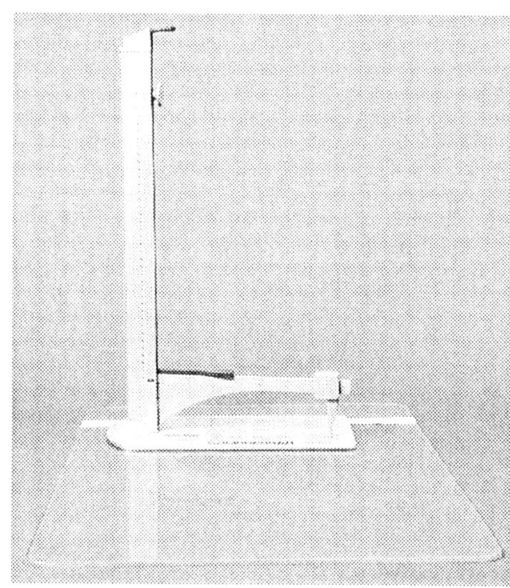

**Figure 6.46 b.** Plexiglas board and C-clamp.

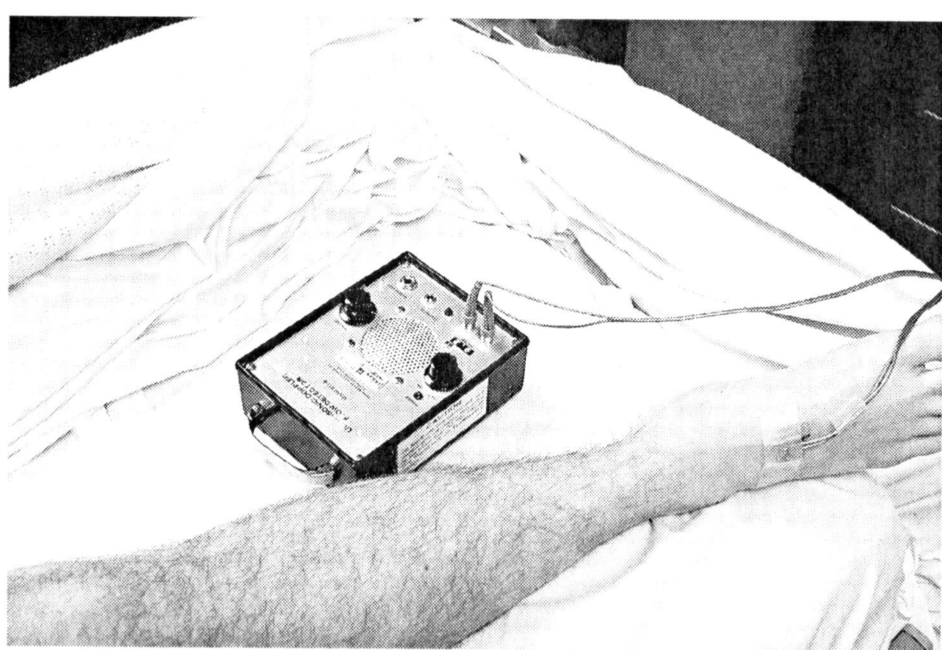

**Figure 6.46 c.** Doppler in place.

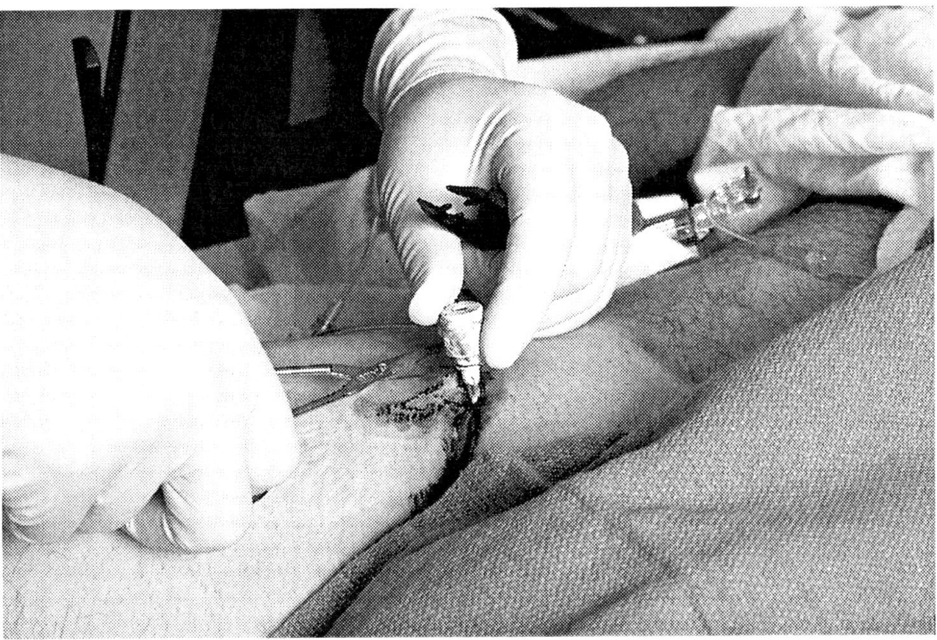

**Figure 6.46 d.** Suture removal.

**14. Manual Method:**

**a.** Apply firm pressure above the puncture site until hemostasis is achieved. The RN will monitor the ECG for vasovagal responses.

**b.** Maintain firm pressure for 15 to 20 minutes.

**c.** Occlude the dorsalis pedis pulse for 3 to 5 minutes. Then release just enough pressure so that you can hear a faint pulse over the Doppler.

**d.** Release pressure *slowly* after 15 to 20 minutes, and watch for bleeding.

**e.** If bleeding continues, reapply pressure for 5 to 10 minutes, then check again for continued bleeding. Continue until bleeding stops.

**C-clamp Method:**

**a.** Apply pressure using the C-clamp.

**b.** Position the Plexiglas board under the patient to provide a firm surface to place the C-clamp on (Figure 6.47a).

**c.** Position the C-clamp on the Plexiglas board but under the patient.

**d.** Attach the sterile disc to the tip of the compressor arm.

**e.** Position the C-clamp disc above the puncture site so that it can be lowered, with pressure applied, while the sheath is removed (Figures 6.47b, c, and d). Take care not to apply too much pressure before the sheath is out. This can cause a milking effect on any clot that is within the sheath.

**f.** Apply firm pressure above the puncture site until hemostasis is achieved. The RN will monitor the ECG for vasovagal responses.

**g.** Occlude the dorsalis pedis pulse for 3 to 5 minutes. Then release just enough pressure to allow some blood flow to the foot. A slight pulse will be audible over the Doppler.

**h.** Release the pressure *slowly*, using the release level on the C-clamp, after 15 to 20 minutes. Watch for bleeding (Figures 6.47e and f).

**i.** If bleeding continues, reapply the C-clamp.

**j.** Apply manual pressure if bleeding cannot be controlled with the C-clamp.

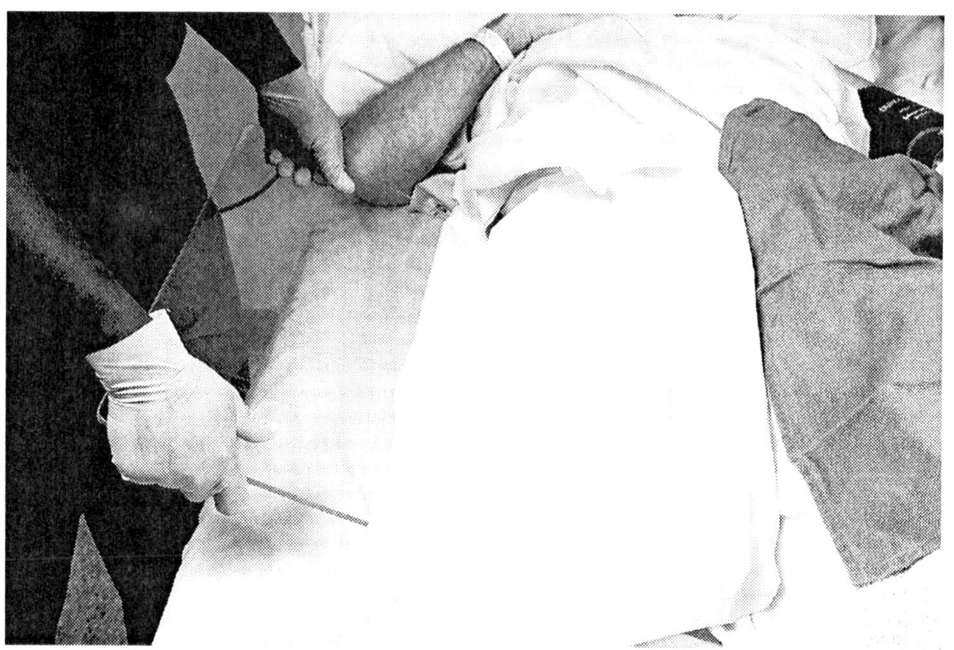

a

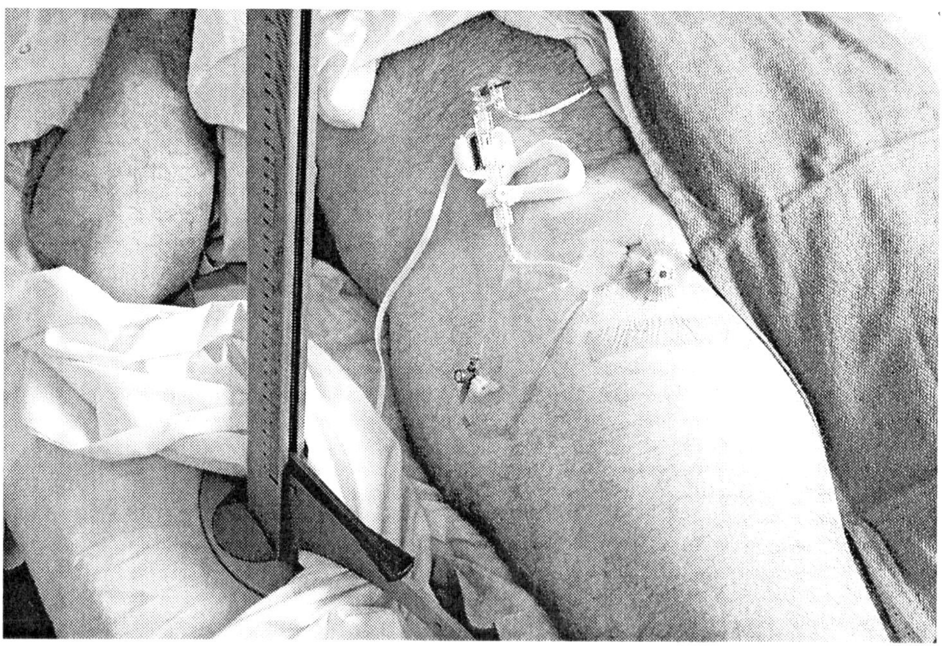

b

**Figure 6.47** Positioning the C-clamp.

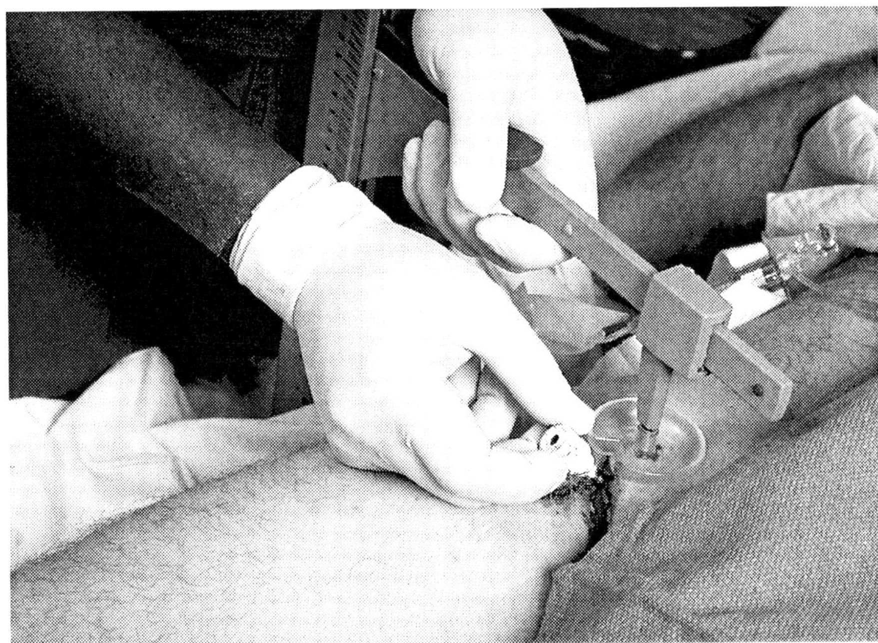

c

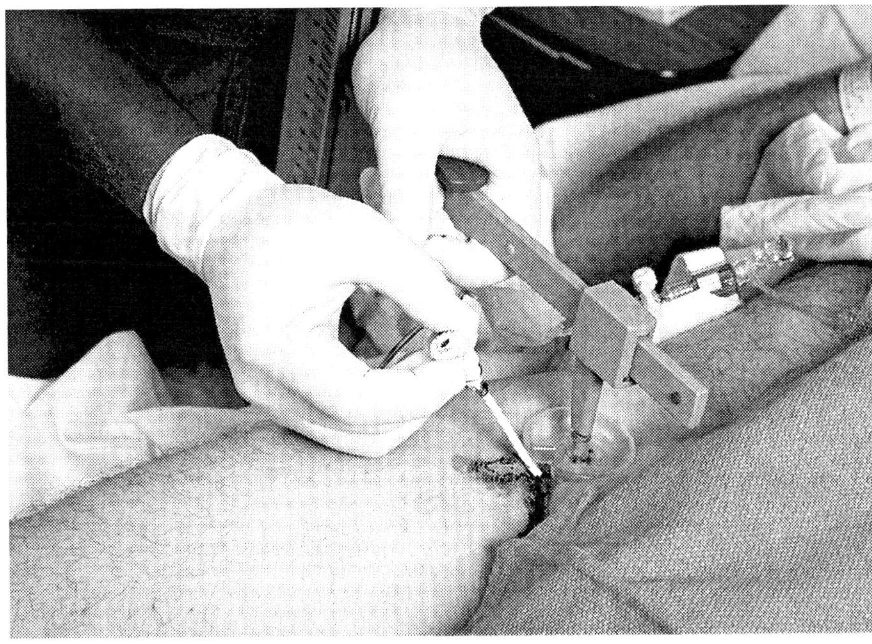

d

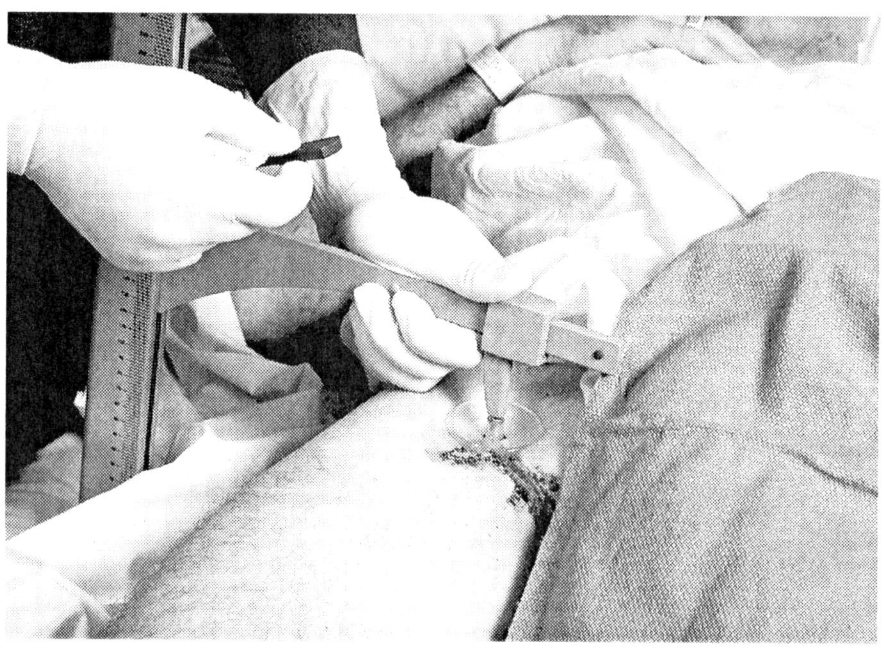

e

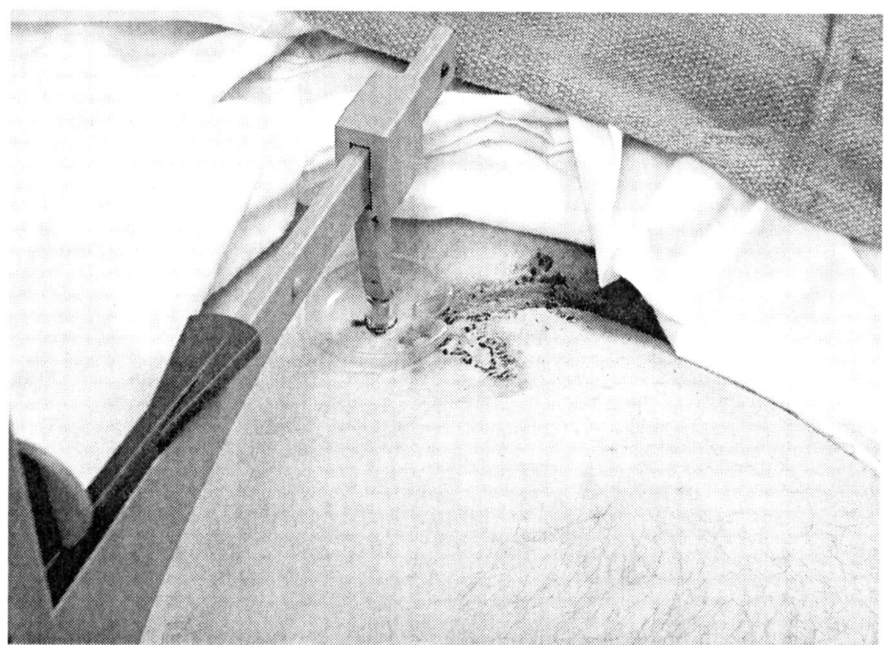

f

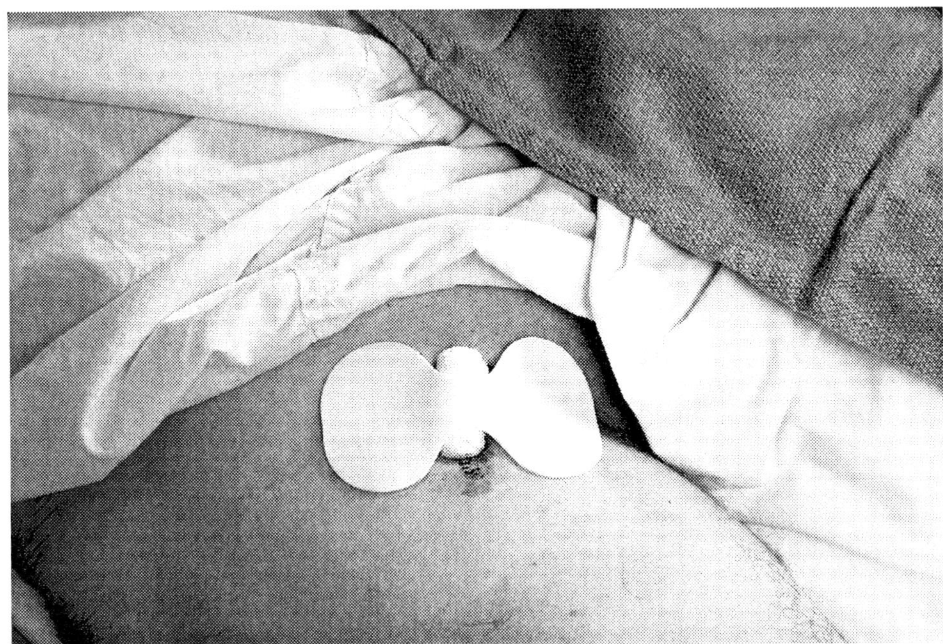

g

15. Observe the site for 3 to 5 minutes before applying the butterfly dressing (Figure 6.47g).
16. Document the patient's vital signs, pedal pulse checks, and dressing checks every 15 minutes for a half hour, then every 30 minutes for an hour, then every hour for 4 hours, and every 4 hours until patient is discharged. Check under the dressing for bleeding. Also check the patient's posterior and buttocks for signs of internal bleeding or hematomas.
17. Notify the RN immediately if you note any of the following: abnormalities in vital signs, chest pain, bleeding on dressing, hematoma, or diminished pedal pulses.
18. Instruct the patient to call for the RN for any of the following signs:
    - **a.** Signs of bleeding, feelings of warm blood oozing, or stickiness
    - **b.** Signs of compromised circulation—coolness, numbness, pain, dizziness
    - **c.** Signs of hematoma
    - **d.** Chest pain
19. Instruct the patient to remain flat in bed (or with the head of the bed up 15 degrees), usually for 4 to 6 hours. Then the patient can be up with assistance. The patient may be logrolled.
20. Remind the patient to apply firm pressure directly on the dressing over the insertion site whenever laughing, coughing, sneezing, bearing down, or tightening the abdominal muscles in any way.
21. Discard the dressings, sheath, and gloves in the appropriate medical waste container.
22. Document and report the results to the RN or preceptor.

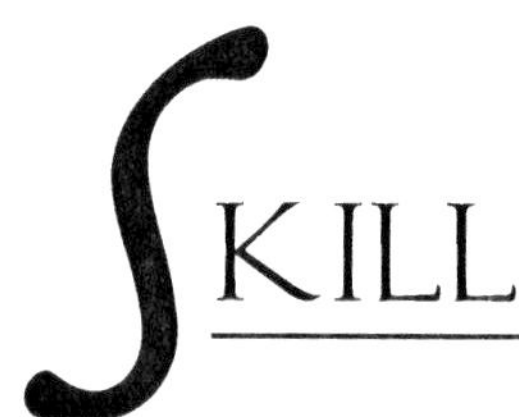

# SKILL

## Performing a Postcardiac Catheterization Check

***Purpose*** A patient might require a cardiac catheterization for any of several reasons. A major purpose of cardiac catheterization is to determine the presence, location, and severity of any blockage to the arteries that supply blood to the heart. Catheterization is also performed to evaluate the function of the heart muscle and of the valves of the heart and to assess any damage to the heart from a heart attack, infection, or trauma. Finally, cardiac catheterization is often performed to assess the status of bypass surgery grafts.

### Objectives

**The caregiver demonstrates the ability to do the following:**

1. Gather the correct supplies.
2. Communicate using a style that reduces the patient's anxiety.
3. Receive the patient after the catheterization.
4. Perform the postcardiac catheterization check.
5. Assist with patient care after the monitoring period is over.
6. Document observations appropriately.
7. Report the results of the procedure to the RN or preceptor.

### Key Term

**Cardiac Catheterization** A common technique for studying the structure and function of the heart. It allows the physician to view the blood supply to the heart and to view the various chambers and valves in the heart. Also called heart cath, coronary angiogram, arteriogram, and angiography.

### Supplies/Equipment

Gloves • Doppler machine • Doppler jelly • Washcloth

### Pertinent Points

- Cardiac catheterization is performed with a soft, narrow, flexible tube or catheter.
- The physician, usually a cardiologist, numbs the area that will be used. (The artery in the groin is usually selected, but the arm is another possible site.) The physician inserts the catheter into the artery and guides it into the heart. An X-ray dye is injected through the catheter into the heart so that the structures of the heart can be seen by X-ray. Patients often feel a warm, flushing feeling during this part of the procedure. When all of the X-ray pictures have been taken, the catheter is removed. Pressure is applied to the artery in the groin or arm for 10 to 20 minutes to allow the artery to close, and then a dressing is placed over the insertion site.
- Patients are not allowed to bend their leg or arm for a period of time after the test, and there will be specific activity restrictions.
- Patients are encouraged to drink fluids after the test to help flush the dye from their systems.

### Age-Specific Considerations

Due to the serious nature of this test, people of all ages are often nervous and anxious. Many of the patients who have this test are older adults. Keep the developmental factors of this age group in mind when providing care. Give step-by-step instructions when providing information. Speak in a low-pitched, clear voice. Be respectful. Provide for the patient's comfort and safety. While technological advances have come to be expected in the medical world, it is still a strange and often frightening environment for many patients.

Key Concept

The most important signs and symptoms to watch for during the post-cardiac catheterization check are discomfort, swelling, or bleeding at the catheter insertion site; chest pain; and numbness or coldness in the limb used for the test. The complications of cardiac catheterization are rare, but they must always be kept in mind. They include bleeding, allergic reaction, blood clot, infection, rhythm disturbance, injury to the heart, and death.

Steps

1. Wash hands.
2. Identify the patient and help move the patient from the stretcher to the bed.
3. Explain the procedure to the patient. Tell the patient what to expect during the postcardiac catheterization check (length of time for the check; frequency of vital signs; observation of the site and dressing, temperature, pallor of legs and feet; checking for pain, tingling in the leg, or chest pain; and the need to keep the leg or arm straight).
4. Obtain the patient's vital signs.
5. Obtain the dorsalis pedis and posterior tibial pulses.
6. Check the dressing for signs of bleeding or dried blood. Tell the patient to notify you or another caregiver immediately if bleeding occurs.
7. Check the insertion site for bleeding, bruising, swelling, and pain.
8. Check the extremity for color, mottling, and warmth. Ask the patient about any numbness or tingling.
9. Instruct the patient to remain on his or her back or supported by pillows toward the side where procedure was performed. The head of the bed may be elevated only to the degree indicated by the physician. Instruct the patient to apply pressure to the site when coughing or sneezing.
10. Help the RN position the patient to sit, stand, and then walk. This is the most common time for bleeding to occur. Patients should ambulate for 10 to 15 minutes before the pressure dressing and the IV are removed.
11. Document all observations on the flow sheet or patient record.
12. Report the following observations and complaints immediately to the nurse: a major change in blood pressure (+/− 20 mm Hg), bleeding at the insertion site, swelling at the site, tenderness or pain at the site, numbness or tingling in the leg or arm, chest pain, and the inability to urinate.

# CHAPTER 7

# OXYGEN THERAPY AND RESPIRATORY THERAPY

## INTRODUCTION

More and more, nurses and many nursing support staff are being asked to perform skills for a growing number of patients with respiratory conditions or diseases. Advanced respiratory skills are becoming necessary tools for caregivers in a variety of settings, from the acute care setting to the home care environment.

This chapter includes information on the basic anatomy and physiology of the organs of the respiratory system. In addition, it prepares caregivers to perform the following skills, which are listed under the relevant section titles:

*Oxygen-Delivery and Monitoring Devices*

Preparing an Oxygen Cylinder for Use

Setting Up a Nasal Cannula

Setting Up a Simple Face Mask

Setting Up the Pulse Oximeter

*Humidity Therapy*

Setting Up an Oxygen Bubble Humidifier

*Pulmonary Hygiene*

Suctioning a Tracheostomy

Performing Tracheostomy Care

Instructing the Patient in the Use of the Incentive Spirometer

Performing Tracheostomy Stoma Care

# SECTION ONE
# Oxygen-Delivery and Monitoring Devices

Objectives

**This section prepares caregivers to do the following:**

1. Describe the basic function of the respiratory system.
2. Acquire a basic understanding of oxygen-delivery devices and their use in the clinical setting.
3. Demonstrate a basic understanding of pulse oximetry as it relates to the evaluation and regulation of oxygen therapy.
4. Demonstrate clinical competence in applying oxygen, pulse oximetry, and oxygen-delivery devices in the patient setting.

## *Introduction to Respiratory Therapy*

Key Terms

**Alveoli** The microscopic units of the lung in which gas exchange takes place. Alveoli have an extensive blood supply.

**Bronchi** The two large airways that branch off the trachea to the right and left lungs.

**Bronchitis** A condition in which the bronchi become inflamed and swollen and produce hypersecretions.

**Chronic Obstructive Pulmonary Disease (COPD)** A category of respiratory ailments that includes bronchitis, asthma, and emphysema. COPD is characterized by bronchospasm, increased secretions, and shortness of breath.

**Cyanosis** A condition characterized by a bluish tint to the mucous membranes, the lips, and the fingernail beds. This physical finding might indicate a low level of oxygen in the blood.

**Epiglottis** A structure within the trachea that acts to cover the trachea when food is swallowed.

**Fraction of Inspired Oxygen ($FiO_2$)** The amount of oxygen delivered, expressed as a percentage.

**Humidity** Molecular water suspended in a gas. Humidity is used to hydrate artificial airways.

**Larynx** A passageway for air between the pharynx (throat) and the trachea (windpipe).

**Lung** The organ responsible for receiving air and transferring gas to the blood.

**Medulla** The portion of the brain that controls respiration.

**Nose** The nose is an organ whose function is smell, and its nasal cavity acts as an air conditioner, humidifying inspired air and warming it to body temperature. The nasal hairs also act as a filter to prevent debris from entering the respiratory tract.

**Pharynx** The back of the mouth; throat. The pharynx serves as a passageway for both food and air. There are three divisions of the pharynx. The nasopharynx consists of the nasal cavity and nasal sinus and ends at the soft palate. The oropharynx lies behind the mouth and serves as a passageway for food. The laryngopharynx consists of the voice box and ends at the esophagus.

**Respiration** The gas exchange between either individual cells or lung tissue and the blood.

**Respiratory Rate** The number of breaths per minute.

**Ventilation** The movement of air into and out of the lungs.

## Basic Anatomy and Physiology of the Respiratory System

The respiratory system provides a pathway through which oxygen moves from the air into the lungs, where it can be picked up by the blood. The structures that make up this system include the nose and mouth, pharynx (throat), trachea (windpipe), larynx (voice box), lungs, and bronchi. Because we must have oxygen to live, it is necessary to keep this pathway open. The structures themselves help to do this. The trachea and bronchi are kept open by incomplete cartilage rings (Figure 7.1). On the top of the trachea, opening from the pharynx, is a structure

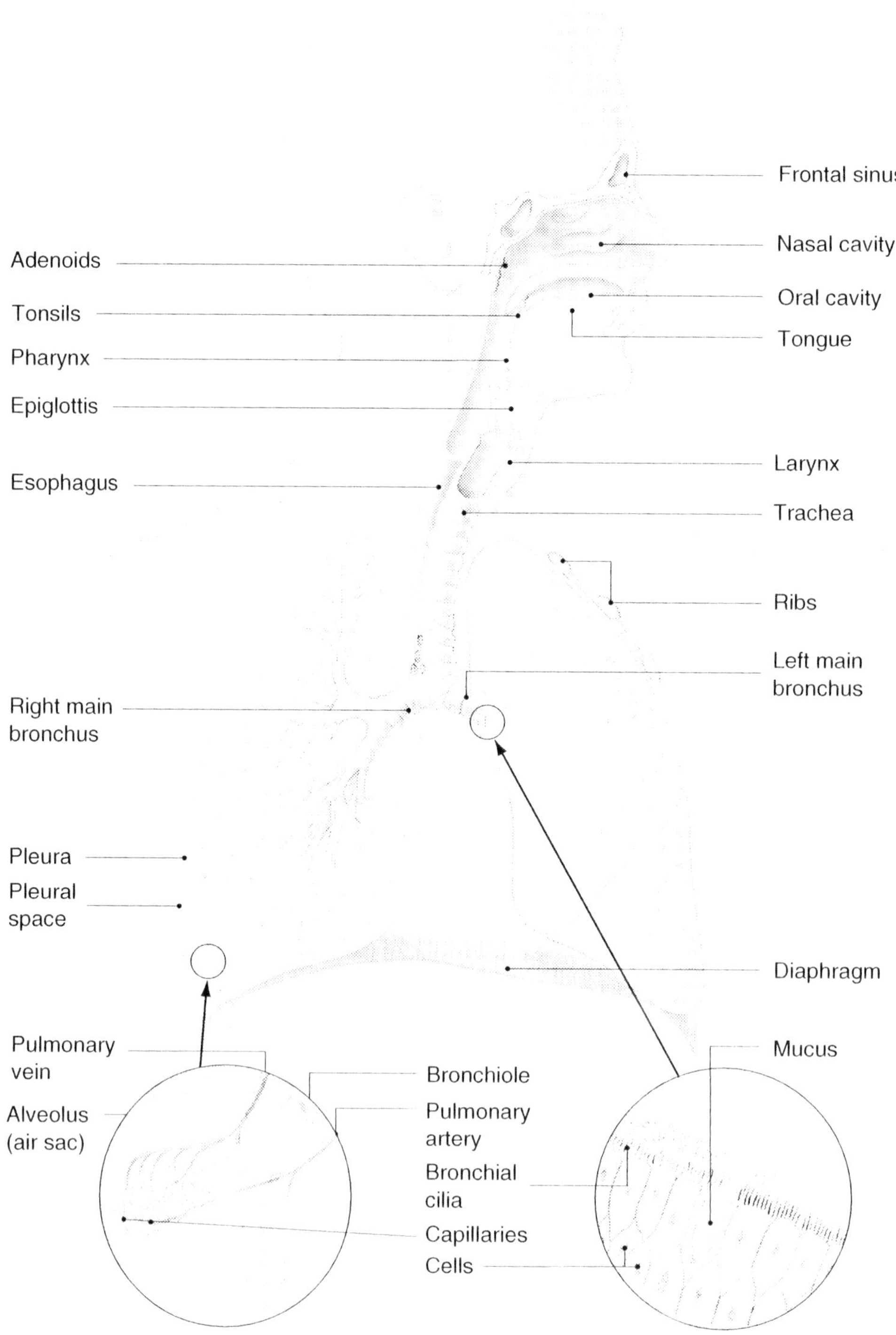


**Figure 7.1** Anatomy of the respiratory system.

known as the larynx. In addition to being the opening to the trachea, it contains the vocal cords, which make it possible for us to talk.

An important piece of cartilage, the epiglottis, covers the opening to the trachea when food is swallowed, preventing the food from getting to the lungs. Very weak patients and those who are having trouble breathing must be watched carefully during feeding so that food does not enter the trachea. This is known as aspiration. An unconscious patient who vomits might also be in danger of aspirating the vomitus. If an unconscious patient vomits, roll the patient to one side at once. You must watch the patient with great care because if the pathway for oxygen is blocked, the patient will die without immediate treatment.

### Oxygen and Carbon Dioxide Exchange

As in the body's other systems, the important work of the respiratory system is done at the cellular level. The exchange of oxygen and carbon dioxide occurs in a unit of the lungs that is so small you would have to use a microscope to see it. At the ends of the last branches of the bronchus—the alveolar ducts—are small sacs called alveoli. Many oxygen molecules fill these sacs after the body breathes air in. The blood has less oxygen, so it can pick up a large amount of oxygen from the alveolar sacs and release the carbon dioxide it is carrying. The blood is then returned to the heart to transport the oxygen around the body.

The respiratory system functions to move oxygen to the blood. Internal respiration occurs when the cells that need the oxygen receive it in exchange for carbon dioxide, which is a cellular waste product. Both functions—the exchange of oxygen and carbon dioxide in the lungs and at the cellular level—are equally important. Breathing is regulated by a center in the medulla, a part of the brain.

### The Respiratory System and the Normal Aging Process

As adults age, the elasticity of the lung tissue decreases, and the airways can become obstructed due to repeated infections or irritants, such as smoking or air pollution. This is known as chronic obstructive pulmonary disease (COPD), which refers to a group of disorders such as bronchitis, asthma, and emphysema.

## Oxygen Therapy

The air we breathe contains two gases: 79 percent is nitrogen, and the remaining 21 percent is oxygen. Supplemental oxygen is widely used for various clinical disorders, both respiratory and nonrespiratory. The administration of oxygen should be based on sound physiological principles. The primary goal of oxygen administration is to prevent hypoxia, a deficiency of oxygen at the tissue level.

*Oxygen therapy* refers to increasing the percentage of oxygen the patient breathes in, technically the fraction of inspired oxygen ($FiO_2$). The goal of oxygen therapy is to relieve hypoxia, decrease the work of breathing, and decrease myocardial work. One objective of oxygen therapy is to improve the oxygenation status of the patient—that is, to increase the amount of oxygen available to the tissues so that the body can function as close to normal as possible. When a hypoxic patient is placed on oxygen, the increased oxygen should relieve the signs and symptoms of hypoxia. In patients suffering from the increased work of breathing, the respiratory muscles work much harder in an attempt to get more air into the lungs. With the use of supplemental oxygen, the patient can breathe with much less effort. When there is inadequate oxygenation, the heart must work harder also. It tries to supply more blood to the tissues; hence, the heart muscles increase their workload to meet the demand for more oxygen. When the amount of inspired oxygen is increased, the heart doesn't have to work as hard to meet the body's demands.

To assess a patient's need for supplemental oxygen, first observe the patient's breathing pattern. Consider the following:

- Are respirations labored?
- Has the respiration rate increased?
- Does the patient report feeling short of breath?
- Is the patient using accessory muscles (neck and intercostal muscles) to assist their ventilation?
- Is the patient wheezing?
- Are there signs of cyanosis—bluish nail beds or a bluish hue to the lips or mucous membranes?

The most reliable method for clinically evaluating the need for oxygen is an arterial blood gas (ABG) performed by a respiratory therapist, nurse, or physician. This test, which involves withdrawing a small amount of blood from the patient's artery, provides the following information:

**pH** A measure of the blood's acidity or alkalinity; the normal range is 7.35 to 7.45.

**$PCO_2$** The amount of carbon dioxide in the blood; the normal range is 35 to 45.

**$PO_2$** The amount of oxygen within the blood; the normal range is 80 to 100.

**Saturation** The amount of oxygen bonded to the red blood cells; the normal range is 96 percent to 98 percent.

The amount of oxygen that the patient will receive is based on the reported values.

Another tool for assessing the patient's need for supplemental oxygen is the noninvasive pulse oximeter, which uses infrared light to determine the patient's oxygen saturation level. It is a very quick method of determining the patient's oxygenation status.

Once it has been decided that the patient would benefit from receiving supplemental oxygen, the correct oxygen-delivery device must be selected.

## Hazards and Complications of Oxygen Therapy

Oxygen is an essential ingredient of life. The air we breathe consists of 21 percent oxygen. Various hazards and complications are associated with oxygen therapy. The use of oxygen poses a considerable fire hazard. Although oxygen is not explosive, it does support combustion and makes flammable items burn much faster and hotter. Never allow an open flame in the presence of oxygen.

There are three complications related to the increased amounts of inspired oxygen:

- *Oxygen-induced hypoventilation or apnea (cessation of breathing).* This complication occurs mainly in the COPD patient who is described as a carbon dioxide retainer—that is, a patient who cannot expel all of the air and carbon dioxide out of the lungs. Carbon dioxide retainers generally have very low oxygen levels and elevated carbon dioxide levels. Their drive to breathe is their chronically low oxygen level. If a carbon dioxide retainer receives supplemental oxygen, the low oxygen level will be elevated, and the drive to breathe might be lost, resulting in cessation of breathing or in a decrease in ventilation or respiratory rate.
- *Absorption atelectasis.* This respiratory condition might develop during inhalation of high oxygen concentrations. If the nitrogen is washed out and replaced by oxygen, the gas volume within the alveoli is reduced because oxygen is rapidly absorbed into the blood, whereas nitrogen is not and maintains a residual volume, helping to keep the alveoli expanded.
- *Oxygen toxicity.* The result of prolonged or continuous high concentrations of supplemental oxygen, oxygen toxicity has been reported to affect the lungs, central nervous system, retina, hematopoietic system, and endocrine organs.

## Oxygen Equipment

Oxygen equipment includes oxygen cylinders, flow meters, and regulators. Safe use, storage, and transport of oxygen equipment are important concepts to incorporate in daily practice.

### Oxygen Cylinders

Oxygen cylinders, or tanks, come in several sizes that are appropriate for various uses and settings. Cylinders are assigned letters to indicate size. The D size cylinder is the smallest. Generally found in the home setting, this cylinder is small enough to carry over one's shoulder in a carrying case. It holds approximately 3 hours of oxygen at a flow rate of 2 liters per minute (l/min). The E size cylinder is found in the hospital setting. At about twice the size of the D cylinder, it holds approximately 5 hours of oxygen at a liter flow rate of 2 l/min. The color code for oxygen cylinders is green, and the international color code for oxygen is white (Figure 7.2).

**Key Concept**

Care must be taken when handling oxygen tanks. The contents are under pressure. Dropping a cylinder might lead to rupture of the flow regulator or the neck of the cylinder, causing a rapid gas leak. For this reason, it is recommended that oxygen cylinders must be transported in an approved carrier.

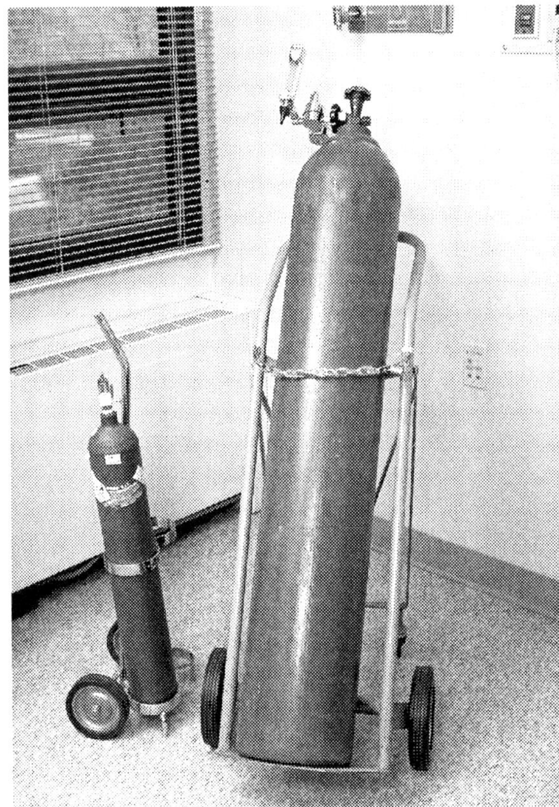

**Figure 7.2** Oxygen cylinders.

*Storage.* The storage area must be permanently posted. Cylinders must be grouped by content, and full and empty cylinders must be segregated. The storage room must be dry, cool, and well ventilated. Cylinders must not be stored near flammable substances and must be protected from being cut or abraded. Cylinders must be protected from extreme weather to prevent rusting, extreme cold, or heat and accumulations of snow and ice. Cylinders should not be stored in an area where the temperature exceeds 125°F. Valves should be kept closed on all empty cylinders at all times.

*Transporting.* If protective valve caps are supplied, they should be used whenever cylinders are in transport and until they are ready for use. Cylinders must not be dropped, dragged, slid, or allowed to strike one another violently. Cylinders must be transported on an appropriate cart and secured by a chain or strap.

*Use.* Before connecting equipment to an oxygen cylinder, be certain that the connections are free of foreign materials. Turn the valve outlet away from personnel, and crack the cylinder valve (open and close the valve to expel a small amount of gas) using an oxygen key (Figure 7.3) to remove any dust or debris from the cylinder valve outlet. Cylinders must be secured at the administration site and not to any movable objects or heat radiators. Outlets and connections must be tightened with only appropriate wrenches and must never be forced on. Equipment designed for one gas should not be used with another. Regulators should be off as the cylinder is turned on, and the cylinder valve should be opened slowly. Before equipment is disconnected from a cylinder, the cylinder valve should be closed and the pressure released from the device. Never lubricate valve outlets or connecting equipment. (Oxygen and oil under pressure cause an explosive oxidation reaction.) A no-smoking sign must be posted conspicuously at the administration site and should be legible from a distance of 5 feet.

An oxygen cylinder contains 2,200 pounds per square inch gauge (psig). As a safety measure, it is advisable to consider a cylinder to be empty when it reaches the 500 psig mark on the pressure gauge. This lessens the possibility that a delay will cause the cylinder to run empty.

### Regulators

All cylinders used for therapy have valves that, in clinical use, are fitted with devices to reduce the pressure (Figure 7.4) going to the patient to a "working pressure," typically 50 psig. Small cylinders (A to F) have a safety system created by the American Standard index called the pin index safety system (PISS; Figure 7.5). The system ensures exact placement with two pins being placed into two holes in the post valve (Figure 7.6).

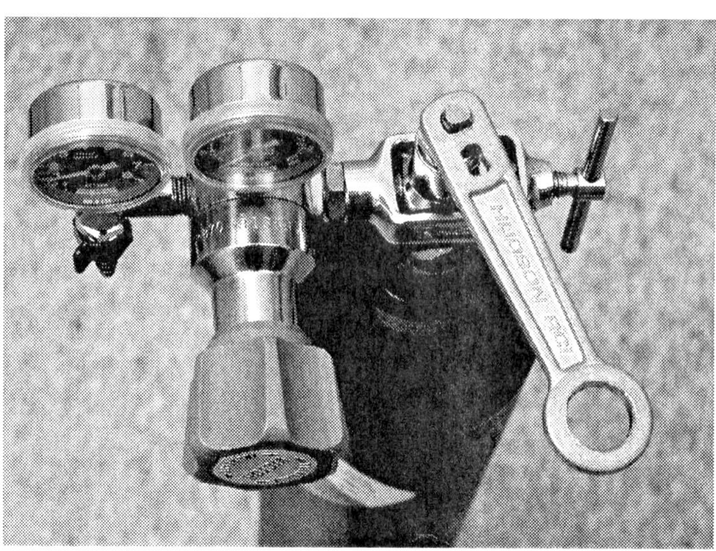

**Figure 7.3** Oxygen key.

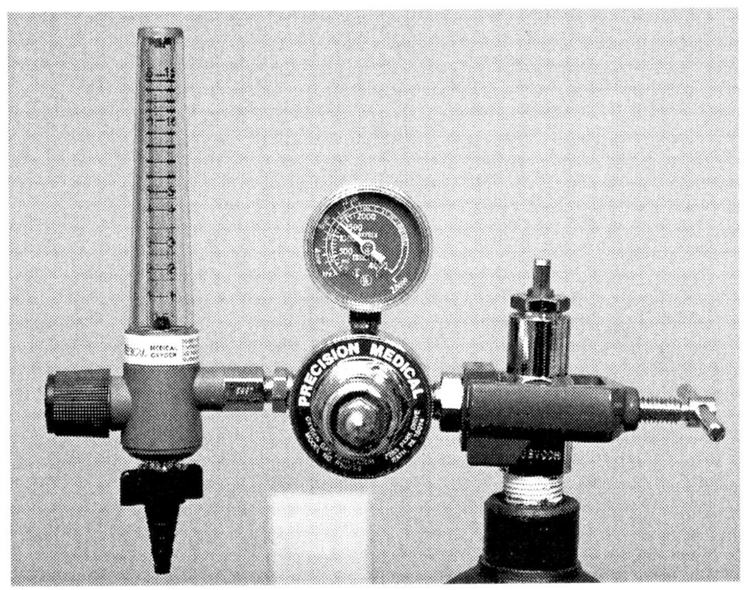


**Figure 7.4** Oxygen E tank, Bourbon regulator, and flowmeter.

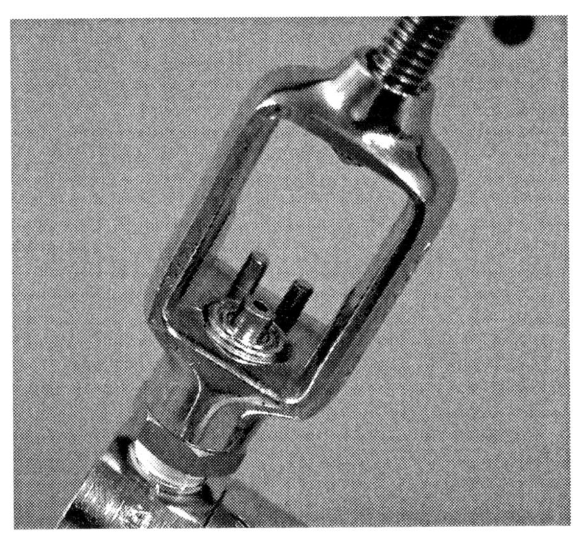

**Figure 7.5** Pins on an oxygen-regulator gauge.

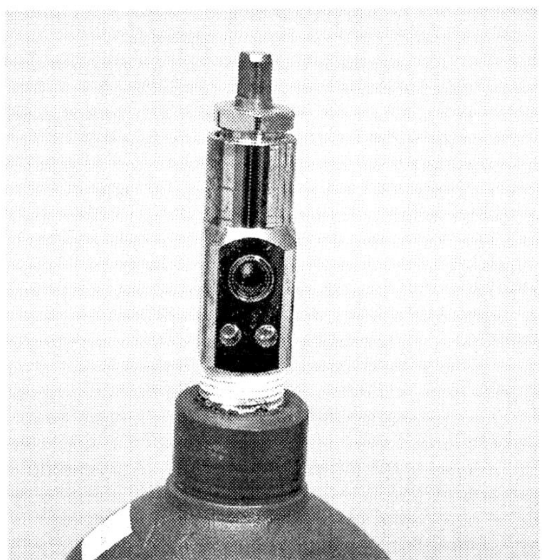

**Figure 7.6** Pin placement on an oxygen tank.

A device attached to the reducing valve, called a flowmeter, controls and indicates flow (see Figure 7.4). As previously described, reducing valves lower gas pressure to a specific working level. A *flowmeter*, by definition, is a device that controls and measures flow. If the two devices, reducing valve and flowmeter, are incorporated into one unit, they become a regulator—a device that reduces high-pressure gas to a safe working pressure as well as controls and measures flow (Figure 7.7).

### Flowmeters

The most common type of flowmeter encountered in respiratory therapy is the Thorpe tube, which incorporates a vertical tube of gradually increasing diameter. The ball float within it is the flow indicator. The liter flow is set by centering the ball with the corresponding line indicating liter flow.

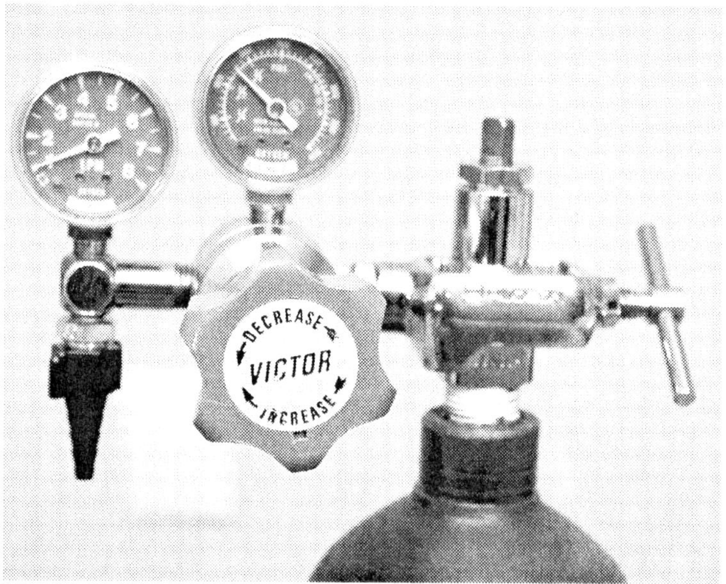


**Figure 7.7** Oxygen E tank and dial gauge.

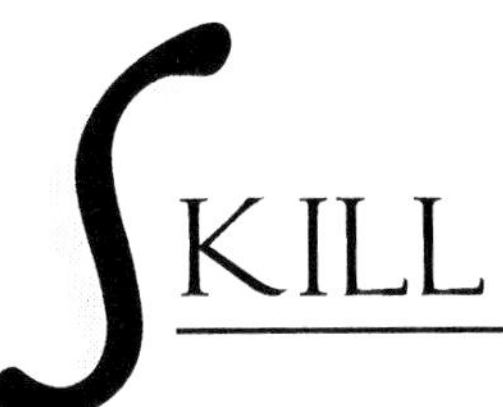

# KILL

## Preparing an Oxygen Cylinder for Use

***Purpose*** Portable oxygen cylinders are used in hospitals when a patient on oxygen must be moved or transported to an area that does not have an oxygen source available. In the home, portable cylinders give the patient greater freedom and mobility.

### Objectives

**The caregiver demonstrates the ability to do the following:**

1. Gather the correct supplies.
2. Communicate using a style that reduces the patient's anxiety.
3. Explain how to set up an oxygen cylinder.
4. Locate the proper regulator to apply to the oxygen cylinder.
5. Attach the Bourbon regulator.
6. Place the cylinder in the appropriate carrier for transport.
7. Document the results of the procedure according to the institution's policy.
8. Report the results of the procedure to the RN or preceptor.

### Key Terms

**Flowmeter** A device used to measure or regulate the amount of oxygen delivered to a patient; expressed in liters per minute.

**Naris** An opening to the nasal cavity; nostril.

**Oxygen Cylinder** An oxygen tank.

**Oxygen Key** A tool used to open the cylinder valve to the regulator.

**Regulator** A device used with an oxygen cylinder to reduce the high pressure of the gas contained in the cylinder to a working pressure suitable for patient care applications.

**Tidal Volume** The amount of air inhaled and exhaled during normal resting breathing.

**Ventilatory Pattern** The rate and depth of respiration.

### Supplies/Equipment

Oxygen E cylinder • Oxygen key • Bourbon regulator with flowmeter • Oxygen tank carrier

### Pertinent Points

- Oxygen is a drug and must be administered as ordered by the physician.
- Never allow an oxygen cylinder to come in close contact with open flames or excessive heat.
- A no-smoking sign should be displayed in a conspicuous location when an oxygen cylinder is in use.
- Special care must be taken in the home to ensure that the patient does not smoke and that all safety measures are being followed.

### Age-Specific Considerations

Oxygen tanks can be difficult for the elderly to handle because they are heavy and cumbersome.

## Key Concepts

- Never leave an oxygen cylinder standing alone. Cylinders must be secured or placed in an appropriate stand.
- When transporting oxygen cylinders, the appropriate carrier must be used.

## Steps

1. Verify the physician's order.
2. Wash hands.
3. Assemble the equipment.
4. Locate the correct cylinder. The universal color code for oxygen cylinders is green.
5. Verify that the cylinder is full.
6. Remove the protective seal or cylinder cap.
7. With an oxygen key, crack the valve open and close the valve cylinder slowly, expelling a small amount of gas to remove any dust or debris. When gas has been expelled, close the valve on the cylinder.
8. Locate a Bourbon regulator.
9. With the gasket in place, align the gauge to the holes of the pin index safety system on the valve of the cylinder.
10. Tighten the thumbwheel screw to secure the Bourbon regulator to the cylinder.
11. Open the valve on the cylinder slowly and observe the pressure gauge. A full cylinder has a pressure of 2,200 psig. Listen for any air leaks coming from the cylinder-gauge attachment. If a leak is present, turn the valve off and reapply, paying close attention to the placement of the gasket.
12. With the valve open, turn the flowmeter to the "on" position, and set the flow as ordered. Set the flow rate by placing the ball at the center line of the desired flow rate.
13. Place the cylinder in an appropriate carrier, and transport it to the area where it will be used.
14. Wash hands.
15. Identify the correct patient.
16. Explain the procedure to the patient.
17. Attach the oxygen tubing or device to the flowmeter, verify that the flowmeter is set to the desired liter flow, and observe the patient to ensure the proper placement of the oxygen device.
18. Wash hands and document and report the results of the procedure to the RN or preceptor.

## Oxygen-Delivery Devices Used in Respiratory Therapy

The many delivery devices available for supplemental oxygen can be divided into two major groups. A low-flow oxygen system is an apparatus whose oxygen flow is not intended to provide the total inspiratory requirements of the patient. For this reason, the inspired oxygen concentration is variable and is influenced by the patient's ventilatory pattern. This remains true even if the oxygen source for the apparatus is set at a high flow rate. A nasal cannula is an example of a low-flow oxygen system. On the other hand, a high-flow system has a reservoir bag and the total gas flow that supplies the entire inspired volume. The patient's ventilatory pattern has no effect on the inspired oxygen concentration. Under most circumstances, a Venturi mask falls into the high-flow category.

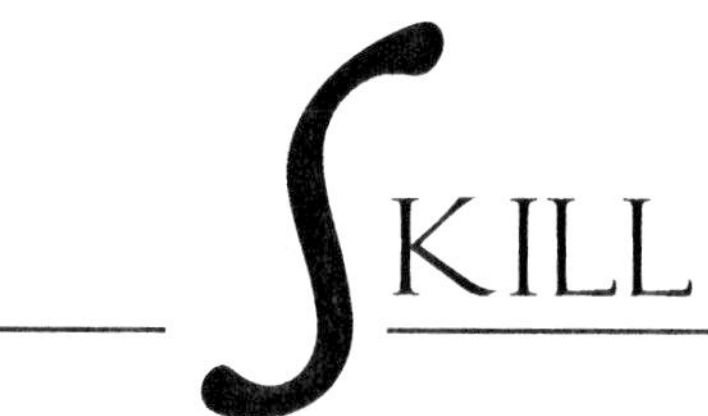

# Skill

## Setting Up a Nasal Cannula

***Purpose*** Low concentrations of inspired oxygen can be provided by nasal cannulas (prongs). Cannulas are generally inexpensive, well tolerated by patients, and one of the most commonly used devices. This simple system delivers 100 percent oxygen through two prongs inserted 1 cm into each anterior naris. The cannulas, made of unobtrusive, soft plastic, are generally comfortable for long-term use (Figure 7.8). The nasal passages should be patent. Mouth breathing does not significantly affect the final oxygen concentration because inspired ambient airflow in the oral pharynx entrains oxygen from the nasopharynx. Because this is a low-flow oxygen system, the final concentration of oxygen received by the patient depends on a mixture of ambient air and oxygen and is therefore sensitive to changes in the tidal volume and the ventilatory pattern. If the tidal volume is large, the fraction of inspired oxygen ($FiO_2$) may be low; if the tidal volume is small, the $FiO_2$ may be higher.

### Objectives

**The caregiver demonstrates the ability to do the following:**

1. Gather the correct supplies.
2. Communicate using a style that reduces the patient's anxiety.
3. Explain how to apply a nasal cannula.
4. Adjust the flowmeter to the prescribed liter flow.
5. Document the results of the procedure according to the institution's policy.
6. Report the results of the procedure to the RN or preceptor.

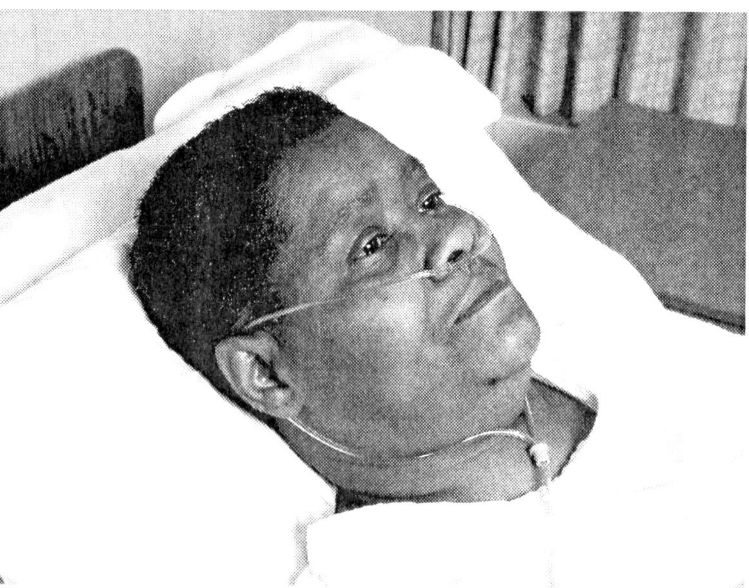

**Figure 7.8** Nasal cannula.

## Key Terms

**Bubble Humidifier** A device used with nasal cannulas to add moisture or humidity to dry medical gases, such as oxygen.

**Flowmeter** A device used to measure or regulate the amount of oxygen delivered to a patient; expressed in liters per minute.

**Liter** A measure of volume; 1 liter equals 1,000 cc.

**Nasal Cannula** A device used to deliver low-dose oxygen to the nares.

**Tidal Volume** The volume of air inhaled and exhaled during normal resting breathing.

## Supplies/Equipment

Nasal cannula • Oxygen flowmeter • Oxygen source—wall or tank • Oxygen tubing

## Pertinent Point

- With nasal cannula liter flows greater than 3 liters, many patients experience nasal mucosal dryness. This might be relieved by adding a bubble humidifier to the nasal cannula setup.

## Age-Specific Considerations

Nasal cannulas can cause irritation to the skin of the ears of elderly patients. The tubing is looped over the ears and tightened under the chin. The constant pressure of the tubing on the ears is the source of irritation and can be relieved by placing cotton or other soft material between the skin and the tubing.

## Key Concept

A nasal cannula is a low-flow oxygen system, an apparatus whose oxygen flow is not intended to meet the total inspiratory requirements of the patient. The inspired oxygen concentration is variable and is influenced by the patient's ventilatory pattern. This remains true even if the oxygen source for the apparatus is set at a high flow rate.

## Steps

1. Verify the physician's order.
2. Identify the correct patient.
3. Explain the procedure to the patient.
4. Wash hands.
5. Assemble the equipment.
6. Carefully insert the nasal prongs into the patient's nares with the prongs facing inward. Loop the tubing over and behind the patient's ears. Snug the tubing under the chin, ensuring the patient's comfort.
7. Attach the oxygen supply tubing to the flowmeter.
8. Adjust the flowmeter to the prescribed liter flow. Set the flow rate by placing the ball at the center line of the desired flow rate.
9. Wash hands and document and report the results of the procedure to the RN or preceptor.

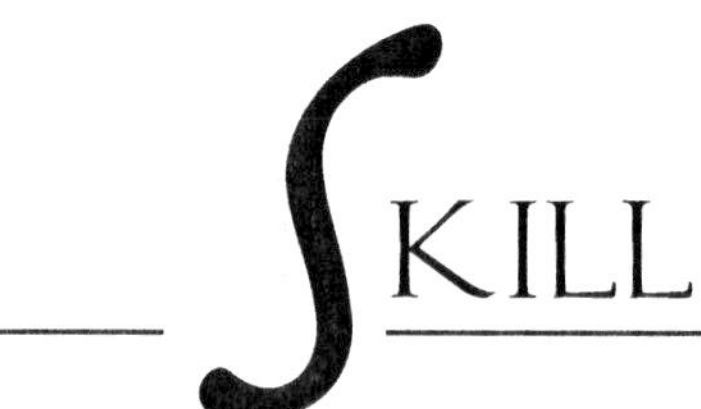

# SKILL

## Setting Up a Simple Face Mask

***Purpose*** The simple face mask is designed to provide a flow of oxygen into a cone-shaped piece that fits over the patient's nose and mouth. It has open ports for exhalation, from which the patient can also draw in some room air during inspiration.

### Objectives

**The caregiver demonstrates the ability to do the following:**

1. Gather the correct supplies.
2. Communicate using a style that reduces the patient's anxiety.
3. Explain how to apply a simple face mask.
4. Adjust the flowmeter to the prescribed liter flow.
5. Document the results of the procedure according to the institution's policy.
6. Report the results to the RN or preceptor.

### Key Terms

**Tidal Volume** The volume of air inhaled and exhaled during normal resting breathing.

**Ventilatory Pattern** Rate and depth of breathing.

### Supplies/Equipment

Oxygen source—wall or tank • Oxygen tubing • Flowmeter • Simple face mask

### Pertinent Points

- In some instances, the cone of the simple face mask acts as a reservoir for accumulated, exhaled carbon dioxide if a minimal flow of gas is not maintained.
- The oxygen percentages delivered through the simple mask approach 35 percent to 55 percent when oxygen flow rates of 6 to 10 l/min are used for adults.
- Oxygen percentages achieved with the simple mask vary greatly, depending on the patient's ventilatory pattern. A patient with a large tidal volume dilutes the oxygen with room air, decreasing the percentage of oxygen. A patient with slow, shallow respirations increases the amount of inspired oxygen.
- If the simple mask will be in place for an extended period of time, care must be taken to clean the area where the mask and skin meet. Inspect the patient's skin for pressure sores or skin breakdown.

### Age-Specific Considerations

Face masks come in both pediatric and adult sizes. Consider the size of the patient when choosing the mask.

### Key Concept

Simple oxygen masks are used when moderate oxygen concentrations are desired for a short period of time. As with all face masks, there is an increased risk of aspiration should the patient vomit and not be able to remove the mask.

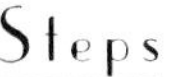

1. Check the physician's order.
2. Identify the correct patient.
3. Explain the procedure to the patient.
4. Wash hands.
5. Assemble the equipment.
6. Attach the oxygen supply tubing to the oxygen flowmeter.
7. Adjust the flowmeter to the desired flow rate (6 to 10 l/min).
8. Place the face mask on the patient. Pull the elastic strap over the patient's head and adjust the mask for a comfortable, secure fit (Figure 7.9).
9. Recheck the ABGs, or confirm with a pulse oximeter that the patient's oxygenation status has improved.
10. Wash hands and document and report the results of the procedure to the RN or preceptor. Document the device used and the liter flow.

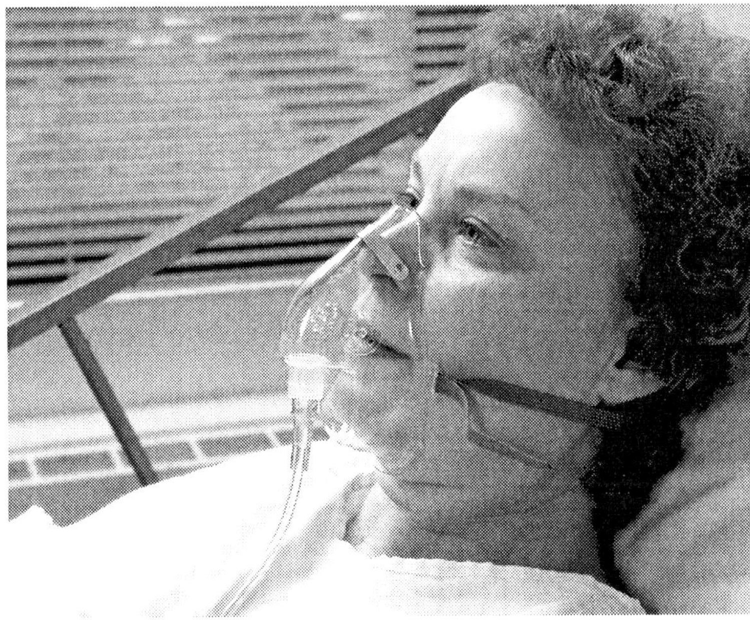

**Figure 7.9** Patient wearing a simple face mask.

## *Assessing the Need for Oxygen*

Oxygen is an essential ingredient for life. For the body to function properly, there must be adequate amounts of oxygen in the blood available to the tissues and body cells. Caregivers use a pulse oximeter to evaluate the patient's oxygenation status. The pulse oximeter is a safe, noninvasive, and simple method used by caregivers. It has the advantage of providing a direct, continuous, yet noninvasive, measure of arterial saturation.

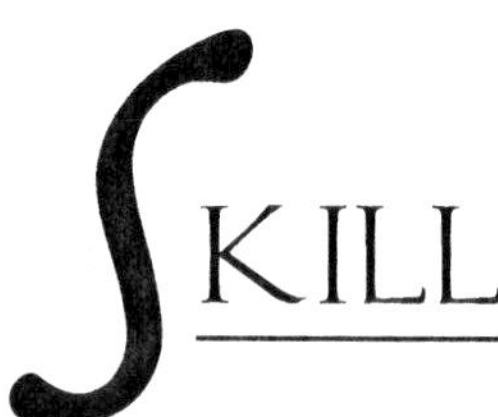

# SKILL

## Setting Up the Pulse Oximeter

***Purpose*** The pulse oximeter is routinely used for noninvasive blood oxygen monitoring to improve oxygen management and to reduce the risk of adverse outcomes (Figures 7.10a and b). The pulse oximeter measures $SpO_2$. By definition, $SpO_2$ is the percentage of hemoglobin that is carrying oxygen to the tissues; it is also commonly referred to as Sat, or saturation. Each red blood cell contains a hemoglobin molecule with four binding sites for oxygen. These binding sites combine with oxygen in an all-or-none fashion. Saturation is the ratio of hemoglobin molecules bound with oxygen to the total amount of hemoglobin molecules available. A normal $SpO_2$ is 95 percent to 100 percent.

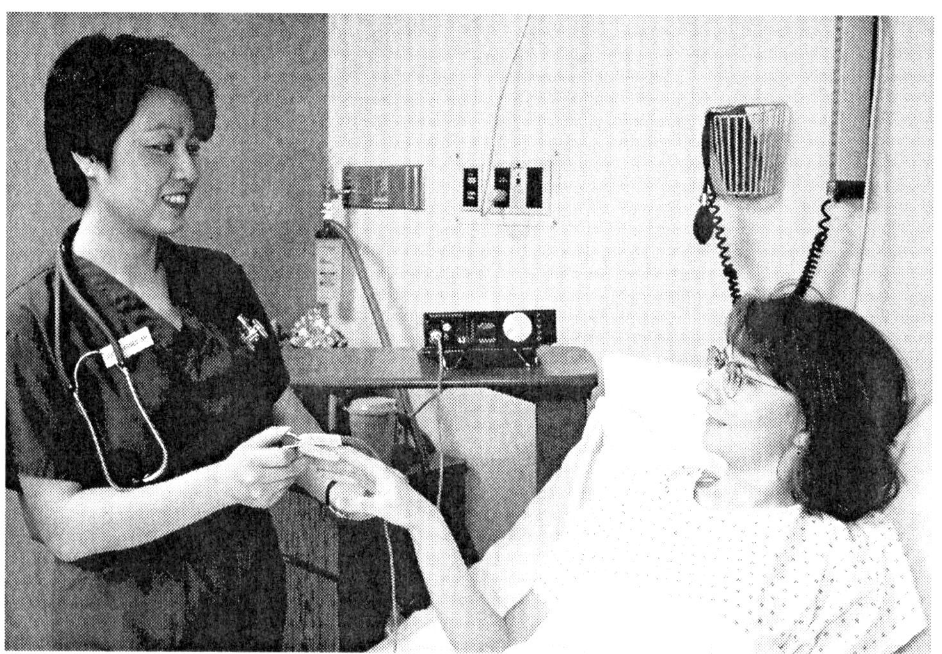

a

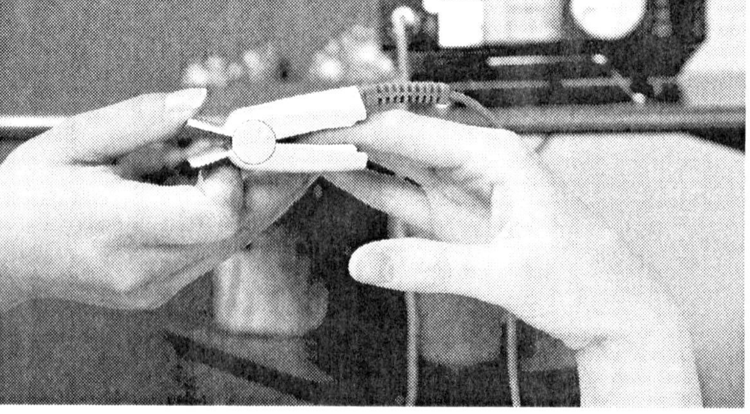

b

**Figure 7.10** Placing a pulse oximeter probe on an adult patient.

## Objectives

**The caregiver demonstrates the ability to do the following:**

1. Gather the correct supplies.
2. Communicate using a style that reduces the patient's anxiety.
3. Explain how to set up a pulse oximeter.
4. Adjust the flowmeter to the prescribed liter flow.
5. Document the results of the procedure according to the institution's policy.
6. Report the results of the procedure to the RN or preceptor.

## Key Terms

**Carboxyhemoglobin** Compound formed when hemoglobin attaches to carbon monoxide, decreasing the functional binding sites for oxygen.

**Finger Probe** An instrument used in conjunction with the pulse oximeter. A clip placed on the finger contains a light source and a photo detector cell to detect the patient's arterial saturation.

**Hypoxia** A reduced or inadequate amount of oxygen in the arterial blood.

**Oxyhemoglobin** Compound formed when hemoglobin combines with oxygen.

**Pulse Oximetry** A noninvasive test to evaluate a patient's oxygenation status by assessing arterial saturation.

**Saturation** The percentage of hemoglobin binding sites that are carrying oxygen to the tissues; also known as $SpO_2$.

**$SpO_2$** The percentage of hemoglobin that is carrying oxygen to the tissues; also known as saturation.

## Supplies/Equipment

Alcohol swab • Finger probe • Pulse oximeter

## Pertinent Points

- The pulse oximeter uses optical, or light, technology to monitor oxygen saturation. It measures the redness or blueness of blood. Well-oxygenated blood appears bright red, whereas poorly oxygenated blood appears blue. The sensor, or probe, that is placed on the patient's finger has two optical components, or light sources: one red and one infrared. The optical components are placed over the patient's fingernail, and the light-sensitive diode lies below the finger. The sensor measures the amount of red or infrared light absorbed during systole and diastole. Heart rate is displayed by the two light sources in the pulsatile capillary artery. When fingers are not an optimal choice, an ear probe can be used.
- Functional, or physiological, saturation is the ratio of oxyhemoglobin to the total amount of hemoglobin available for binding with oxygen. Dysfunctional hemoglobin is hemoglobin that is not available to bind with oxygen. This situation presents itself when carboxyhemoglobin is present and carbon monoxide binds to the hemoglobin sites. Dysfunctional hemoglobin should be suspected whenever a patient presents with coma, cyanosis of unknown etiology, or smoke inhalation.
- Optical shunt occurs when the light from the light-emitting diode (LED) pulse oximeter reaches the photo detector without passing through a pulsatile arterial bed. This event occurs with improper finger probe placement. An important clinical situation is presented by the patient with a low blood count (a decreased number of red blood cells). This patient might have a saturation of 100 percent, but because of the decreased carrying capacity for oxygen resulting from the low red blood cell count, the patient might report shortness of breath. When oxygen saturation falls below 90 percent, physiological changes occur, and the oxygen supply decreases rapidly.

## Age-Specific Considerations

Check the fingernails of teens and women for artificial nails and fingernail polish. Blue, rust, and green polish especially can give a false reading. Young children are sometimes fearful of having their finger restricted by the probe and need to be reassured that it will not be painful (Figure 7.11).

## Key Concepts

The pulse oximeter is not without its limitations. Factors that affect the reliability of readings include the following:

1. Motion while the probe is in use on a patient. Motion might interfere with the true arterial pulses.
2. Low perfusion. A patient with low blood pressure might have an undetectable arterial pulse.
3. Venous pulsation. In patients with right-sided heart failure, the pulse oximeter might detect both arterial and venous pulsation and give an erroneous reading.
4. Artificial nails and fingernail polish. Some colors of polish—especially blue, rust, and green—can give a false reading.
5. Ambient light. Interference from an external light source due to poor placement of the probe might give an inaccurate reading.

## Steps

1. Check the physician's order if your institution requires one for this procedure.
2. Identify the correct patient.
3. Explain the procedure to the patient.
4. Wash hands.
5. Assemble the equipment.
6. With an alcohol swab, clean the portion of the finger probe that will come in contact with the patient's skin.
7. Place the finger probe on the patient's finger so that the light-emitting source is on top of the fingernail. Check for correct placement, and turn the pulse oximeter on.
8. Ask the patient to remain still while you note the saturation number displayed.
9. Wash hands and document and report the results of the procedure to the RN or preceptor.
10. Remove the probe from the patient's finger, use an alcohol pad to swab skin contact area, and turn off the pulse oximeter unit.
11. Store the pulse oximeter unit plugged into a wall socket, allowing it to charge its internal battery while not in use.

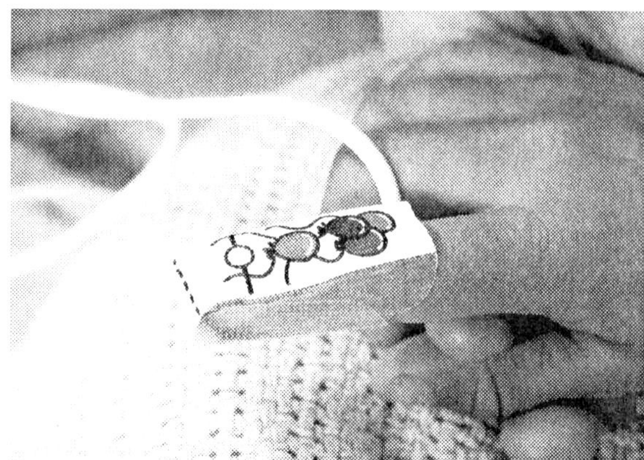

**Figure 7.11** Finger probe on a child.

# SECTION TWO
# Humidity Therapy

Objectives

**This section prepares caregivers to do the following:**

1. Describe the properties of humidity and the equipment associated with its use.
2. Identify the goals of humidity therapy.
3. Relate the hazards associated with humidity therapy.

Key Terms

**Saline** Of or pertaining to a salt solution. Normal saline is 0.9 percent sodium chloride.

**Upper Airway** The structures in the respiratory tract that are above the trachea.

## Humidification Devices Used in Respiratory Therapy

The nasal and oral cavities form the gateway to the respiratory system. Warming and humidification of air begins as soon as it starts its two-way journey through the respiratory tract. The mucous membranes are supplied with a large amount of blood flow, particularly in the nasal cavity, where moving air first enters the respiratory system and humidification begins. This helps to warm the incoming air rapidly. This process continues throughout the respiratory tract. If one considers how brief one respiration is and notes how warm and wet the air is on its return to the outside, it is apparent that these processes are very effective.

In an extremely dry environment, the wetting function might be overpowered, and a person might note drying of the nose and mouth. For these reasons, it is important to add humidity to the air we breathe. In the hospital, medical gases provide no humidity at all. In patients with artificial airways, the respiratory system's normal humidification process is bypassed. Therefore, the amount of humidity must be supplemented for these patients. Clinical uses for humidity, or molecular water, can be divided into two broad classes: (a) to humidify dry therapeutic gases to make them more comfortable to breathe and (b) to provide near-body-humidity levels of inspired gases for patients with artificial airways.

Water is available to the respiratory tract in two forms. *Humidity* is water in its vapor form. It is the invisible, gaseous state of water, sometimes referred to as molecular water. The capacity of gas to hold water in its vapor state increases as temperature increases. In an *aerosol,* particles of liquid or solids are suspended in gas. These particles could be cigarette smoke, dust, fog, aerosolized water or medication, and so forth. To contrast, humidity is water in a gaseous state, whereas an aerosol is water in a liquid state (water droplets suspended in a gas).

### Simple Humidifiers

Simple humidifiers do not employ heat. They are designed to add only enough humidity to make the gas being administered more comfortable to breathe. As the gas enters the patient's airways, the normal humidification mechanism of the nose supplies the balance of moisture not provided by the humidifier.

There are three types of simple, nonheated humidifiers. The first has been used in respiratory therapy for many years: the pass-over, or blow-by, humidifier. In this unit, the gas merely passes over the water surface and then flows to the patient. The second type of simple humidifying device is the bubble humidifier (Figure 7.12). Probably the most common, this unit introduces the gas to be

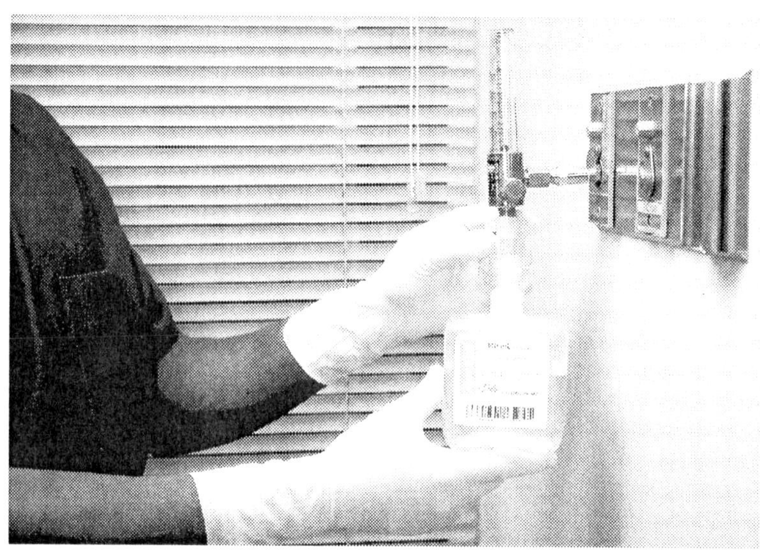

**Figure 7.12** Bubble humidifier in place on a wall.

inspired below the surface of the water to allow it to bubble back to the top. The third type is a jet humidifier. This humidifier actually produces an aerosol, but it employs a baffle system that removes large particles and sweeps the smaller particles away within the airstream.

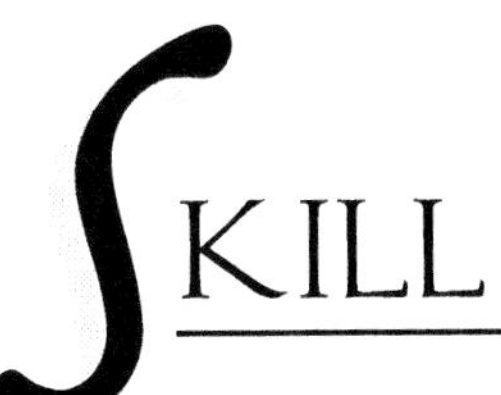

# Skill

## Setting Up an Oxygen Bubble Humidifier

***Purpose*** Bubble humidifiers are used as a comfort measure with nasal cannulas to add humidity to the dry medical gas.

### Objectives

**The caregiver demonstrates the ability to do the following:**

1. Gather the correct supplies.
2. Communicate using a style that reduces the patient's anxiety.
3. Explain how to set up a bubble humidifier.
4. Adjust the flowmeter to the prescribed liter flow.
5. Document the results of the procedure according to the institution's policy.
6. Report the results of the procedure to the RN or preceptor.

### Key Terms

**Humidity** Molecular water suspended in a gas.

**Nasal Cannula** A device used to deliver low-flow oxygen to the nares.

**Pop-off Valve** A device that relieves pressure.

**Resistance** A force that impedes or slows forward movement.

### Supplies/Equipment

Bubble humidifier • Sterile water labeled for respiratory use • Oxygen flowmeter • Oxygen source—wall or tank • Oxygen supply tubing • Nasal cannula

### Pertinent Points

- When a bubble humidifier is added to a nasal cannula setup, the resistance to the flow of oxygen is increased. It is therefore advisable to maintain a nasal cannula liter flow of 6 liters or less.
- Many bubble humidifiers have a factory-installed pop-off valve that whistles when the resistance to flow is too high.
- When administering a medicated nebulized mist treatment, the bubble humidifier must be removed and a Christmas tree adapter applied to the nebulizer, or there will be too much resistance to flow.
- To reduce the risk of infection, many institutions have policies to change all bubble humidifiers in use every 71 hours or 3 days.

### Age-Specific Considerations

The elderly sometimes suffer adverse effects from breathing dry medical gas. The addition of humidity can be very comforting.

### Key Concept

The amount of humidity added to the gas depends on the amount of time the gas is in contact with the water. As the water level decreases, so too does the amount of humidity being added to the gas. Change the device as the water level approaches an unacceptable level.

## Steps

1. Identify the correct patient.
2. Explain the procedure to the patient.
3. Wash hands.
4. Assemble the equipment. Remove the humidifier from its container, and screw the top onto the bottle containing the water (Figure 7.13).
5. Remove the Christmas tree adapter from the oxygen flowmeter, and attach the screw-on portion of the humidifier to the oxygen flowmeter with the water bottle attached.
6. Select the desired liter flow on the oxygen flowmeter.
7. Attach the oxygen supply tubing from the nasal cannula to the oxygen outlet adapter on the bubble humidifier, being careful not to tip the bottle and introduce water into the oxygen supply tubing.
8. Observe the equipment and ensure that the oxygen is bubbling through the system (see Figure 7.12).
9. Wash hands and document and report the results of the procedure to the RN or preceptor.

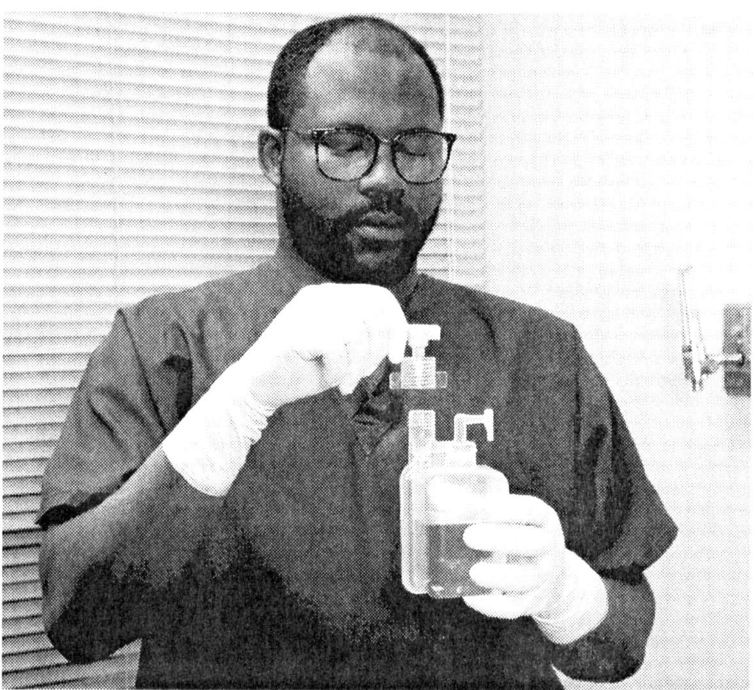

**Figure 7.13** Assembling the parts of a bubble humidifier.

## Heated Humidifiers

The second type of humidifier used in respiratory therapy requires control of a third ingredient, heat, to increase humidifier efficiency. Heated humidifiers are used when the inspired air needs to be 100 percent saturated at body temperature. They are used when artificial respiration from a breathing machine (ventilator) is needed. The heated humidifier is usually incorporated into a ventilator circuit. If the patient requires total or partial support of ventilation, a heated humidifier is used.

# Section Three
## Pulmonary Hygiene

### Introduction

Pulmonary hygiene includes tracheal suctioning and respiratory care after surgery. Often, especially after surgery, a patient must be encouraged to breathe deeply in order to keep all the air sacs open and inflated. Caregivers encourage the patient to cough, especially if there is inflammation of the lung tissue. In many of the larger health care institutions, the Pulmonary Medicine Department (Respiratory Therapy) will, by a doctor's order, institute a treatment that will encourage the patient to breathe deeply and cough. An incentive spirometer is used postoperatively for this in most hospitals.

After a patient has had abdominal surgery, she may, fearing pain, resist coughing. One way to make the patient more comfortable is to place a pillow over the patient's abdomen and instruct the patient to hold it firmly against the abdomen when she coughs. The patient is usually instructed to breathe in and out slowly and deeply twice. After breathing in deeply a third time, the patient should cough twice instead of letting the air out slowly. Make sure she covers her mouth with a tissue and turns her head away from you.

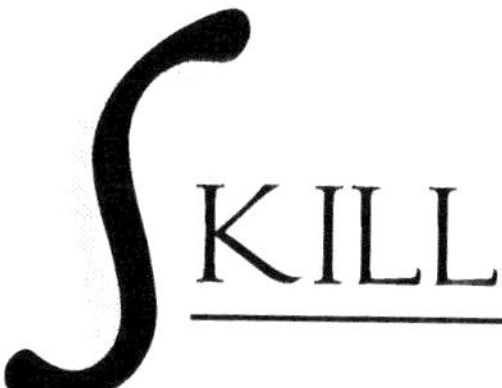

## SKILL

## Suctioning a Tracheostomy

**Purpose** Tracheal suctioning is an important procedure that removes thick secretions that have accumulated in a patient's lungs (Figure 7.14). Because a patient with a tracheostomy has lost the protective filtering function usually performed by the nose, irritants in the air can directly enter the lungs. This often leads to increased secretions, mucus, and the formation of crusts. The lungs are challenged to remove these extra particles on their own. Tracheostomy patients might also have underlying medical conditions that increase secretions and mucus or make it difficult for patients to expel them on their own. Failure to remove these irritants can lead to infection, pneumonia, or severe respiratory distress.

Suctioning with a soft rubber catheter assists the tracheostomy patient by removing these secretions, mucus, and small crusts. The caregiver inserts the catheter into the trachea for a short time and then withdraws it. Suctioning removes some secretions from the lungs and stimulates the patient to cough violently. This coughing also helps the patient expel secretions, debris, and mucus.

Because suctioning is a difficult procedure for the patient, it must only be performed when necessary. Indications that a patient might need to be suctioned include an increased rate of respiration; more difficult, labored respiration; and noisy, gurgling respirations.

### Objectives

**The caregiver demonstrates the ability to do the following:**

1. Gather the correct supplies.
2. Communicate using a style that reduces the patient's anxiety.
3. Explain when to suction a patient.

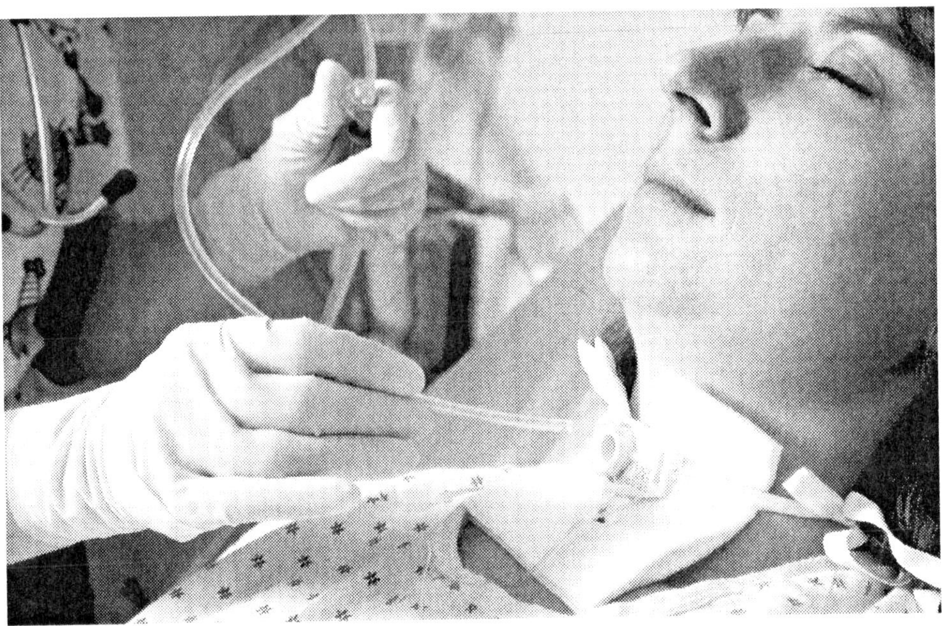

**Figure 7.14** Suctioning a tracheostomy.

4. Describe ways to minimize complications from tracheal suctioning.
5. Perform the suctioning procedure correctly.
6. Document the results of the procedure according to the institution's policy.
7. Report the results of the procedure to the RN or preceptor.

## Key Terms

**Hypoxia** An inadequate amount of oxygen in the blood.

**Tracheostomy** A surgical opening in the trachea (windpipe) that leads directly to the lungs.

## Supplies/Equipment

Wall suction • Goggles or face shield • Catheter and glove kit (sterile gloves, sterile basin, 14–16F suction catheter) • 500-cc bottle of normal saline (sterile)

## Pertinent Points

- Patients consider procedures that interfere with breathing to be very invasive. Suctioning is a traumatic experience for the patient because the catheter removes air from the lungs as well as any secretions. Help relieve the patient's anxiety by describing every step you take.
- Take time and care while performing this procedure. Although suctioning is routine for caregivers, it is not routine for patients.
- Be prepared, and have all of the equipment and supplies ready.
- Maintaining sterile technique is very important. Suctioning introduces a foreign object (the catheter) deep into a body cavity.
- Safe suction pressure for an adult is 80 to 140 mm Hg.
- The size of the suction catheter should not be more than one-half the diameter of the tracheostomy. Remember, the larger the catheter, the more oxygen will be removed during suctioning.
- As you insert the catheter into the patient's airway, do not apply any suction. This helps prevent trauma to the mucosal tissue of the lungs.
- Keep the suction catheter in the airway for no more than 10 to 15 seconds.
- When you withdraw the catheter, twirl it and apply suction intermittently to prevent the catheter from adhering to the tissue..

- Do not introduce the catheter into the patient's lungs more than three times. After this point, the rinse (normal saline) will be fairly contaminated. This precaution helps prevent infection for the patient.

## Age-Specific Considerations

Patients of all ages will have concerns about suctioning. Being unable to breathe is a frightening experience. Explain the procedure in language that the patient can understand. Show respect and concern for patients by addressing them using the name they have asked you to use.

As people age, the lungs become less elastic, or able to expand. The membranes become thicker, making the exchange of oxygen more difficult. For these reasons, suctioning is a more traumatic process for the elderly. Allow elderly patients more time to catch their breath between insertions of the suction catheter into the tracheostomy.

## Key Concepts

- Suctioning is a traumatic procedure for the patient. Only suction when it is necessary.
- Infection and lack of oxygen are two common complications of suctioning that can be minimized.
- The patient cannot breathe while being suctioned. The whole process must last no longer than 10 to 15 seconds. This time limit will help prevent hypoxia, or lack of oxygen, for the patient. Putting the oxygen back on the patient as soon as the suction is out of the tracheostomy will also help prevent hypoxia.
- Hold your breath while you insert the catheter into the tracheostomy. This will give you an indication of how long the patient will be without oxygen during the suctioning process. Remember that patients who are compromised by illness or age usually cannot hold their breath as long as you can.

## Steps

1. Identify the correct patient.
2. Explain the procedure to and provide privacy for the patient.
3. Wash hands.
4. Assemble the equipment.
5. Turn the wall suction on to achieve a pressure of between 80 and 140 mm Hg for patient safety.
6. Put on goggles shilling face shield.
7. Loosen the patient's oxygen mask. Leave it in place until ready to suction.
8. Open the catheter kit in a sterile manner.
9. Apply gloves. Determine which hand will guide the catheter into the tracheostomy; this hand must remain sterile to the patient.
10. Attach the catheter to the suction tubing from the wall suction, holding the tubing with the nonsterile hand and the suction catheter with the sterile hand.
11. Remove the patient's oxygen mask with your nonsterile hand.
12. With your sterile hand, insert the catheter in the airway, without applying suction, until a cough reflex is stimulated or resistance is felt (approximately 6 inches).
13. Withdraw the catheter $\frac{1}{2}$ to 1 inch before applying suction. Withdraw by twisting the catheter with your forefinger and thumb, and apply intermittent suction with other thumb over suction valve.

14. Apply suction for no more than 10 to 15 seconds.
15. Repeat steps 12 to 14 until secretions are minimal and the patient breathes easily. Allow time between suction episodes for the patient to reoxygenate. (Apply oxygen mask with your nonsterile hand.) Between suction episodes, rinse the end of the catheter in the sterile saline basin. Apply suction to rinse the normal saline through the entire suction catheter tubing.
16. Remove and discard gloves.
17. Wash hands and document and report the results of the procedure to the RN or preceptor. Report the color and amount of secretions, as well as how the patient tolerated the procedure.

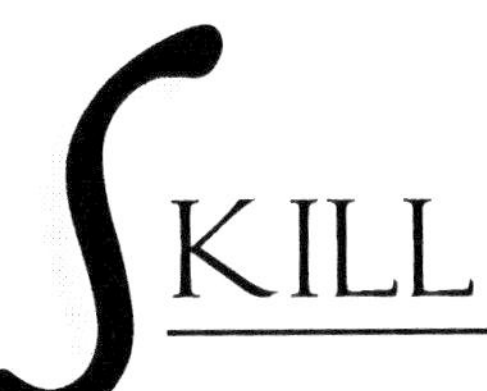

# SKILL

## Performing Tracheostomy Care

**Purpose** Tracheostomy care is given to prevent a buildup of secretions and crustations from forming on the trach. This helps prevent infection and clogging of the trach. A clogged trach will prevent the patient from breathing. There are two types of trach care. One type is used when the patient has a nondisposable (metal or plastic) inner cannula (Figure 7.15), and the other is used when the patient has a disposable (plastic) inner cannula (Figure 7.16).

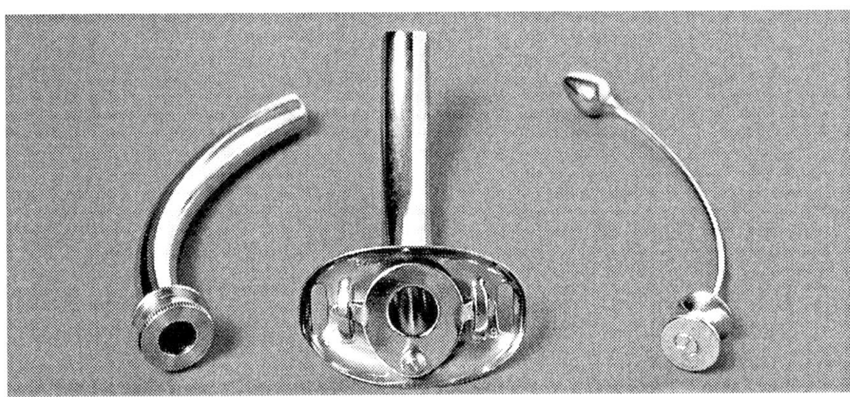

**Figure 7.15** Nondisposable trach.

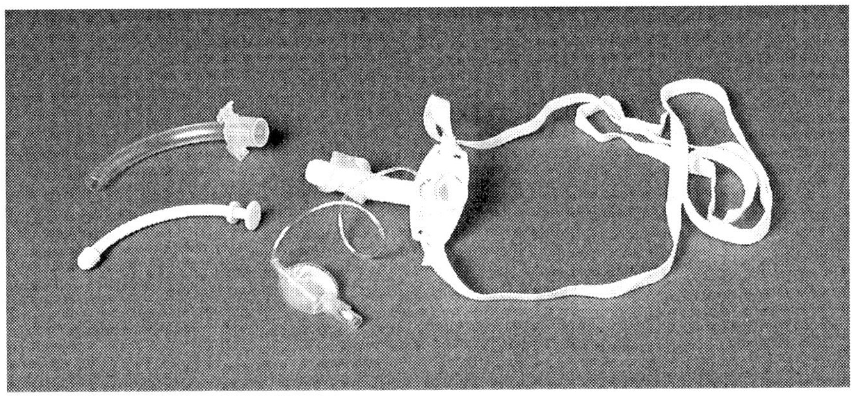

**Figure 7.16** Disposable trach.

### Objectives

**The caregiver demonstrates the ability to do the following:**

1. Gather the correct supplies.
2. Communicate using a style that reduces the patient's anxiety.
3. State when to perform trach care.
4. Maintain sterile technique.
5. Perform the procedure correctly.
6. Report the results of the procedure to the RN or preceptor.

### Key Terms

**Disposable Inner Cannula** The inner tube of the trach set that is thrown away and replaced with a clean one during trach care.

**Flange** The metal or plastic plate section of the trach that holds the trach set flush to the skin. The trach ties attach to the flange.

**Nondisposable Inner Cannula** The inner tube of the trach set that is cleaned and replaced using sterile technique when performing trach care.

**Obturator** The wire or plastic guide that is used when first inserting the trach set.

**Outer Cannula** The larger tube of the trach set that stays in the patient.

## Supplies/Equipment

### Nondisposable Inner Cannula

Trach care kit • Peroxide and saline solutions (sterile) • Sterile gloves • 4-by-4-inch gauze • Sterile cotton-tip applicators • Trach pants (drain sponge) • Pipe cleaners

### Disposable Inner Cannula

Trach care kit, with a replacement inner cannula • Peroxide and saline solutions (sterile) • Sterile gloves • Sterile cotton-tip applicators • Trach pants (drain sponge) • 4-by-4-inch gauze

## Pertinent Points

- Trach care is a very important procedure for keeping the patient's airway clean and protecting against infection.
- Sterile technique must be maintained throughout the procedure.
- Because the patient's oxygen will not be on during the procedure, speed is important.

## Age-Specific Considerations

Patients of all ages will have concerns about tracheostomy care. Explain the procedure so that the patient can understand. Show respect and concern for patients by addressing them using the name they have asked you to use. Take time and care while performing the procedure. Although trach care is routine for caregivers, it is not routine for patients or their families.

Tracheostomy care is an invasive procedure. Children may not understand why it is necessary or what is happening when caregivers perform the procedure. Adolescents, adults, and the elderly will understand the need for cleanliness but may still fear the procedure. Be understanding of the feelings of your patients.

## Key Concept

Some patients need extra oxygen to assist with breathing, and many also need it to help humidify the air, a function that is lost when the air is not filtered and warmed by the nose. Both functions are compromised during trach care. If at any time the patient's respiratory status is compromised, check that the inner cannula is in place. Stop the process and call for assistance.

## Steps for Performing Tracheostomy Care with a Nondisposable Inner Cannula

1. Wash hands.
2. Explain the procedure to the patient.
3. Provide for privacy.
4. Assemble the equipment (Figure 7.17). Open the trach care kit and prepare the sterile field. Organize your supplies and equipment.
5. Pour the peroxide solution into one container and the saline solution into the other.
6. Put on gloves.
7. Hold the flange with one hand and unlock the inner cannula by twisting it to the open position. Carefully withdraw the inner

cannula with an upward arc without touching the inside of the cannula.

8. Inspect the inner cannula for crustations and mucus, then put it in the peroxide solution.
9. Use the wire brush to clean the inner cannula, then put the cannula in the saline solution to rinse. Dry it thoroughly with the gauze (Figure 7.18a). A pipe cleaner may be used to dry the inside.
10. Holding the outer rim, gently reinsert the cannula and twist it to lock it into place (Figure 7.18b).
11. Pour peroxide in the third section of the basin. Clean the flange with the peroxide and rinse it with the saline solution, using the cotton-tip applicators. Apply the trach pants (drain sponge) around the flange (Figure 7.18c).
12. Dispose of the supplies. Remove and discard gloves; wash hands.
13. Document and report the results to the RN or preceptor.

Note: You may want to use a clean pair of exam gloves to remove the inner cannula in step 7; then put on a new pair of sterile gloves before performing step 9.

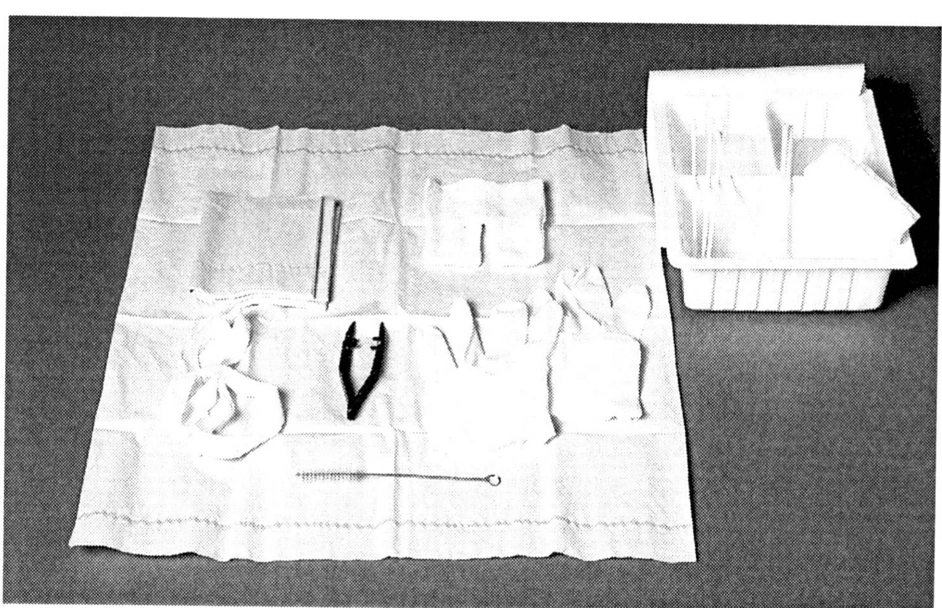

**Figure 7.17** Trach care kit.

## Steps for Performing Tracheostomy Care with a Disposable Inner Cannula

1. Wash hands.
2. Explain the procedure to the patient.
3. Provide for privacy.
4. Assemble the equipment (Figure 7.17). Open the trach care kit and prepare the sterile field.
5. Pour the peroxide solution into one container and the saline solution into the other.
6. Put on gloves.
7. Hold the flange with one hand and unlock or pinch open the inner cannula. Carefully withdraw the inner cannula with an upward arc.
8. Inspect the inner cannula for crustations and mucus, then dispose of it.
9. Insert the new inner cannula by grasping the outer rim and inserting gently. Clip the inner cannula onto the rim.
10. Clean the flange with peroxide and rinse it with the saline solution, using the cotton-tip applicators.
11. Dispose of the supplies. Remove and discard gloves; wash hands.
12. Document and report the results to the RN or preceptor.

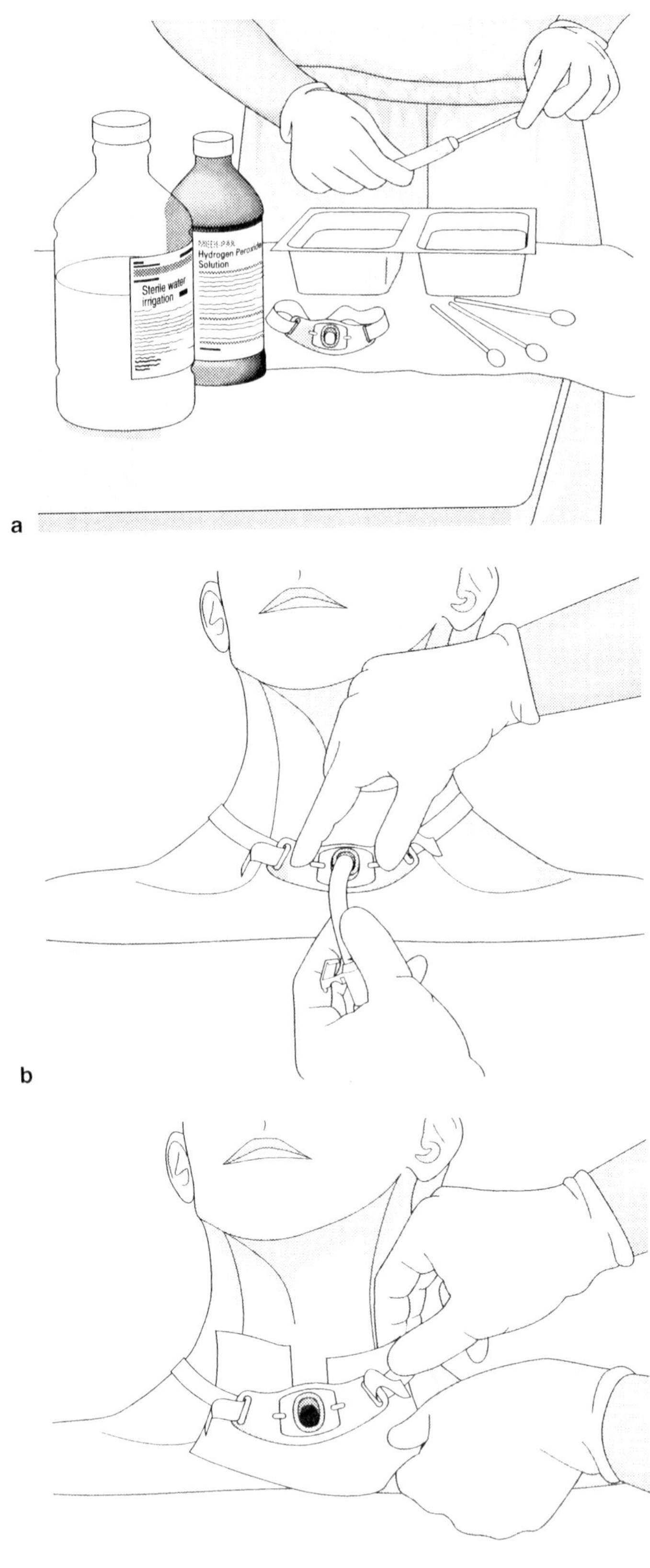


Figure 7.18 Steps in trach care: (a) cleaning and drying the inner cannula, (b) reinserting the inner cannula, (c) replacing the trach pants.

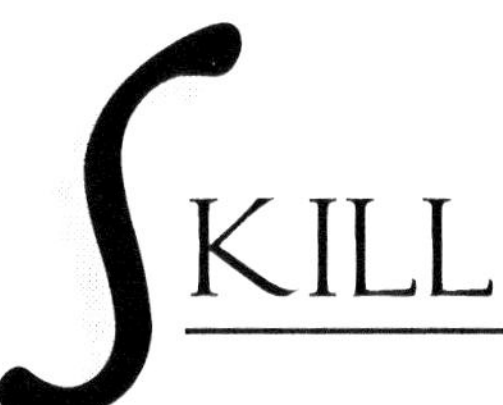

# SKILL

## Instructing the Patient in the Use of the Incentive Spirometer

***Purpose*** The incentive spirometer is a simple device that comes in many different shapes and sizes. The primary use of the device is to increase alveolar inflation. The goal is to expand collapsed alveoli and maintain lung volumes or return them to normal (Figure 7.19). Normally, we all take several deep breaths each hour, usually without being aware of it. They are spontaneous and automatic and take the form of sighs and yawns. After surgery or illness, a patient's breathing pattern might change due to pain or other causes. This is when breathing becomes shallow. An incentive spirometer gives patients an easy way to do breathing exercises and monitor their own progress. By simply taking several slow, deep breaths each hour, the patient will begin to see an increase in her inspiratory volume while preventing the possibility of respiratory complications.

### Objectives

**The caregiver demonstrates the ability to do the following:**

1. Gather the correct supplies.
2. Communicate using a style that reduces the patient's anxiety.
3. Explain how to use an incentive spirometer.
4. Perform the procedure correctly.
5. Document the results of the procedure according to the institution's policy.
6. Report the results of the procedure to the RN or preceptor.

### Key Term

**Atelectasis** Closure or collapse of the alveoli, leading to decreased gas exchange.

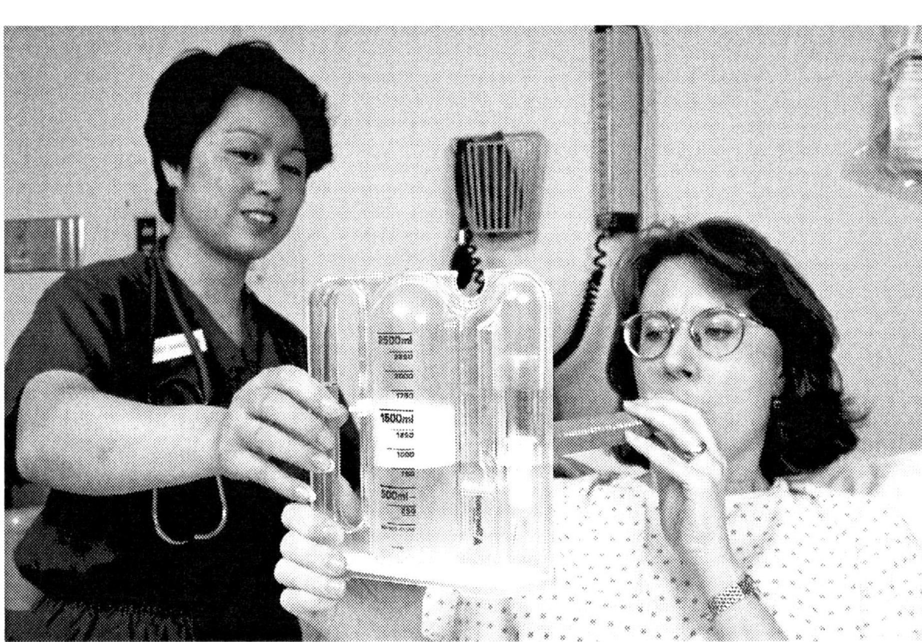


**Figure 7.19** Patient using an incentive spirometer.

## Supplies/ Equipment

Incentive spirometer • Mouthpiece

## Pertinent Points

- Encourage the patient to use the spirometer ten times per hour.
- A pause between breaths should avoid hyperventilation.
- Mark the patient's progress and set reasonable goals for the patient to achieve.

## Age-Specific Considerations

Some elderly patients might have difficulty understanding the instructions and might need frequent reminders to use the instrument hourly.

## Key Concept

The incentive spirometer gives patients an easy way to do breathing exercises and monitor their progress to relieve or prevent postoperative atelectasis.

## Steps

1. Identify the correct patient.
2. Explain the procedure to the patient.
3. Wash hands.
4. Assemble the equipment.
5. Position the patient in an upright position, as tolerated, for optimal chest expansion.
6. Instruct the patient to place the mouthpiece in the mouth, making a tight seal around it with the lips. Encourage the patient to suck in on the mouthpiece in a manner similar to sucking on a straw.
7. Have the patient take slow, deep breaths through the mouthpiece. At full inspiration, have the patient try to hold the breath for several seconds.
8. Instruct the patient to exhale normally. Observe the volume level achieved with the last breath. Have the patient pause for several moments between breaths to avoid hyperventilating. Repeat ten times.
9. Wash hands, and document and report the results of the procedure to the RN or preceptor.

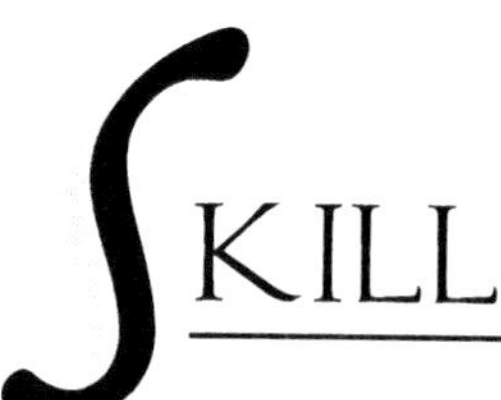

# SKILL

## Performing Tracheostomy Stoma Care

**Purpose** Patients who have tracheostomies often experience a buildup of secretions or crusts around their stoma. Built-up secretions can interfere with the patient's ability to breathe. This may occur with either a disposable or a nondisposable trach (see Figures 7.15 and 7.16). Stoma care is the process of removing these secretions, crusts, or other debris from under the flange of the trach and from around the stoma.

### Objectives

**The caregiver demonstrates ability to do the following:**

1. Gather the correct supplies.
2. Communicate using a style that reduces the patient's anxiety.
3. State when to perform stoma care.
4. Maintain sterile technique.
5. Perform the procedure correctly.
6. Report the results of the procedure to the RN or preceptor.

### Key Term

**Stoma** A surgically created opening to the trachea that serves as an airway.

### Supplies/Equipment

Peroxide and saline solutions • Two small sterile containers • Sterile cotton-tip applicators • Trach pants (drain sponge)

### Pertinent Points

- Trach care is a very important procedure for keeping the patient's airway clean and protecting against infection.
- Sterile technique must be maintained throughout the procedure.
- If at any time the patient's respiratory status is compromised, check that the inner cannula is in place. Stop the procedure and call for assistance.

### Age-Specific Considerations

Patients of all ages will have concerns about tracheostomy stoma care. Explain the procedure so that the patient can understand. Show respect and concern for patients by addressing them using the name they have asked you to use. Take time and care while performing the procedure. Although stoma care is routine for caregivers, it is not routine for patients or their families.

Tracheostomy stoma care is a potentially irritating procedure. Children may not understand why it is necessary or what is happening when caregivers begin to clean the area. Adolescents, adults, and the elderly will understand the need for cleanliness but may still fear the procedure.

### Key Concept

In most people, the nose serves as a filter during the breathing process. In tracheostomy patients, the stoma provides direct access to the bronchi and the lungs. Therefore, accidentally pushing secretions or crustrations into the trach tube when swabbing around the stoma may cause obstruction of the airway or breathing difficulties.

## Steps

1. Wash hands.
2. Explain the procedure to the patient.
3. Provide for privacy.
4. Assemble the equipment.
5. Pour the peroxide solution into one container and the saline into the other.
6. Put on gloves.
7. Remove the old, soiled trach pants.
8. Note the condition of the skin and stoma (Figure 7.20). Report any unusual findings to the nurse or preceptor.
9. Apply sterile gloves.
10. Clean the stoma with sterile cotton applicators dipped in peroxide, and then rinse with sterile cotton applicators dipped in saline solution. Rinse the skin thoroughly to prevent irritation. Use each applicator only once. Use a rolling motion to apply the peroxide and to rinse with the saline.
11. Apply the sterile trach pants (Figure 7.18c).
12. Remove and discard gloves; wash hands.
13. Document and report the results to the RN or preceptor.

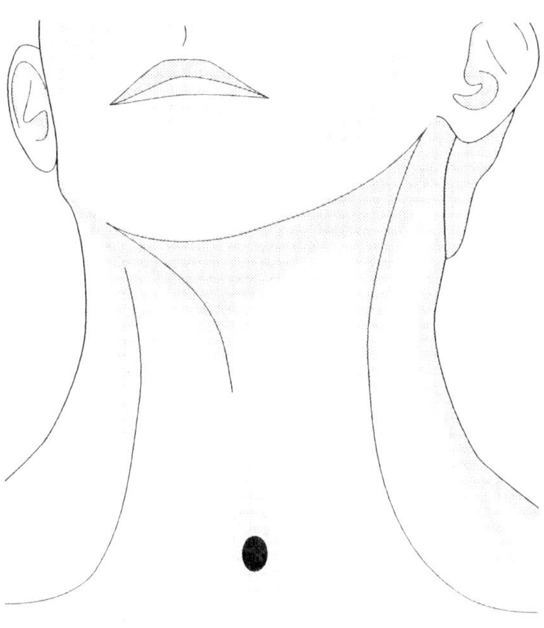

**Figure 7.20** Patient with a tracheostomy stoma.

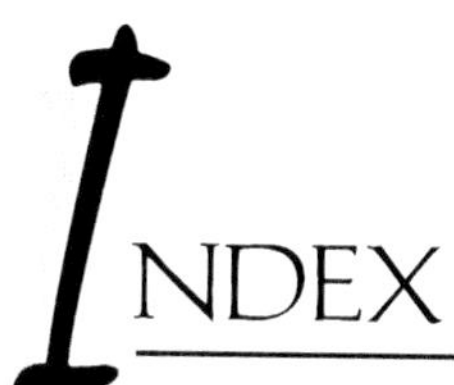

# INDEX

## J



## K



## L



## M



## N



## O



## P





GRIDLINE SET IN 1ST -PP TO INDICATE SAFE AREA: TO BE REMOVED AFTER 1ST-PP

## Q



## R



## S



## T



## U



## V



## W



## X